ADVANCES IN RENAL PHYSIOLOGY

ADVANCES IN RENAL PHYSIOLOGY

Edited by Christopher J. Lote, PhD
Senior Lecturer, Physiology Department,
University of Birmingham, UK

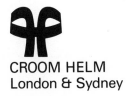

CROOM HELM
London & Sydney

Croom Helm Ltd, Provident House, Burrell Row,
Beckenham, Kent BR3 1AT

Croom Helm Australia Pty Ltd, Suite 4, 6th Floor,
64-76 Kippax Street, Surry Hills, NSW 2010, Australia

British Library Cataloguing in Publication Data

Advances in physiology
  1. Kidneys
  I. Lote, Christopher J.
  612'.463   QP249

    ISBN 0-7099-1682-5

41 ed 1708 £40.00 7.90

Phototypeset by Words & Pictures Ltd, Thornton Heath, Surrey
Printed and bound in Great Britain

CONTENTS

To Patsy, Nicholas and Hazel

PREFACE

The explosion of knowledge over the past thirty years or so has made it difficult for scientists to be 'experts' over a broad area, and it is a truism that, as individuals, we tend to know 'more and more about less and less'. In my opinion, renal physiologists have been fighting a valiant rearguard action against this trend, and still see the subject as a coherent whole, even though it is now almost impossible to keep up with the research literature on *all* aspects of renal physiology.

Accordingly, the aim of this book is to help those physiologists and medical practitioners who wish to keep abreast of recent developments over a broad area of renal physiology; there has been enormous progress over the past decade, but many of the new findings, ideas and concepts have yet to find a place in standard textbooks of physiology. The type of review that has become popular in recent years — the conference report — usually suffers from the fact that it is written from a standpoint a little too close to the frontiers of knowledge, where controversy reigns supreme!

This book is not a conference report: it is the old-style review. I selected areas of renal physiology in which there have been major advances, and invited review contributions in these areas from experts in their respective fields. The early chapters of the book deal with fundamental renal mechanisms of filtration and ion handling, whereas the later chapters cover aspects of renal homeostatic mechanisms.

I am grateful to the contributors for their enthusiastic and co-operative response to the concept of the book; my hope is that it will help to keep renal physiologists up to date, and will also make the subject accessible to those postgraduate students just entering the field.

C.J. Lote

LIST OF CONTRIBUTORS

Christine Baylis, Department of Medicine, Division of Nephrology, V.A. Medical Center, University of California at San Diego, California 92093, USA.

J.M. Davis, Physiologisches Institut der Universität München, Pettenkofer-strasse 12, D 8-Munich 2, Federal Republic of Germany.

Roger Green, Department of Physiology, University of Manchester, The Medical School, Stopford Building, Oxford Road, Manchester M13 9PT, England.

Rainer Greger, Max Planck Institut für Biophysik, Kennedyallee 70, D6000 Frankfurt 70, Federal Republic of Germany.

D.A. Häberle, Physiologisches Institut der Universität München, Petten-koferstrasse 12, D8-Munich 2, Federal Republic of Germany.

J. Haylor, Department of Pharmacology, University of Sheffield, Sheffield S10 2TN, England.

M.R. Lee, Department of Therapeutics and Clinical Pharmacology, University of Edinburgh, Edinburgh EH8 9AG, Scotland.

C.J. Lote, Department of Physiology, The Medical School, University of Birmingham, Vincent Drive, Birmingham B15 2TJ, England.

Graeme B. Ryan, Department of Anatomy, University of Melbourne, Parkville, Victoria 3052, Australia.

Eberhard Schlatter, Max Planck Institut für Biophysik, Kennedyallee 70, D 6000 Frankfurt 70, Federal Republic of Germany.

H. Sonnenberg, Department of Physiology, University of Toronto, Medical Sciences Building, Toronto, Ontario M5S 1A8, Canada.

J.D. Swales, Department of Medicine, University of Leicester, Leicester Royal Infirmary, Leicester LE2 7LX, England.

TERMINOLOGY AND ABBREVIATIONS

In general, abbreviations are defined on first usage in the text.

AII	Angiotensin II
ACE	Angiotensin converting enzyme
ADH	Antidiuretic hormone, vasopressin
ANRL	Antihypertensive neutral renomedullary lipid
AVP	Arginine vasopressin
CTAL	Cortical thick ascending limb of Henle's loop
Da	Dalton, molecular weight
DOCA	Deoxycorticosterone acetate
EPFR	Early proximal flow rate
ERPF	Effective renal plasma flow
GFR	Glomerular filtration rate
HRP	Horseradish peroxidase
IgG	Immunoglobulin G
NaD	Salt deprived
PG	Prostaglandin
PR	Pars recta (of proximal tubule)
RBF	Renal blood flow
RPF	Renal plasma flow
SNFF	Single nephron filtration fraction
SNGFR	Single nephron glomerular filtration rate
TAL	Thick ascending limb of Henle
tALH	Thin ascending limb of Henle
tDLH	Thin descending limb of Henle
TF/P	Tubular fluid to plasma ratio
TX	Thromboxane

1 THE GLOMERULAR FILTRATION BARRIER

Graeme B. Ryan

Introduction

In the first comprehensive description of the renal nephron and its blood supply in 1842, William Bowman gave a remarkably accurate account of the structural relationship of the glomerulus to the renal tubule. Bowman believed that the glomerular capillary wall acted to separate water and salts from the blood, and that the other components of urine were secreted by tubular cells. In 1844, Carl Ludwig proposed that a protein-free ultrafiltrate of plasma was forced out of the glomerular capillaries by the hydrostatic pressure of blood, and that the subsequent transfer of water and solutes across the tubular epithelium occurred by passive diffusion mechanisms. Ludwig's 'mechanical' theory of glomerular filtration was later challenged by Rudolf Heidenhain who, in 1874, suggested that glomeruli actively secreted water and salts, and that the process was complemented by major secretory activity in the tubules. A long period of controversy ensued between proponents of the views of Ludwig and Heidenhain until, in 1917, Arthur Robertson Cushny put forward his 'modern' theory in which he agreed with Ludwig that the initial step in urine formation is the hydrostatically regulated ultrafiltration of plasma across the glomerular capillary wall, but proposed that active reabsorption of water and solutes occurs in the tubules. Subsequently, the classical micropuncture studies of Richards and Walker and their collaborators (see review, Smith, 1951) clearly confirmed the concepts of glomerular ultrafiltration and tubular reabsorption, with additional modifications of the final urine being attributable to tubular secretory processes.

Although the idea that the glomerulus functions as a sieve is well over a hundred years old, there remains considerable controversy as to how the glomerulus solves the problem of retaining plasma proteins in the capillary lumen in the face of the high rates of ultrafiltration flux that operate across the glomerular capillary wall. Glomerular capillaries show water permeability of the order of 100 times that across muscle capillaries (Pappenheimer, 1953). At the same time, molecules the size of albumin or larger are normally prevented from reaching the urinary space. This chapter is particularly concerned with identifying the nature of the barriers in the glomerular capillary wall responsible for restricting the passing of plasma proteins during normal glomerular function, and how such barriers may be disturbed in proteinuric states.

1

Morphology of the Glomerular Capillary Wall

The glomerulus consists of a network of capillaries encased by an unusually prominent basement membrane. Three cell types are present in the glomerulus: visceral or podocytic epithelial cells outside the basement membrane; endothelial cells lining the capillaries; and mesangial cells occupying the axial or mesangial region between the capillaries and in continuity with the extraglomerular mesangium or lacis region in the juxtaglomerular apparatus.

Podocytic Epithelium

The cell bodies of the podocytic epithelial cells lie in Bowman's capsular space, extending tentacle-like major processes that partially encircle the outside of the glomerular capillary basement membrane. Along the capillary wall (Figure 1.1), these major processes alternate at regular distances with other major processes from different podocytes extending around the capillary from the opposite direction. The area of basement membrane between these major processes is covered by multiple, narrow cytoplasmic extensions, called foot processes, that project across the basement membrane from each major process and interdigitate closely with one another. When viewed from the urinary space with the scanning electron microscope, the foot processes give an appearance resembling interlocking fingers applied to the outside of the glomerular basement membrane. The podocytic cytoplasm contains prominent microtubules that may be significant in maintaining the complex shape of such cells. Microfilaments are also abundant in such cells, suggesting that they may have contractile properties.

Between the interdigitating foot processes are narrow gaps called the epithelial or filtration slits. At their base, close to the basement membrane, such slits are 20-30 nm wide and are bridged by a thin membrane, 4-6 nm thick, called the epithelial or filtration slit diaphragm. When examined *en face*, following tannic acid-glutaraldehyde fixation, the slit diaphragm shows a regular substructure composed of a zipper-like arrangement of offset cross-bridges extending inwards from the foot-process plasmalemma to a central filament (Rodewald and Karnovsky, 1974). This arrangement results in a highly ordered array of rectangular pores, with dimensions approximately 4×14 nm, which is about the dimensions of an albumin molecule. Freeze-cleaving and etching techniques confirm that the slit diaphragm is composed of a row of pores on each side of a central filament (Karnovsky and Ryan, 1975). When there is disruption of glomerular foot-process architecture in glomerular disease, the slit diaphragm coils up and fractures (Ryan *et al.*, 1975b), indicating that it is a real structure rather than an artefactual condensation of material between the foot processes.

Figure 1.1: Electron Micrograph of Rat Glomerular Capillary Wall Showing Capillary Lumen (C), Fenestrated Endothelium (E), Basement Membrane (B), Epithelial Foot Processes (F), Podocytic Cell Body (P) and Urinary Space (U). Note epithelial slit diaphragm (arrows). x 40 000

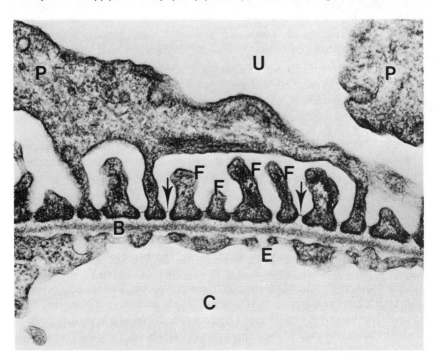

Glomerular Basement Membrane

The basement membrane is located between the podocytic epithelium and the capillary endothelial layer (Figure 1.1). In man, it is approximately 300 nm thick, compared with 150 nm in rats and mice. It consists of a central, electron-dense zone called the lamina densa, flanked on each side by electron-lucent zones: the lamina rara externa, beneath the epithelium, and the lamina rara interna, beneath the endothelium. The lamina densa appears to be composed of a feltwork of closely packed fibrils, whereas the laminae rarae contain fewer fibrils, mostly extending perpendicularly between the lamina densa and the epithelial foot processes in the lamina rara externa and the endothelium in the lamina rara interna.

The glomerular basement membrane contains type IV and V collagens, laminin, entactin and various proteoglycans (Kanwar, 1984). The most significant proteoglycan in the basement membrane, apparently concentrated in the lamina rara interna and externa, is heparan sulphate (Kanwar and Farquhar, 1979b,c; Kanwar, 1984), a molecule characterised by high net negative charge density as well as a capacity to promote steric exclusion effects within membranes (Kanwar *et al.*, 1980; Rosenzweig and Kanwar,

1982). Accordingly, it has been suggested that proteoglycans in the basement membrane are involved in establishing the proposed 'charge-selective and/or size-selective' properties of the glomerular capillary wall (Rosenzweig and Kanwar, 1982) (see below).

Endothelium

The attached glomerular endothelium is characterised by the presence of multiple round fenestrae, 40-100 nm in diameter (Figure 1.1). These fenestrae are open in most species, exposing the lamina rara interna of the basement membrane to the capillary lumen, although a diaphragm across the fenestrae was reported in the mouse in early studies by Rhodin (1962).

Negative Charge in the Glomerular Capillary Wall

The glomerular capillary wall contains intrinsic negatively charged molecules. Staining with colloidal iron reveals the presence of a thick polyanionic sialoglycoprotein cell coat on epithelial foot processes, especially on the exposed urinary surface (Jones, 1969; Latta *et al.*, 1975). A much thinner cell coat is present on the endothelial surfaces. In the basement membrane, colloidal iron staining has been described in the lamina rara externa and lamina rara interna, including within the endothelial fenestrae, whereas the lamina densa is unstained (Latta *et al.*, 1975). However, if superficial glomeruli in Munich-Wistar rats are fixed rapidly by *in situ* drip fixation during good blood flow, heavy colloidal iron staining is present on cell surfaces but is virtually absent in the lamina rara interna and within endothelial fenestrae (Ryan *et al.*, 1978b). This suggests that colloidal iron staining in the lamina rara interna and endothelial fenestrae in immersion-fixed material may be an artefact resulting from local clumping of albumin and other plasma polyanions following their diffusion into the glomerular capillary wall as blood flow stops (Ryan and Karnovsky, 1976; Ryan *et al.*, 1976).

More convincing evidence of staining of fixed anionic sites in both laminae rarae of the basement membrane was obtained by Farquhar and her colleagues using a variety of perfused anionic probes, e.g. lysozyme (Caulfield and Farquhar, 1976), Alcian blue (Caulfield, 1979), cationised ferritin or ruthenium red (Kanwar and Farquhar, 1979a). Kanwar and Farquhar (1979b, c) also presented cytochemical and biochemical data indicating that such anionic sites are predominantly composed of the proteoglycan heparan sulphate. There is controversy concerning the significance of these anionic proteoglycans in the laminae rarae of the basement membrane. In assigning to these molecules an important role in controlling permselectivity of plasma proteins across the glomerular capillary wall, a simple view is that they form a space-occupying matrix that is size-selective, tending to prevent the entry of macromolecules by means of steric-hindrance effects (Kanwar, 1984). A currently more fashionable theory is that, because of their negative electrostatic charge, such proteoglycans may be a major factor in limiting the penetration of plasma albumin (a polyanion in physiological solution) across the normal glomerular capillary wall (Kanwar *et al.*, 1980). In a variation of this theory, Kanwar and Rosenzweig (1982a) suggested that heparan sulphate molecules in the lamina rara interna act as anticlogging agents by preventing hydrogen bonding and absorption of plasma proteins on to the basement membrane, thereby permitting the maintenance of efficient ultrafiltration through the basement membrane pores. Alternatively, anionic sites in the glomerular capillary wall may be simply involved in the attachment of the endothelial and epithelial layers to the basement membrane.

Functional Permselectivity of the Glomerular Capillary Wall

During normal glomerular ultrafiltration, the fractional clearance of a solute (the ratio of its concentration in Bowman's space to its concentration in plasma) is affected by various parameters. These include molecular size, molecular charge, molecular shape and deformability, and haemodynamic factors. Failure to take full account of the range of such parameters affecting solute permeability has not only caused difficulties in estimating the dimensions of pores in the glomerular capillary wall, but has also significantly compromised the development of rational theories to explain glomerular barrier function.

Molecular Size

Inulin, which has an Einstein-Stokes effective radius of 1.4 nm, suffers no measurable restriction during its passage across the glomerular capillary wall. It therefore has a fractional clearance of 1.0. With larger molecules, the fractional clearance progressively decreases, approaching zero for molecules the size of albumin (effective radius 3.55 nm) or larger. This implies that the pores restricting the passage of macromolecules across the glomerular capillary wall have a radius of approximately 3.55 nm. However, the results of clearance studies using molecules such as dextrans or polyvinylpyrrolidone (Renkin and Gilmore, 1973; Chang *et al.*, 1975b) suggest that such pores are significantly larger than predicted from the size of the albumin molecule. Chang *et al.* (1975b) found that the fractional clearance values for graded fractions of neutral dextran molecules did not approach zero until their effective radii exceeded 4.2 nm. This indicates that neutral dextran molecules of the same apparent radius as albumin penetrate the glomerular capillary wall more readily than albumin. This phenomenon has been explained on the assumption that the glomerular capillary wall contains significant numbers of intrinsic anionic groups that can restrict the passage of negatively charged molecules such as albumin but not neutral molecules such as dextrans. However, as shown by Rennke and Venkatachalam (1979), a more likely alternative explanation for such a phenomenon lies in the fact that, in contrast to the relatively compact albumin molecule, dextrans and polyvinylpyrrolidone are extremely flexible linear polymers with the ability to deform and unfold, and may therefore display markedly different size characteristics under ultrafiltration conditions (see below).

Molecular Charge

Because albumin is a polyanion in physiological solution (isoelectric point pI 4.7), it seemed logical to attribute its very low fractional clearance value of 0.001 to the presence of intrinsic negative groups in the glomerular capillary wall, causing electrostatic repulsion of the albumin molecules. Again, studies using graded dextran molecules appeared to support this concept. Chang *et al.* (1975a) found that the addition of sulphate groups to produce anionic dextran sulphate molecules gave rise to dramatically lower clearance values compared with uncharged dextran molecules. Thus, wherever the clearance value for neutral dextran of the same apparent size as albumin was 0.14, the clearance of a comparably sized dextran sulphate fraction was 0.01. However, as with comparing the clearances of albumin and neutral dextran, a potential flaw in this argument lies in the diminished deformability of the sulphated dextran molecule under ultrafiltration conditions (see below). Somewhat more convincing in this respect are the studies of Rennke *et al.* (1978) who, seeking to examine the behaviour of variously charged globular protein molecules rather than flexible polymers, found reduced clearance values for succinylated anionic horseradish peroxidase compared with neutral horseradish peroxidase. However, even here, the results could be explained by minor changes in molecular flexibility, in combination with the observed small increase in the effective radius of the anionic molecule following succinylation.

In contrast to such studies using anionic tracers, the clearances of fractions of DEAE dextran, a highly cationised derivative of dextran, were relatively increased compared with neutral dextran fractions, giving a value of 0.4 for DEAE dextran of an effective radius comparable with that of albumin (Bohrer *et al.*, 1978). Similarly, Rennke *et al.* (1978) found that the clearance of a hexanediamine-cationised form of horseradish peroxidase exceeded that of neutral horseradish peroxidase. Purtell *et al.* (1979) compared the clearances in rats of human albumin derivatives that were cationised to produce isoelectric points of 5.5-6.6 or 7.2-8.2 (compared with a normal albumin pI of 4.9 in these studies); they found that the cationised derivatives showed clearance values that were higher than those obtained for normal albumin, although they drew attention to the possibility that such results could be due to the reduced effective radius of the albumin derivatives (i.e. 3.3 nm compared with 3.5 nm for normal albumin). It should be appreciated that the increased clearances of cationised preparations of dextran, horseradish peroxidase, albumin or other derivatives may reflect an abnormality in glomerular permeability induced by binding of the cationised derivative to cell surfaces. Thus, in the above studies of Purtell *et al.* (1979), the cationised albumin derivative with the higher pI value, 7.2-8.2, showed higher clearance values but also provoked prominent leakage of the rat's own albumin into the urine. In these experiments, extensive binding of the cationised albumin could be demonstrated in the mesangium and glomerular capillary walls. The potential nephrotoxic effect of cationised derivatives was demonstrated by the development of acute renal failure and impaired oxidative phosphorylation in response to DEAE dextran but not neutral dextran (Weinberg *et al.*, 1979). Such findings make it difficult to interpret the results of clearance studies using cationised derivatives. A similar difficulty may compromise the ultrastructural tracer studies of the glomerular distribution of hexanediamine-cationised ferritin molecules (Rennke *et al.*, 1975; Rennke and Venkatachalam, 1979) (see below).

Under diffusion conditions *in vitro*, the penetration of albumin molecules into artificial membranes is reduced if a membrane is negatively charged (Laurent, 1966) and enhanced if the membrane is positively charged, such as following treatment with the polycation protamine (Larsen, 1967). Attempts have been made to extend such studies to the glomerular capillary wall but with equivocal results. For instance, with the rationale that infused polycations should neutralise intrinsic anionic groups in the glomerular capillary wall and thus cause proteinuria, Hunsicker *et al.* (1981) infused the polycation hexadimethrine into rats and provoked heavy albuminuria. In the same studies, however, it was noted that substantial quantities of plasma immunoglobulin G (a virtually uncharged molecular species in physiological solution) also entered the urine, indicating that there was an induced abnormality of size-selective permeability. There were also significant morphological abnormalities of glomerular epithelial foot processes similar to those described as occurring in response to the infusion of the polycation protamine by Seiler *et al.* (1975, 1977) and resembling to some extent the changes seen in proteinuric states. Vehaskari *et al.* (1982) reported that albuminuria occurred in rats infused via the renal artery with protamine or other polycations. These workers noted 'patchy foot process fusion' in such animals but attributed the albuminuria to 'neutralization of glomerular polyanion'. In recent studies in our laboratory (Messina, Davies and Ryan, in preparation), infusion of the renal artery with protamine was found to cause more severe morphological changes than those reported by Vehaskari *et al.* (1982). In particular, podocytic epithelium showed extensive damage, leaving focal areas of externally bare glomerular basement membrane. These appearances resembled those seen in aminonucleoside nephrosis (Ryan and Karnovsky, 1975), a model of proteinuria in which the areas of bare basement membrane are sites of leakage of plasma proteins from the glomerular capillary lumen to the urinary space (Ryan and Karnovsky, 1975; Ryan *et al.*, 1978b) (see below).

Molecular Shape and Deformability

The higher fractional clearance values for neutral dextran and polyvinyl-pyrrolidone when compared with albumin are probably due to the linear polymeric nature of the dextran and polyvinylpyrrolidone molecules. Renkin and Gilmore (1973) and Laurent *et al.* (1975) pointed out that such polymers form loose and randomly coiled hydrated spheres in free solution, the state in which their Einstein-Stokes effective radii are calculated using gel chroma-tography. Under such conditions, these molecules have an apparently larger radius than compact globular proteins of equivalent molecular weight. The unexpectedly high glomerular clearance of these polymers probably results from their extreme flexibility, and hence their ability to unfold in response to the deforming forces of pressure and solvent flow under ultrafiltration conditions (Renkin and Gilmore, 1973). Such unfolding would enable relatively large molecules to elongate and thereby wriggle end-on through the interstices of the glomerular capillary wall. This reptile-like movement has been called 'reptation' (DeGennes, 1971). Such unfolding cannot occur with globular proteins such as albumin because of the firm internal cross-linking of the folded polypeptide chains.

The relatively reduced clearance values for dextran sulphate molecules when compared with neutral dextrans of apparently equivalent radius (Chang *et al.*, 1975a) may be explained on the basis of reduced molecular flexibility. The addition of sulphate groups to produce the anionic dextran molecule will, by the introduction of mutually repulsive electrostatic forces into the polymer, result in a tendency to stretch the macromolecule and open up the random coil (Katchalsky, 1964). This will lead to conversion of the flexible dextran polymer into a relatively more rigid rod-like dextran sulphate molecule which, under ultrafiltration conditions, may be less able to penetrate the glomerular capillary wall by reptation. Because it is less flexible, such a molecule will presumably tend to become impacted within the glomerular capillary wall, either in the fibrillary meshwork of the lamina densa or between the glycosaminoglycan molecules in the laminae rarae. In other words, sulphation of the dextran polymer may result in reduced glomerular clearance because of decreased deformability of the molecule rather than, as first proposed (Chang *et al.*, 1975a), its induced negative charge.

Rennke and Venkatachalam (1979) obtained data on renal clearance that emphasised the significance of reptation in affecting such data. These workers compared the clearance of globular protein molecules (horseradish peroxidase) with the clearance of neutral dextran molecules with an effective radius equivalent to that of horseradish peroxidase (i.e. 2.845 nm). Horseradish peroxidase and neutral dextran are similarly charged, with an isoelectric point (*c.* 7.4) in the physiological pH range. They found that the clearance of neutral dextran was more than seven times that of horseradish peroxidase, thus confirming the important role of molecular shape and deformability as well as molecular size in the permselectivity of the glomerular capillary wall.

Haemodynamic Factors

Local haemodynamic factors are important determinants of glomerular permselectivity. Thus, increased glomerular plasma flow rates, induced by volume expansion wth isotonic plasma, resulted in a fall in the dextran clearance profile (Chang *et al.*, 1975b). Conversely, decreased glomerular flow rates, induced by the infusion of angiotensin II, resulted in an increase in the dextran clearance profile, as well as proteinuria (Bohrer *et al.*, 1977b). These findings conform with the predictions of Pappenheimer (1953) based on the theory of 'molecular sieving' across capillary walls. According to this concept, macromolecules suffer increasing restriction in their passage through pores with increasing rates of solvent flux. Conversely, at abnormally low rates of filtration, such macromolecules will approach diffusion equilibrium with the ultrafiltrate. Thus, the concentration of macromolecules in the filtrate will be lower at high filtration rates, and higher at lower filtration rates. This phenomenon may have considerable relevance in explaining, first, how plasma proteins are retained within the glomerular capillary lumen during normal ultrafiltration, and, secondly, why such proteins, including albumin (Ryan and Karnovsky, 1976), penetrate the glomerular capillary wall during reduced glomerular blood flow (see below).

Ultrastructural Tracer Studies

To determine which layer of the glomerular capillary wall is responsible for restricting the penetration of plasma proteins, the usual approach has been to study the glomerular distribution of circulating macromolecular tracers that are of known size and amenable to identification by electron microscopy. If the tracer is held up at a certain level in the wall, it seems a reasonable assumption that a barrier to the tracer is present at that level. This approach has been used in two kinds of studies: first, those examining the distribution of intravenously administered exogenous tracers, and secondly, those examining the distribution of endogenous plasma proteins (Figure 1.2).

Exogenous Tracer Studies

The first major exogenous tracer studies were those of Farquhar *et al.* (1961), who found that ferritin (molecular weight 480 000; effective radius a_e 6.1 nm), a molecule which is intrinsically electron-opaque because of its high iron content, entered the endothelial fenestrae but did not penetrate significantly beyond the lamina rara interna. On the basis of this result, it was proposed that the basement membrane, in particular the lamina densa, is the major filtration barrier for plasma proteins. However, because ferritin is a particularly large molecule, it was apparent that its distribution might not reflect the normal distribution of endogenous plasma albumin (molecular weight 68 000; a_e 3.55 nm). In 1966, Graham and Karnovsky introduced the use of

Figure 1.2: Scheme Depicting Distribution of Endogenous Albumin and IgG, and Intravenously Administered Ferritin, Catalase and Horseradish Peroxidase in the Rat Glomerular Capillary Wall; in the Left Panel, under Normal Conditions with *in situ* Fixation of Glomeruli ('Good blood flow'); in the Right Panel, Following the Diffusion of Tracer Molecules that Occurs with Cessation of Blood Flow such as with Immersion Fixation of Glomeruli ('no blood flow'). In each panel, the capillary lumen is on the left and the urinary space is on the right. In the left panel ('good blood flow'), all tracer molecules except horseradish peroxidase are held up at the endothelial fenestrae, whereas horseradish peroxidase, being a smaller molecule, is found in the glomerular basement membrane (GBM) and penetrates the epithelial slit diaphragm to reach the urinary space. In the right panel ('no blood flow'), albumin, IgG and catalase enter the GBM, but, whereas albumin penetrates to the urinary space, IgG and catalase are held up by the epithelial slit diaphragm; ferritin, being a larger molecule, shows very little penetration beyond the endothelial fenestrae under such conditions. These data are based upon the experiments of Ryan and Karnovsky (1976), Ryan *et al.* (1976) and Ryan (1979)

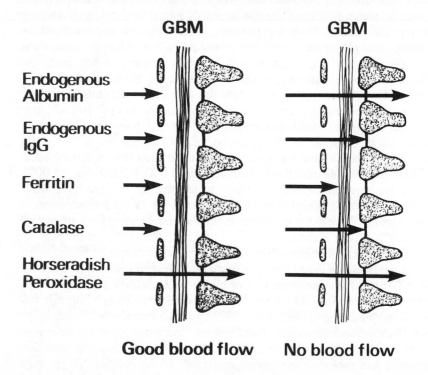

peroxidatic enzyme tracers to the investigation of this issue. After intravenous injection such tracers can be visualised histochemically by means of a peroxidase reaction with diaminobenzidine in the presence of hydrogen peroxide, leading to the oxidation of diaminobenzidine to an osmiophilic, electron-dense, insoluble polymer at the site of the enzyme reaction. First it was found that horseradish peroxidase (molecular weight 40 000; a_e 3.0 nm) passed rapidly into the urinary space with only slight restriction being offered by the basement membrane (Graham and Karnovsky, 1966). Myeloperoxidase (molecular weight 160 000; a_e 4.4 nm) suffered only minor restriction within the basement membrane, filling the capillary wall up to the epithelial slit diaphragm but showing very little penetration into the urinary space (Graham and Karnovsky, 1966). Catalase (molecular weight 240,000; a_e 5.2 nm) showed only partial restriction within the basement membrane but was completely blocked by the slit diaphragm; in this case no tracer was detectable in the urinary space (Venkatachalam *et al.*, 1970a). Since little or no plasma albumin enters the urinary space under normal conditions (Oken and Flamenbaum, 1971), and because albumin is smaller than catalase, these catalase results suggested that the epithelial slit diaphragm should act as the major barrier to the penetration of albumin across the glomerular capillary wall. Taken together, the ferritin and catalase results led to the 'double barrier' hypothesis which proposed that the basement membrane acts as a coarse, primary filter that restricts the passage of large plasma proteins such as globulins, and that the epithelial slit diaphragm acts as an additional, fine, final filter which is the major barrier for relatively smaller plasma proteins, including albumin (Karnovsky and Ainsworth, 1972; Venkatachalam *et al.*, 1970a). The subsequent finding that the slit diaphragm has a regular substructure, delineating pores of a size close to the dimensions of the albumin molecules (Rodewald and Karnovsky, 1974), seemed to support the concept that the slit diaphragm was the definitive barrier for albumin.

In 1974, Caulfield and Farquhar studied the distribution of three graded fractions of neutral dextran (molecular weights 32 000, 62 000 and 125 000) using a heavy-metal staining technique to identify the dextran molecules. Particles were found filling the capillary lumen and in the lamina rara interna, but no particles were detected deeper in the basement membrane with any of the fractions. It was claimed that these findings confirmed that the basement membrane is the major permeability barrier to plasma proteins. However, with each of the fractions tested, dextran particles were also found in the urinary space. To reach the urinary space, such molecules must traverse the basement membrane. To do this, the molecules may unfold and wriggle through the interstices by reptation (DeGennes, 1971) as described above. Presumably, when the dextran molecule is stretched out and surrounded by basement membrane material, it is not amenable to the staining reaction that identifies the coiled and probably aggregated molecules in the capillary lumen and urinary space.

In tracer studies designed to assess the role of intrinsic negative charge in glomerular barrier function, Rennke and colleagues (Rennke *et al.*, 1975; Rennke and Venkatachalam, 1977) compared the distribution of native anionic ferritin and hexanediamine-cationised derivatives of ferritin. Whereas anionic ferritin showed little penetration into the basement membrane, the cationised derivatives penetrated deeply into the basement membrane, the degree of penetration being greatest for the most cationic molecules. This seemed to favour the concept that molecular charge is an important factor in glomerular permselectivity but, as discussed above, the results require cautious interpretation in view of the nephrotoxic, permeability-provoking effects of exogenous cationised derivatives (Purtell *et al.*, 1979). If, under the conditions of such experiments (Rennke *et al.*, 1975; Rennke and Venkatachalam, 1977), there is increased leakage of macromolecules across the glomerular capillary wall due to an induced size-selective defect, the prominent aggregation of cationised ferritin in the lamina rara externa in such experiments may simply reflect a 'staining' reaction resulting from the binding of the charged tracer molecules to intrinsic anionic groups in this region. Recently, Barnes *et al.* (1984) reported the results of experiments indicating that cationic ferritin 'by itself' can provoke a size-selective defect in glomerular permselectivity by distorting glomerular basement membrane structure; these authors commented that the use of such tracers involves 'an inherent artifact in the study of their filtration characteristics'.

In an interesting series of experiments, Kanwar and his colleagues (Kanwar *et al.*, 1980; Rosenzweig and Kanwar, 1982; Kanwar, 1984) found that removal of heparan sulphate from the rat glomerular basement membrane by means of enzyme digestion resulted in increased penetration of perfused native anionic ferritin into the basement membrane and into the urinary space. Incidentally, such treatment also resulted in abolition of binding of cationised ferritin to anionic sites in the lamina rara interna and externa (Kanwar *et al.*, 1980). Similarly, when ^{125}I-bovine serum albumin was infused into rat kidneys, autoradiographic studies showed that increased leakage of the labelled albumin tracer occurred from the capillary lumen to the urinary space across glomerular basement membranes that had been digested with enzymes that removed a range of glycosaminoglycans (Rosenzweig and Kanwar, 1982). It was concluded from these studies that heparan sulphate and hyaluronic acid, and possibly chondroitin sulphates, play a role in determining the permeability characteristics of the glomerular basement membrane to albumin. Rosenzweig and Kanwar (1982) suggested that these glycosaminoglycans 'are involved in establishing the charge-selective and/or size-selective properties of the glomerular basement membrane'. Until recently there has been considerable emphasis upon the potential charge-selective effects of such basement membrane components in limiting the penetration of plasma albumin across the glomerular capillary wall. It is worth noting that the above results are equally compatible with the concept that basement membrane glycosaminoglycans contribute to glomerular barrier function by restricting plasma protein penetration on a size-selective basis due to steric exclusion effects (Comper and Laurent, 1978).

Endogenous Plasma Protein Studies

In contrast to the use of injected exogenous tracers, a more direct approach has been the development of ultrastructural immunoperoxidase techniques to delineate the glomerular distribution of endogenous plasma proteins such as albumin (Ryan and Karnovsky, 1976). As it turned out, an important innovation in these studies was the use of Munich-Wistar rats in which superficial glomeruli were rapidly fixed *in situ* in anaesthetised animals by dripping fixative on to the kidney surface during good renal blood flow. In such glomeruli, it was found that dense reaction product specific for albumin (molecular weight 68 000) uniformly filled the capillary lumen but did not penetrate beyond the endothelial fenestrae (Figure 1.2). On the other hand, if renal blood flow was stopped by ligating the renal artery before *in situ* drip fixation, albumin completely filled the basement membrane and was also found in small amounts in the urinary space (Figure 1.2). A similar pattern of staining was found in glomeruli subjected to the conventional immersion fixation techniques used for the previous exogenous tracer experiments. If drip fixation was performed *in situ* after simultaneous ligation of the renal artery and vein, albumin was present in the basement membrane and, in large amounts, in the urinary space. If blood flow was restored after ligation of the renal artery and vein, the glomerular distribution of albumin rapidly returned to normal, i.e. showing no penetration beyond the endothelial fenestrae. It is difficult to explain such results on the basis of the concept that the penetration of plasma albumin across the glomerular capillary wall is normally prevented by the presence of fixed anionic groups in the basement membrane.

The same approach was used to examine the effect of comparable haemodynamic changes on the distribution of endogenous immunoglobulin G (IgG) in Munich-Wistar rats (Ryan *et al.*, 1976). This larger plasma protein (molecular weight 150 000) showed the same distribution as albumin during good blood flow, i.e. it was held up at the endothelial fenestrae following *in situ* drip fixation (Figure 1.2). After ligation of the renal artery (or following immersion fixation), IgG filled the basement membrane but, unlike albumin, did not penetrate to the urinary space (Figure 1.2). If fixation was performed *in situ* after simultaneous ligation of the renal artery and vein, IgG was found in the basement membrane and, in small amounts, in the urinary space. If blood flow was restored by removing the ligature on the renal artery and vein, the distribution of IgG rapidly returned to normal. These results suggested that the earlier studies of the glomerular distribution of exogenous catalase using immersion fixation (Venkatachalam *et al.*, 1970a) may not reflect the true distribution of the tracer under normal haemodynamic conditions. To test this possibility, it was decided to re-examine the distribution of catalase using the *in situ* drip-fixation method. In these experiments (Ryan *et al.*, 1976), it was found that intravenously administered catalase showed precisely the same pattern of distribution as endogenous IgG. Thus, catalase did not penetrate beyond the endothelial fenestrae during good blood flow, but filled the basement membrane up to, but not beyond, the epithelial slit diaphragm after either renal artery ligation or immersion fixation (Figure 1.2). As with IgG, penetration of catalase to the urinary space was detected only following simultaneous ligation of the renal artery and vein. Here again, the distribution of the tracer returned to normal if blood flow was restored by removing the ligature on the renal vessels.

The penetration of albumin, IgG and catalase into the basement membrane following cessation of blood flow, such as was seen in immersion-fixed glomeruli, probably results from artefactual diffusion of the proteins into the basement membrane following breakdown of a haemodynamically dependent barrier that operates at the endothelial fenestrae (Ryan and Karnovsky, 1976; Ryan *et al.*, 1976). The penetration of IgG and catalase to the urinary space in kidneys fixed after ligation of the renal artery and vein presumably resulted from occlusion of the vein slightly ahead of the renal artery as the ligature was tightened around both vessels, thereby resulting in a transient increase in intravascular pressure, causing the tracer molecules to pass through stretched pores in the epithelial slit diaphragm. Such a mechanism might also help to explain the finding by Caulfield and Farquhar (1974) of unexpectedly large tracer molecules in the urinary space after the injection of various dextran fractions: these investigators clamped the renal artery and vein simultaneously with injecting fixative into the substance of the kidney.

It could be argued that the method of *in situ* drip fixation during good blood flow somehow causes circulating proteins to be either abnormally excluded from entering the basement membrane, or artefactually pushed out of the basement membrane, or rendered histochemically undetectable within the basement-membrane matrix. That none of these arguments is likely is indicated by the finding that intravenously administered horseradish peroxidase, a tracer that normally passes readily through the glomerular capillary wall to the urinary space, is clearly demonstrable histochemically in the basement membrane as well as in the capillary lumen and urinary space under identical drip-fixation conditions during good blood flow (Ryan, 1979) (Figure 1.2).

Thus, these ultrastructural studies of the distribution of endogenous albumin and IgG and exogenous catalase under different conditions of renal blood flow call into question the interpretation of previous studies of the distribution of exogenous tracers in immersion-fixed glomeruli. The data emphasise that glomerular barrier function cannot be attributed solely to fixed structural or charged elements in the glomerular capillary wall but that normal haemo-dynamic conditions are somehow critically important in restricting the penetration of plasma proteins beyond the endothelial fenestrae.

Mechanisms Involved in Normal Glomerular Permselectivity

Since the demonstration that albumin and other plasma proteins are normally held up by a functionally dependent barrier that operates at the level of the endothelial fenestrae (Ryan and Karnovsky, 1976; Ryan *et al.*, 1976), interest has centred on the nature of this barrier. Attempts to detect diaphragms across the fenestrae in superficial glomeruli of Munich-Wistar rats drip-fixed using a variety of fixatives during good blood flow have been unsuccessful (Ryan,

1979). In view of their large diameter, the fenestrae can offer no significant structural restriction to plasma-protein penetration. Any hypothesis as to the nature of the functional barrier at this level needs to explain not only how albumin is retained within the capillary lumen during normal ultrafiltration but also what change occurs in the capillary wall to allow albumin to leak across the basement membrane to the urinary space as blood flow stops. At least four major factors may each contribute to some extent towards the maintenance of normal glomerular barrier function. These are: (a) structural pores in the basement membrane; (b) molecular sieving; (c) concentration-polarisation phenomena; (d) charge effects.

Structural Pores in the Basement Membrane

The earliest and most basic hypothesis to explain glomerular barrier function is that plasma proteins are held up by steric hindrance effects within structural pores in the basement membrane. It has been suggested that the fine fibrillary meshwork of the basement membrane, particularly the lamina densa, delineates an array of multiple slit-like pores (Renkin and Gilmore, 1973). More recently, it has been proposed that glycosaminoglycans, such as heparan sulphate, form a sterically significant array in the laminae rarae (Rosenzweig and Kanwar, 1982; Kanwar, 1984). To explain the above results, i.e. the penetration of plasma proteins beyond the endothelial fenestrae with cessation of blood flow, it is conceivable that the intraluminal hydrostatic pressure that is present during normal blood flow may cause relative compaction of the basement membrane, effectively narrowing the interfibre or interglycosamino-glycan spaces. As the intraluminal pressure falls with cessation of blood flow, these spaces may open, allowing penetration of macromolecules from the capillary lumen. Schurer *et al.* (1980) have proposed a structural model of the glomerular basement membrane that would be consistent with this view. However, despite its attractive simplicity, it is unlikely that steric hindrance effects alone can explain all of the experimental data relating to glomerular permselectivity. Any or perhaps all of the following factors may be involved additionally in determining such permselectivity.

Molecular Sieving

According to the molecular-sieving hypothesis (Pappenheimer, 1953), the structural pores in the basement membrane may be sufficiently large to allow the passage of albumin molecules by diffusion, but during normal glomerular blood flow and ultrafiltration, the penetration of albumin and other plasma proteins may be significantly limited by the high rates of water flux through the same structural pores. With decreased glomerular blood flow and hence low rates of water flux across the capillary wall, plasma proteins are more readily able to diffuse into and through the basement membrane pores. It is very likely that molecular sieving operates, at least to some degree, during normal glomerular ultrafiltration (Chang *et al.*, 1975b; Pappenheimer, 1953; Landis and Pappenheimer, 1963;). It is less clear, however, whether molecular sieving alone could be entirely responsible for restricting the penetration of albumin through the structural pores in the basement membrane during normal blood flow.

The finding that IgG molecules (effective radius 5.5 nm) penetrate beyond the lamina rara interna and lamina densa under diffusion conditions, i.e. with cessation of ultrafiltration (Ryan *et al.*, 1976), indicates that the structural pores in the basement membrane have an effective radius of at least 5.5 nm under such conditions. Data from artificial ultrafiltration systems indicate that, during ultrafiltration, a filter with a pore radius of 5.5 nm will efficiently retain IgG molecules whereas, in the absence of IgG or other plasma proteins, albumin molecules pass freely into the filtrate (Blatt *et al.*, 1970). These results suggest that factors additional to simple molecular sieving must be operating during normal ultrafiltration to effectively reduce the structural pore size of the basement membrane and thereby limit the penetration of albumin. Such factors may relate to concentration-polarisation phenomena or charge effects or both.

Concentration-Polarisation Phenomena

The basement membrane may have structural pores that are sufficiently large to allow the passage of albumin under diffusion conditions except that, during normal blood flow and ultrafiltration, an additional barrier (with pores smaller than those in the basement membrane) is set up between the endothelial layer and the basement membrane. Such a functionally dependent barrier could arise if larger plasma proteins were held up by the basement membrane during ultrafiltration and formed a 'concentration-polarisation' layer (Blatt *et al.*, 1970) in a narrow, relatively unstirred zone immediately beneath the endothelium or possibly within the endothelial fenestrae, i.e. in areas protected from the sweeping effect of erythrocytes in the flowing blood. This phenomenon has been shown to occur in artificial ultrafiltration systems with mixtures of macromolecules (Blatt *et al.*, 1970). Thus, returning to the example mentioned above (i.e. ultrafiltration through an artificial filter with a pore radius of 5.5 nm), the addition of IgG or other larger proteins to a solution of albumin dramatically decreases the flux of albumin molecules through such a filter (Blatt *et al.*, 1970). Because concentration-polarisation depends upon the maintenance of a hydrostatic pressure difference across the filtering membrane (Blatt *et al.*, 1970), macromolecules composing the concentration-polarisation barrier against the basement membrane would become dispersed as blood flow stopped. Albumin molecules could then gain unrestricted access to the relatively coarse structural pores in the basement membrane and diffuse across the capillary wall to reach the urinary space.

From a theoretical analysis of the possible effects of concentration-polarisation upon hydraulic permeability of glomerular capillaries, Deen *et al.* (1974) concluded that some degree of concentration-polarisation of proteins could be present during glomerular ultrafiltration. The significance of the presence of the normal complement of plasma proteins in maintaining normal glomerular permselectivity is highlighted by the albuminuria that occurs in the isolated kidney perfused with a solution containing albumin and no other macromolecules (Stolte *et al.*, 1979). Although it is conceded that there is a range of possible explanations for this phenomenon (Swanson *et al.*, 1981), the finding that the addition of globulin and erythrocytes to the perfusate markedly suppresses the level of proteinuria in the isolated kidney (Swanson *et al.*, 1981) is consistent with the concept that concentration-polarisation phenomena contribute significantly to normal glomerular barrier function. From their studies of the filtration of protein solutions at high pressure across basement membranes *in vitro*, Robinson and Cotter (1980) concluded that concentration-polarisation effects can dramatically modify the permselectivity of the membranes: 'when proteins of different sizes are filtered together, the larger proteins tend to form a polarisation layer which prevents small proteins escaping through the filter'.

The concentration-polarisation concept provides an attractive explanation for the *in vivo* endogenous tracer results of Ryan and Karnovsky (1976), particularly if it is considered to operate in conjunction with molecular-sieving phenomena. The concept has also been linked with the charge hypothesis in a proposal that large negatively charged plasma glycoproteins may form a major component of a labile concentration-polarisation layer, thereby operating particularly to limit the penetration of albumin (Ryan and Karnovsky, 1976). On the other hand, a clearly defined labile concentration-polarisation layer, either uncharged or charged, has yet to be identified morphologically within or beneath the endothelial fenestrae during normal blood flow. Until the molecular composition of such a layer is elucidated, and until more appropriate super-rapid fixation methods are devised, its morphological demonstration will be difficult.

Charge Effects

In recent years there has been considerable, commonly uncritical, enthusiasm for the idea that albumin molecules, being polyanionic, suffer restriction in passing through the structural pores in the basement membrane because the latter contains considerable quantities of fixed anionic groups. The lines of evidence relating to this concept are discussed above, along with alternative interpretations, and have been reviewed recently (Kanwar, 1984). If charge effects are significant factors in glomerular permselectivity, they are most likely to be due to the presence of heparan sulphate in the laminae rarae of the basement membrane (Kanwar and Farquhar, 1979b,c; Kanwar, 1984), especially in the lamina rara interna in view of the fact that albumin is normally held up at the level of the endothelial fenestrae (Ryan and Karnovsky, 1976). It remains difficult, however, for intrinsic charge effects alone to explain why endogenous IgG, a molecule with an isoelectric point spanning neutrality, shows a glomerular distribution identical to that of albumin during good blood flow (Ryan and Karnovsky, 1976; Ryan *et al.*, 1976).

In summary, then, the functionally dependent barrier which normally operates to restrict plasma-protein penetration beyond the endothelial fenestrae during good blood flow may be attributed in part to molecular-sieving phenomena through pores in the basement membrane, perhaps in association with ultrafiltration-dependent concentration-polarisation effects and/or possibly with some contribution from intrinsic, negatively charged, sterically significant glycosaminoglycans in the basement membrane.

Control of Water Flux across the Glomerular Capillary Wall

The structural pores in the podocytic epithelial layer of the glomerular capillary wall appear not to be directly involved in restricting the passage of the major plasma proteins under normal conditions because, under these conditions, such plasma proteins do not penetrate this far into the wall. However, the epithelial layer may exert a major influence upon trans-glomerular water flux during ultrafiltration. This possibility is suggested by the finding that IgG and catalase cross the basement membrane up to the epithelial layer but do not reach the urinary space under diffusion conditions, i.e. following cessation of blood flow (Ryan *et al.*, 1976). This implies that the epithelial slit diaphragm contains the smallest structurally defined pores in the glomerular capillary wall. Furthermore, estimates from quantitative morphological studies indicate that the slit diaphragm pores occupy only 2 to 3 per cent of the total glomerular capillary surface area (Rodewald and Karnovsky, 1974; Shea and Morrison, 1975), a value that corresponds closely with estimates of effective pore area based upon hydraulic conductivity data (Landis and Pappenheimer, 1963; Renkin and Gilmore, 1973). Because it seems likely that the functional barrier to macromolecular penetration at the endothelial level depends critically upon the balance between convective and diffusive forces operating at the endothelial fenestrae, the epithelial layer may make an important, perhaps crucial, contribution to maintaining this equilibrium by controlling water flux between the capillary lumen and the urinary space. It might be predicted, therefore, that focal damage and loss of the epithelial layer, by allowing a focal increase in water flux across the wall at such sites, will cause a disturbance of the equilibrium at the endothelial fenestrae and therefore lead to the penetration of plasma proteins to the urinary space. As discussed below, such focal leakage of plasma proteins at sites of epithelial loss occurs in some important forms of glomerular disease associated with significant proteinuria.

Abnormal Glomerular Permselectivity: Mechanisms of Proteinuria

Proteinuria results from a breakdown in the normal permselectivity barrier in the glomerulus. The idea that proteinuria is caused by a failure of tubules to reabsorb normally filtered albumin was firmly refuted by Oken and Flamenbaum (1971) whose micropuncture studies revealed extremely low concentrations of albumin in the normal glomerular filtrate compared with increased concentrations of albumin in the glomerular filtrate of nephrotic rats. However, the nature of the glomerular permselectivity defect that leads to proteinuria is an issue that has provoked much debate over several years. There are two major schools of opinion. The first, led by Farquhar and Brenner and their associates (Farquhar and Palade, 1961; Brenner *et al.*, 1977; Caulfield and Farquhar, 1978), considers that proteinuria is caused by a generalised increase in permeability of the glomerular capillary wall due to a generalised abnormality of the basement membrane. More specifically, in recent years, data have been adduced by these workers in support of the notion that the key abnormality in proteinuric states is a generalised loss of intrinsic negative charge from the glomerular basement membrane (Brenner *et al.*, 1977; Caulfield and Farquhar, 1978). The second school of opinion, led by Ryan and Karnovsky and their colleagues (Ryan and Karnovsky, 1975; Ryan *et al.*, 1978a), is of the view that most forms of experimental and clinically significant proteinuria result primarily from focal leakage of plasma proteins across the glomerular capillary wall, particularly at sites of loss of the podocytic epithelial covering on the outside of the basement membrane. As will be discussed below, this latter view, placing considerably less emphasis on the proposed loss of intrinsic negative charge from the glomerulus, has recently been endorsed by Kanwar and his colleagues (Kanwar *et al.*, 1981; Kanwar and Rosenzweig, 1982b; Kanwar, 1984; Kanwar and Jakubowski, 1984).

Structural Abnormalities Associated with Proteinuria

Clinically significant forms of proteinuria are associated with prominent structural abnormalities in the glomerulus. On the other hand, in view of the functional dependence of the glomerular filtration barrier (Ryan and Karnovsky, 1976; Ryan *et al.*, 1976), it would not be surprising if milder more episodic proteinuria could occur in the absence of structural changes, particularly in response to significant reduction in glomerular blood flow. The importance of haemodynamic changes in causing proteinuria is supported by the finding that proteinuria induced by angiotensin II infusion is associated with reduced glomerular blood flow (Bohrer *et al.*, 1977b). It has been proposed that inappropriate reduction in renal blood flow may be responsible for postural proteinuria (Robinson, 1970) or exercise proteinuria (Poortmans, 1970) with no detectable abnormalities in glomerular structure. Furthermore the possibility that proteinuria may result from increased glomerular capillary pressure, perhaps by expanding basement-membrane pore size, has been

Figure 1.3: Electron Micrograph of Portions of Two Adjacent Glomerular Capillaries in a Rat with Proteinuria due to Aminonucleoside Nephrosis. Normal epithelial foot processes are replaced by extensive expanses of epithelial cytoplasm (arrows) applied to the outside of the basement membrane (B). Note prominent focal defect (asterisks) in epithelial layer, leaving externally denuded area of basement membrane directly exposed to urinary space (U). It has been proposed that such denuded areas of basement membrane are major sites of leakage of plasma proteins from the capillary lumen (C) to the urinary space in proteinuric states (Ryan and Karnovsky, 1975; Ryan *et al.*, 1978a). R, erythrocyte in capillary lumen; E, fenestrated endothelium.   x 25 000

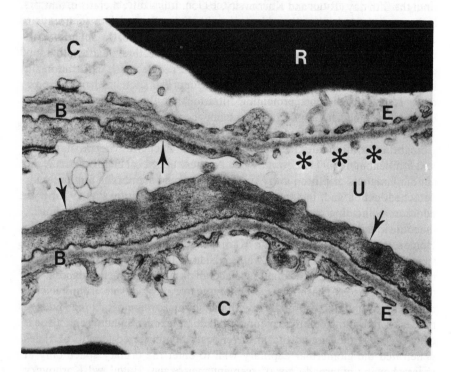

raised in respect of the proteinuria that occurs following subtotal nephrectomy in rats (Shea *et al.*, 1980).

The most extensively studied experimental model of severe proteinuria is puromycin aminonucleoside nephrosis in rats. In this model, rats injected with puromycin aminonucleoside show progressive replacement of glomerular epithelial foot processes by flattened expanses of epithelial cytoplasm (Feldman and Fisher, 1959; Vernier *et al.*, 1959; Farquhar and Palade, 1961; Ryan and Karnovsky, 1975) (Figure 1.3). This epithelial change, previously called 'foot process fusion', closely resembles the abnormality seen in glomeruli of patients with minimal change disease or focal glomerulosclerosis and hyalinosis. In detailed electron microscopic studies of aminonucleoside nephrosis, it has been demonstrated that true 'fusion' of foot processes does not occur (Ryan and Karnovsky, 1975; Ryan *et al.*, 1975a). Instead, the changes result from progressive spreading of epithelial cells on the outside of the glomerular capillaries, leading to replacement of interdigitating foot processes. It was formerly believed that this change occurred as a secondary response to the presence of plasma proteins in Bowman's capsular space. That this is incorrect was shown as follows: after a single intravenous injection of puromycin aminonucleoside into rats, epithelial spreading was present within two days and was extensive by four days although proteinuria did not develop until the fifth day (Ryan and Karnovsky, 1975). It is likely, therefore, that the lesion results from injury to podocytic epithelial cells caused by puromycin aminonucleoside itself or a toxic derivative. The epithelial cell responds to this injury by undergoing a simplification of its architecture, leading to foot-process retraction. As this occurs, there is a marked decrease in filtration slit length associated with loss of foot-process interdigitation, and furthermore there is closure of most remaining filtration slits by the development of incomplete tight junctional complexes between adjacent cells (Ryan *et al.*, 1975a). This loss of available filtration slits presumably explains the reduced glomerular filtration rates seen in rats with aminonucleoside nephrosis (Oken and Flamenbaum, 1971; Lewy, 1976). As these epithelial changes occur, the slit diaphragm is displaced away from the basement membrane and becomes detached, coiled and, in some instances, fractured (Ryan *et al.*, 1975b). In addition, coinciding precisely with the onset and persistence of proteinuria, there are found focal areas of complete absence of the epithelial covering of the glomerular capillaries (Ryan and Karnovsky, 1975) (Figure 1.3). At such sites, the glomerular capillary wall consists only of the endothelium and basement membrane, the outer surface of which is directly exposed to the urinary space. These areas probably develop as a result of imprecisely co-ordinated epithelial spreading, with the slit diaphragm detaching and foot processes retracting before firm junctional complexes form between adjacent cells. Because they found that intravenously administered ferritin particles penetrated the glomerular capillary wall to enter the urinary space only at areas showing externally bare basement membrane, Ryan and Karnovsky (1975) postulated that such areas represent focal sites of leakage of plasma proteins across the glomerular capillary wall in aminonucleoside nephrosis. This was subsequently confirmed by the detection of endogenous albumin and IgG crossing the basement membrane in such bare areas in glomeruli that were drip-fixed during good blood flow; no albumin or IgG penetration was detected beyond the endothelial fenestrae at sites of epithelial spreading (Ryan *et al.*, 1978a).

The mechanism of focal leakage of plasma proteins across the glomerular capillary wall at sites of epithelial denudation awaits elucidation. It may result from an increase in porosity of the basement membrane due to a biochemical compositional change wherever it is deprived of 'nourishment' from the overlying epithelium. It should be noted, however, that no ultrastructural change has been detected in the basement membrane in such sites;

incidentally, nor has any reduction in staining for intrinsic negative charge been detected in or on either side of the basement membrane in these areas (Alcorn and Ryan, 1981; Kanwar *et al.*, 1981). A more attractive possibility, taking account of the proposed important role of the intact epithelial layer in controlling water flux across the glomerular capillary wall (see above), is that loss of the epithelial layer may allow a focal increase in bulk flow of water across the denuded basement membrane (Ryan and Karnovsky, 1975). The increased transmural hydraulic driving force in such areas may either cause stretching and physical dilatation of structural pores in the unsupported basement membrane, or may simply lead to disturbance of the functionally dependent equilibrium that normally restricts the passage of plasma proteins beyond the endothelial fenestrae. In other words, focal epithelial loss may lead to a focal 'blow-out' in water flux that 'drags' plasma proteins across the basement membrane to the urinary space.

Glomerular epithelial defects have been detected by other investigators in aminonucleoside nephrosis (Venkatachalam *et al.*, 1969, 1970b; Caulfield *et al.*, 1976; Olson *et al.*, 1981; Kanwar and Rozenzweig, 1982b). In the early studies of Venkatachalam *et al.* (1969, 1970b), intravenously administered tracer molecules (horseradish peroxidase, catalase) were found in 'pockets' between the basement membrane and epithelium, as well as within intraepithelial vacuoles. No through-and-through communications of vacuoles from the basal to the urinary surface were encountered, presumably because the glomeruli were relatively collapsed as a result of immersion fixation. From their studies, Venkatachalam *et al.* (1970b) postulated that proteinuria in this model resulted from 'increased permeability of the basement membrane' in combination with an epithelial 'vacuolar pathway' whereby the tracer is 'transported across altered epithelial cells into the urinary space through a system of vacuoles'. This 'vacuolar pathway' concept differs substantively from the 'focal blow-out' concept of Ryan and Karnovsky (1975). Caulfield *et al.* (1976) described epithelial cell detachment in aminonucleoside nephrosis but only as a 'late change' (10-15 days) following a protocol of daily injections of a low dose of puromycin aminonucleoside in which proteinuria was first detected at 5-8 days. Recent studies in our laboratory (Messina, Davies and Ryan, in preparation), reproducing precisely the low-dose protocol of Caulfield *et al.*, have clearly demonstrated the presence of epithelial defects coincident with the onset of proteinuria at 5 days. More recently, Olson *et al.* (1981) and Kanwar and Rosenzweig (1982b) confirmed the finding of Ryan and Karnovsky (1975) that intravenously administered ferritin molecules traverse the basement membrane at sites of epithelial denudation. Kanwar and Rosenzweig (1982b) supported the 'focal blow-out' concept as follows: 'epithelial detachment could lead to major glomerular haemodynamic changes that effectively over-ride the barrier properties of the GBM (glomerular basement membrane), leading to enhanced bulk flow of plasma macro-molecules from capillary lumina through the GCW (glomerular capillary wall) into the urinary spaces'.

Similar glomerular epithelial defects, leaving segments of externally bare basement membrane, have been described in other experimental models of the nephrotic syndrome in rats. These include the lesions seen in response to N,N'-diacetylbenzidine (Carroll *et al.*, 1974), antiglomerular basement membrane nephritis (Kühn *et al.*, 1977), protein overload nephropathy (Davies *et al.*, 1978, 1985), autologous immune complex nephritis (Schneeberger *et al.*, 1979), extreme renal ablation nephropathy (Olson *et al.*, 1982) and Adriamycin nephrosis (Weening and Rennke, 1983). Of special interest are the findings of Olson *et al.* (1982) in rats subjected to extreme ablation of renal mass. Such animals showed glomerular epithelial detachment and proteinuria if fed a normal laboratory diet but not if fed a low-protein diet. Because low-protein feeding substantially modulates the increased glomerular pressures and flows which normally occur in the remnant kidney in this model (Olson *et al.*, 1982), it was suggested that glomerular hyperfiltration may trigger glomerular damage, possibly leading eventually to glomerulosclerosis. This concept is of considerable significance in relationship to the pathogenesis of progressive destruction of surviving glomeruli following a range of causes of primary renal damage.

Although glomerular epithelial defects appear likely to play a major role in the pathogenesis of proteinuria, it should be appreciated that any structural abnormality that affects the equilibrium of forces that operate at the endothelial fenestrae is a potential additional candidate for such a role. For instance, endogenous albumin has been found penetrating the basement membrane at sites of focal endothelial loss in antiglomerular basement membrane nephritis in rats (Kühn *et al.*, 1977), possibly as a result of disruption of a concentration-polarisation layer or whatever functional barrier normally operates at the endothelial level. In this experimental model, as can be found in human proliferative glomerulonephritis, some capillary loops also show endothelial swelling and leukocytic accumulation, either of which could cause patchy plasma protein leakage due to interference with blood flow in such capillaries.

Role of Glomerular Charge

As a corollary of the hypothesis that intrinsic negative charge in or associated with the basement membrane is the major factor responsible for restricting the penetration of plasma albumin across the normal glomerular capillary wall, it has been widely thought that proteinuria occurs in glomerular disease as a result of loss of such negative charge from the glomerulus (Michael *et al.*, 1970; Chiu and Drummond, 1972; Roy *et al.*, 1972; Blau and Haas, 1973; Bennett *et al.*, 1976; Bohrer *et al.*, 1977a; Brenner *et al.*, 1977, 1978; Caulfield and Farquhar, 1978; Caulfield, 1979; Kreisberg *et al.*, 1979). Permselectivity studies in antiglomerular basement membrane nephritis in rats indicated that, whereas fractional clearances of neutral dextran molecules were reduced when compared with normal values (Chang *et al.*, 1976), fractional clearances of anionic dextran sulphate molecules over the corresponding range of effective radii were greater than normal (Bennett *et al.*, 1976). In the same model, reduced clearances of cationic DEAE dextran molecules were detected (Bohrer *et al.* 1978). In aminonucleoside nephrosis, Bohrer *et al.* (1977a) reported a reduction in the clearances of neutral dextran molecules, accompanied by a slight, just significant, increase in the clearances of dextran sulphate molecules, but in the larger size range only. These findings seemed to support the idea of a significant role for loss of intrinsic negative charge from the glomerulus in the development of proteinuria. Subsequently, however, Olson *et al.* (1981) used a broader range of fractions to show that although the clearances of neutral dextran molecules with an effective radius smaller than 3.0 nm were decreased in rats with aminonucleoside nephrosis when compared with control animals, the clearances of molecules with an effective radius larger than 3.8 nm were increased in nephrotic as compared with control rats. The latter findings shifted the emphasis to the view that a loss of size-selective barrier function is of special importance in this model. The reduced clearance of the smaller neutral dextran fractions presumably results from the extreme loss of filtration slits that occurs in such glomeruli, correlating with the reduction in glomerular filtration rate. The increased clearance of the larger neutral dextran fractions simply reflects the loss of size-selective barrier function that results in proteinuria. Similarly, the increased clearance values for dextran sulphate molecules reflect their behaviour as relatively larger molecules under ultrafiltration conditions, due to their impaired flexibility (as discussed earlier). Olson *et al.* (1981) also reported increased fractional clearances for anionic and neutral horseradish peroxidase (HRP) and some decrease in the clearance of cationic HRP in aminonucleoside nephrosis. The anionic and neutral HRP results can be explained by the loss of size-selective barrier function in such animals. The reduced clearances of cationic DEAE dextran (see above, Bohrer *et al.*, 1978) and cationic HRP in proteinuric animals are difficult to interpret in conjunction with the associated data. However, as discussed earlier, the use of cationised derivatives needs to be treated with caution: the apparently reduced clearances of the cationised molecules in aminonucleoside nephrosis may result from a relatively lessened susceptibility of the architecturally abnormal glomeruli (i.e. with extensive epithelial spreading) to respond to the proteinuria-provoking effects seen with such derivatives in normal animals (Purtell *et al.*, 1979).

There have been various claims that there is a reduction in the amount of stainable glomerular polyanion in proteinuric states (Michael *et al.*, 1970; Chiu and Drummond, 1972; Roy *et al.*, 1972; Blau and Haas, 1973; Bennett *et al.*, 1976; Brenner *et al.*, 1977, 1978; Bohrer *et al.*, 1978; Caulfield and Farquhar, 1978; Caulfield, 1979; Kreisberg *et al.*, 1979;). Such reports have been regularly cited as providing evidence favouring the key role for generalised loss of intrinsic negative charge from the glomerulus in the pathogenesis of proteinuria. However, many of the reports are based largely upon light microscopic studies and therefore provide inadequate information concerning the ultrastructural distribution of the charged molecules in the glomerular capillary wall. Indeed when superficial glomeruli of Munich-Wistar rats with antiglomerular-basement membrane nephritis or aminonucleoside nephrosis were examined electron microscopically following rapid *in situ* drip fixation during good blood flow, no reduction in the amount of colloidal iron staining for negative groups was detected on podocytic epithelial cell surfaces, in the basement membrane or on endothelial surfaces (Alcorn and Ryan, 1981). Similar results were obtained more recently in protein-overload nephropathy (Davies *et al.*, 1985). In each of these models, however, there was the usual extensive replacement of the normal multiple foot processes by flattened expanses of epithelial cytoplasm. This resulted in a great decrease in podocytic epithelial surface area, the site of heaviest binding of colloidal iron. It appears, then, that the reduced glomerular polyanionic staining detected light microscopically in glomerular disease may be an epiphenomenon of simplified glomerular epithelial architecture rather than necessarily being an explanation for proteinuria. A similar conclusion was reached by Weening and Rennke (1983) as a result of their studies of Adriamycin nephrosis in rats.

The use of a variety of other cationic stains in various experimental models has produced variable results. Caulfield and Farquhar (1978) reported reduced binding of perfused lysozyme to podocytic epithelium and glomerular basement membrane in aminonucleoside nephrosis. However, because free ultrafiltration flux will not occur at sites of extensive epithelial spreading in this model, such a decrease in lysozyme binding under the perfusion conditions operating in these studies could result from reduced penetration of lysozyme into the glomerular capillary wall. This may also explain the reduced podocytic binding of perfused Alcian blue reported by Caulfield (1979) in the same model. In a subtotal nephrectomy model in rats, Shea *et al.* (1980) found that proteinuria was not accompanied by changes in the ultrastructural distribution of anionic sites in the glomerular basement membrane, as determined by perfusion with cationised ferritin or ruthenium red. Similarly, Kanwar *et al.* (1981) detected no change in the binding of cationised ferritin, cytochrome-*c* or ruthenium red to the glomerular basement membrane in rats with aminonucleoside nephrosis. In contrast, using an immunoperoxidase technique, Mynderse *et al.* (1983) reported a loss of heparan sulphate from the glomerular basement membrane of nephrotic rats although, because the investigators used an intravenous route to administer the antibodies to the glomeruli, there must again be a serious question as to whether the antibody molecules had comparable access to the basement membrane in the nephrotic versus the normal animals in view of the reduced glomerular filtration rates in nephrotic animals. Finally, in a recent elegant study, Kanwar and Jakubowski

(1984) used quantitative autoradiographic techniques to demonstrate that there was no reduction in the binding of radiolabelled cationised ferritin to the glomerular basement membrane of rats with aminonucleoside nephrosis. Nor was there any reduction in binding of this probe to areas of basement membrane that were denuded of podocytic epithelium. These workers concluded that there are 'no significant alterations in the anionic sites rich in heparan sulphate proteoglycan' during the course of aminonucleoside nephrosis. On the other hand it is possible that changes in anionic sites may be relevant in other circumstances. For instance, minor changes in the synthesis of heparan sulphate have been reported in streptozotocin-induced diabetic nephropathy (Kanwar *et al.*, 1983).

In view of the prominence of glomerular epithelial changes, i.e. spreading and detachment, in proteinuric states, consideration needs to be given to the possibility that such changes result from abnormalities of the substratum to which the epithelial cells are attached, i.e. the glomerular basement membrane. The components of the basement membrane that are involved in epithelial attachment are not yet known, although there are suggestions that anionic molecules are significant factors in view of the finding by Kanwar and his colleagues (Kanwar and Farquhar, 1980; Kanwar and Rosenzweig, 1982b; Kanwar, 1984) that treatment of kidneys with protease-free neuraminidase resulted in the detachment of epithelial foot processes from the basement membrane. In such kidneys, ferritin passed from the capillary lumen to the urinary space across areas of basement membrane denuded of epithelium (Kanwar and Rosenzweig, 1982b). Further studies are clearly required to investigate this aspect of the potential role of intrinsic anionic sites in the glomerular basement membrane.

Relevance of Experimental Models to the Pathogenesis of Severe Proteinuria in Human Glomerular Disease

What is the relationship of the ultrastructural changes found in experimental models of the nephrotic syndrome to the pathogenesis of proteinuria in human glomerulonephritis? Glomerular epithelial spreading is a well-known lesion in nephrotic patients, particularly those with minimal change disease or focal glomerulosclerosis and hyalinosis. Grishman and Churg (1975) described epithelial defects with bare areas of basement membrane in nephrotic patients with focal glomerulosclerosis. Detailed ultrastructural examination of renal biopsy specimens has revealed the presence of such epithelial defects in a broad range of nephrotic patients including those with minimal change disease, focal glomerulosclerosis and hyalinosis, membranous glomerulo-nephritis, diabetic glomerulopathy and amyloidosis (G.B. Ryan, unpublished observations).

In studies of glomerular filtration dynamics and fractional clearances of neutral dextrans, albumin and IgG in patients with a variety of causes of proteinuria (including diabetic nephropathy), Myers and his colleagues

(Myers *et al.*, 1982a, b; Friedman *et al.*, 1983, 1984) concluded that severe proteinuria was associated with the development of a subpopulation of enlarged pores in the glomerular capillary wall through which large as well as small macromolecules are able to penetrate. They regarded these enlarged pores as being in a 'defective region of the membrane, not normally present in healthy individuals' (Friedman *et al.*, 1984). The focal areas of externally bare basement membrane may represent the morphological counterpart of these 'large-pore regions'. These findings, in conjunction with the experimental data in animal models, suggest that the podocytic epithelial lesion, producing areas of denuded basement membrane, is likely to be a major site of clinically significant plasma protein leakage from the glomerulus in human glomerular disease.

Summary

Plasma proteins are normally retained within the glomerular capillary lumen by a functionally dependent barrier that operates at the level of the endothelial fenestrae. This barrier depends critically upon the maintenance of normal haemodynamic and ultrafiltration conditions in the glomerulus, such conditions providing an appropriate balance between convective and diffusive forces across the glomerular capillary wall. Molecular sieving phenomena in association with the effects of concentration-polarisation and perhaps intrinsic glycosaminoglycans are likely to contribute to normal glomerular perm-selectivity. The podocytic epithelial layer, by significantly controlling water flux across the capillary wall, may play a key role in such permselectivity. In proteinuric states, podocytic epithelial cells show prominent changes characterised by cytoplasmic spreading and areas of detachment from the basement membrane. Except insofar as anionic groups may be involved in the attachment of the podocytic epithelial layer to the basement membrane, generalised loss of intrinsic negative charge from the glomerulus does not appear to be a major determining factor in the pathogenesis of proteinuria. Rather, plasma proteins cross the basement membrane to enter the urinary space at sites of epithelial denudation, possible as a result of a focal 'blow-out' of ultrafiltration flux causing a breakdown of the normal equilibrium of forces that operate at the endothelial fenestrae.

Acknowledgements

The author's work in this field since 1976 has been funded by grants from the National Health and Medical Research Council of Australia. The author thanks Mrs M. Mackie for drawing Figure 1.2; Dr D. Alcorn, Miss A. Messina and Mrs G. Kelly for Figures 1.1 and 1.3; Ms P. Brown for photographic assistance; and Mrs J. Bennett and Miss F. Bowers for typing the manuscript.

References

Alcorn, D. and Ryan, G.B. (1981) 'Distribution of Anionic Groups in the Glomerular Capillary Wall in Rat Nephrotoxic Nephritis and Aminonucleoside Nephrosis', *Pathology, 13*, 37–50

Barnes, J.L., Radnik, R.A., Gilchrist, E.P. and Venkatachalam, M.A. (1984) 'Size and Charge Selective Permeability Defects Induced in Glomerular Basement Membrane by a Polycation', *Kidney Int., 25*, 11–19

Bennett, C.M.,Glassock, R.J., Chang, R.L.S., Deen, W.M., Robertson, C.R. and Brenner, B.M. (1976) 'Permselectivity of the Glomerular Capillary Wall: Studies of Experimental Glomerulonephritis in the Rat Using Dextran Sulfate', *J. Clin. Invest., 57*, 1287–94

Blatt, W.F., Dravid, A., Michaels, A.S. and Nelsen, L. (1970), 'Solute Polarization and Cake Formation in Membrane Ultrafiltration: Causes, Consequences and Control Techniques, in J.E. Flinn (ed.), *Membrane Science and Technology. Industrial, Biological and Waste Treatment Processes*, Plenum Press, New York, pp. 47–97

Blau, E.B. and Haas, J.E. (1973) 'Glomerular Sialic Acid and Proteinuria in Human Renal Disease', *Lab. Invest., 28*, 477–81

Bohrer, M.P., Baylis, C., Robertson, C.R. and Brenner, B.M. (1977a) 'Mechanisms of the Puromycin-induced Defects in the Transglomerular Passage of Water and Macromolecules', *J. Clin. Invest., 60*, 152–61

Bohrer, M.P., Deen, W.M., Robertson, C.R. and Brenner, B.M. (1977b) 'Mechanisms of Angiotensin II-induced Proteinuria in the Rat', *Am. J. Physiol., 233*, F13–21

Bohrer, M.P., Baylis, C., Humes, H.D., Glassock, R.J., Robertson, C.R. and Brenner, B.M. (1978) 'Permselectivity of the Glomerular Capillary Wall: Facilitated Filtration of Circulating Polycations', *J. Clin. Invest., 61*, 72–8

Bowman, W. (1842) 'On the Structure and Use of the Malpighian Bodies of the Kidney, with Observations on the Circulation through that Gland', *Phil. Trans. Roy. Soc. Lond. (Biol. Sci.), 132*, 57–80

Brenner, B.M., Bohrer, M.P., Baylis, C. and Deen, W.M. (1977) 'Determinants of Glomerular Permselectivity: Insights Derived from Observations *in vivo*', *Kidney Int., 12*, 229–37

Brenner, B.M., Hostetter, T.H. and Humes, H.D. (1978) 'Glomerular Permselectivity: Barrier Function Based on Discrimination of Molecular Size and Charge', *Am. J. Physiol., 234*, F455–60

Carroll, N., Crock, G.W., Funder, C.C., Green, C.R., Ham, K.N. and Tange, J.D. (1974) 'Glomerular Epithelial Cell Lesions Induced by N,N'-Diacetylbenzidine', *Lab. Invest., 31*, 239–45

Caulfield, J.P. (1979) 'Alterations in the Distribution of Alcian Blue-staining Fibrillar Anionic Sites in the Glomerular Basement Membrane in Aminonucleoside Nephrosis', *Lab. Invest., 40*, 503–11

Caulfield, J.P. and Farquhar, M.G. (1974) 'The Permeability of Glomerular Capillaries to Graded Dextrans', *J. Cell Biol., 63*, 883–902

Caulfield, J.P. and Farquhar, M.G. (1976) 'Distribution of Anionic Sites in Glomerular Basement Membranes: their Possible Role in Filtration and Attachment', *Proc. Natl Acad. Sci. USA, 73*, 1646–50

Caulfield, J.P. and Farquhar, M.G. (1978) 'Loss of Anionic Sites from the Glomerular Basement Membrane in Aminonucleoside Nephrosis', *Lab. Invest., 39*, 505–12

Caulfield, J.P., Reid, J.J. and Farquhar, M.G. (1976) 'Alterations of Glomerular Epithelium in Acute Aminonucleoside Nephrosis: Evidence for Formation of Occluding Junctions and Epithelial Detachment', *Lab. Invest., 34*, 43–59

Chang, R.L.S., Deen, W.M., Robertson, C.R. and Brenner, B.M. (1975a) 'Permselectivity of the Glomerular Capillary Wall: III Restricted Transport of Polyanions', *Kidney Int., 8*, 212–18

Chang, R.L.S., Ueki, I.F., Troy, J.L., Deen, W.M., Robertson, C.R. and Brenner, B.M. (1975b) 'Permselectivity of the Glomerular Capillary Wall: II Experimental Studies in Rats Using Dextran', *Biophys. J., 15*, 887–906

Chang, R.L.S., Deen, W.M., Robertson, C.R., Bennett, C.M., Glassock, R.J. and Brenner, B.M. (1976) 'Permselectivity of the Glomerular Capillary Wall: Studies of Experimental Glomerulonephritis in the Rat Using Neutral Dextran', *J. Clin. Invest., 57*, 1272–86

Chiu, J. and Drummond, K.N. (1972) 'Chemical and Histochemical Studies of Glomerular Sialoprotein in Nephrotoxic Nephritis in Rats', *Am. J. Pathol., 68*, 391–406

Comper, W.D. and Laurent, T.C. (1978) 'Physiological Function of Connective Tissue Polysaccharides', *Physiol. Rev.*, *58*, 255–315

Cushny, A.R. (1917) *The Secretion of the Urine*, Longmans, Green, London

Davies, D.J., Brewer, D.B. and Hardwicke, J. (1978) 'Urinary Proteins and Glomerular Morphometry in Protein Overload Proteinuria', *Lab. Invest.*, *38*, 232–43

Davies, D.J., Messina, A., Thumwood, C.M. and Ryan, G.B. (1985) 'Glomerular Podocytic Injury in Protein Overload Proteinuria', *Pathology*, in press

Deen, W.M., Robertson, C.R. and Brenner, B.M. (1974) 'Concentration Polarization in an Ultrafiltering Capillary', *Biophys. J.*, *14*, 412–31

DeGennes, P.G. (1971) 'Reptation of a Polymer Chain in the Presence of Fixed Obstacles', *J. Chem. Phys.*, *55*, 572–9

Farquhar, M.G. and Palade, G.E. (1961) 'Glomerular Permeability. II Ferritin Transfer across the Glomerular Capillary Wall in Nephrotic Rats', *J. Exp. Med.*, *114*, 699–715

Farquhar, M.G., Wissig, S.L. and Palade, G.E. (1961) 'Glomerular Permeability: I Ferritin Transfer across the Normal Glomerular Capillary Wall', *J. Exp. Med.*, *113*, 47–66

Feldman, J.D. and Fisher, E.R. (1959) 'Renal Lesions of Aminonucleoside Nephrosis as Revealed by Electron Microscopy', *Lab. Invest.*, *8*, 371–85

Friedman, S., Jones, H.W. III, Golbetz, H.V., Lee, J.A., Little, H.L. and Myers, B.D. (1983) 'Mechanisms of Proteinuria in Diabetic Nephropathy II. A Study of the Size-selective Glomerular Filtration Barrier', *Diabetes*, *32* (*Suppl. 2*), 40–6

Friedman, S., Strober, S., Field, E.H., Silverman, E. and Myers, B.D, (1984) 'Glomerular Capillary Wall Function in Human Lupus Nephritis', *Am. J. Physiol.*, *246*, F580–91

Graham, R.C. and Karnovsky, M.J. (1966) 'Glomerular Permeability. Ultrastructural Cytochemical Studies Using Peroxidases as Protein Tracers', *J. Exp. Med.*, *124*, 1123–34

Grishman, E. and Churg, J. (1975) 'Focal Glomerular Sclerosis in Nephrotic Patients: an Electron Microscopic Study of Glomerular Podocytes', *Kidney Int.*, *7*, 111–22

Heidenhain, R. (1874) 'Versuche über den Vorgang der Harnabsonderung', *Arch. F. D. Ges. Physiol.*, *9*, 1–27

Hunsicker, L.G., Shearer, T.P. and Shaffer, S.J. (1981) 'Acute Reversible Proteinuria Induced by Infusion of the Polycation Hexadimethrine', *Kidney Int.*, *20* 7–17

Jones, D.B. (1969) 'Mucosubstances of the Glomerulus', *Lab. Invest.*, *21*, 119–25

Kanwar, Y.S. (1984) 'Biology of Disease. Biophysiology of Glomerular Filtration and Proteinuria', *Lab. Invest.*, *51*, 7–21

Kanwar, Y.S. and Farquhar, M.G. (1979a) 'Anionic Sites in the Glomerular Basement Membrane. *In vivo* and *in vitro* Localization to the Laminae Rarae by Cationic Probes', *J. Cell Biol.*, *81*, 137–53

Kanwar, Y.S. and Farquhar, M.G. (1979b) 'Presence of Heparan Sulfate in the Glomerular Basement Membrane', *Proc. Natl Acad. Sci. USA*, *76*, 1303–7

Kanwar, Y.S. and Farquhar, M.G. (1979c) 'Isolation of Glycosaminoglycans (Heparan Sulfate) from Glomerular Basement Membranes', *Proc. Natl Acad. Sci. USA*, *76*, 4493–7

Kanwar, Y.S. and Farquhar, M.G. (1980) 'Detachment of Endothelium and Epithelium from the Glomerular Basement Membrane Produced by Perfusion with Neuraminidase', *Lab. Invest.*, *42*, 375–84

Kanwar, Y.S. and Jakubowski, M.L. (1984) 'Unaltered Anionic Sites of Glomerular Basement Membrane in Aminonucleoside Nephrosis', *Kidney Int.*, *25*, 613–18

Kanwar, Y.S. and Rosenzweig, L.J. (1982a) 'Clogging of the Glomerular Basement Membrane to Ferritin after Removal of Glycosaminoglycans (Heparan Sulfate) by Enzyme Digestion', *J. Cell Biol.*, *86*, 688–93

Kanwar, Y.S. and Rosenzweig, L.J. (1982b) 'Altered Glomerular Permeability as a Result of Focal Detachment of Visceral Epithelium', *Kidney Int.*, *21*, 565–74

Kanwar, Y.S., Linker, A. and Farquhar, M.G. (1980) 'Increased Permeability of the Glomerular Basement Membrane to Ferritin after Removal of Glycosaminoglycans (Heparan Sulfate) by Enzyme Digestion', *J. Cell Biol.*, *86*, 688–93

Kanwar, Y.S., Rosenzweig, L.J. and Kerjaschki, D.I. (1981) 'Glycosaminoglycans of the Glomerular Basement Membrane in Normal and Nephrotic States', *Renal Physiol.*, *4*, 121–30

Kanwar, Y.S., Rosenzweig, L.J., Linker, A. and Jakubowski, M.L. (1983) 'Decreased *de novo* Synthesis of Glomerular Proteoglycan in Diabetes: Biochemical and Autoradiographic Evidence', *Proc. Natl Acad. Sci. USA*, *80*, 2272–5

Karnovsky, M.J. and Ainsworth, S.K. (1972) 'The Structural Basis of Glomerular Filtration', in J. Hamburger, J. Crosnier and M.H. Maxwell (eds), *Advances in Nephrology*, vol. 2,Yearbook Medical Publishers, Chicago, pp.35–60

Karnovsky, M.J. and Ryan, G.B. (1975) 'Substructure of the Glomerular Slit Diaphragm in Freeze-fractured Normal Rat Kidney', *J. Cell Biol.*, *65*, 233–6

Katchalsky, A. (1964) 'Polyelectrolytes and their Biological Interactions', *Biophys. J.*, *4 (Suppl. to Jan. issue)*, 9–31

Kreisberg, J.I., Wayne, D.B. and Karnovsky, M.J. (1979) 'Rapid and Focal Loss of Negative Charge Associated with Mononuclear Cell Infiltration Early in Nephrotoxic Nephritis', *Kidney Int.*, *16*, 290–300

Kühn, K., Ryan, G.N., Hein, S.J., Galaske, R.G. and Karnovsky, M.J. (1977) 'An Ultrastructural Study of the Mechanisms of Proteinuria in Rat Nephrotoxic Nephritis', *Lab. Invest.*, *36*, 375–87

Landis, E.M. and Pappenheimer, J.R. (1963), 'Exchanges of Substances through the Capillary Wall', in W.F.Hamilton and P. Dow (eds) *Handbook of Physiology*, Section 2, *Circulation*, vol. 2, American Physiological Society, Washington, DC, pp. 961–1034

Larsen, B. (1967) 'Increased Permeability to Albumin Induced with Protamine in Modified Gelatin Membranes', *Nature (Lond.)*, *215*, 641–2

Latta, H., Johnston, W.H. and Stanley, T.M. (1975) 'Sialoglycoproteins and Filtration Barriers in the Glomerular Capillary Wall', *J. Ultrastruct. Res.*, *51*, 354–76

Laurent, T.C. (1966) '*In vitro* Studies on the Transport of Macromolecules through the Connective Tissue', *Fed. Proc.*, *25*, 1128–34

Laurent, T.C., Preston, B.N., Pertroft, H., Gustafsson, B. and McCabe, M. (1975) 'Diffusion of Linear Polymers in Hyaluronate Solutions', *Eur. J. Biochem.*, *53*, 129–36

Lewy, J.E. (1976) 'Micropuncture Study of Fluid Transfer in Aminonucleoside Nephrosis in the Rat', *Pediat. Res.*, *10*, 30–4

Ludwig, C. (1844) 'Nieren und Harnbereitung'. *Wagner's Handb. Physiol.*, *2*, 628–40

Michael, A.F., Blau, E. and Vernier, R.L. (1970) 'Glomerular Polyanion: Alteration in Aminonucleoside Nephrosis', *Lab. Invest.*, *23*, 649–57

Myers, B.D., Okarma, T.B., Friedman, S., Bridges, C., Ross, J., Asseff, S. and Deen, W.M. (1982a) 'Mechanisms of Proteinuria in Human Glomerulonephritis', *J. Clin. Invest.*, *70*, 732–46

Myers, B.D., Winetz, J.A., Chui, F. and Michaels, A.S. (1982b) 'Mechanisms of Proteinuria in Diabetic Nephropathy: a Study of Glomerular Barrier Function', *Kidney Int.*, *21*, 633–41

Mynderse, L.A., Hassell, J.R., Kleinman, H.K., Martin, G.R. and Martinez-Hernandez, A. (1983) 'Loss of Heparan Sulfate Proteoglycan from Glomerular Basement Membrane of Nephrotic Rats', *Lab. Invest.*, *48*, 292–302

Oken, D.E. and Flamenbaum, W. (1971) 'Micropuncture Studies of Proximal Tubule Albumin Concentrations in Normal and Nephrotic Rats', *J. Clin. Invest.*, *50*, 1498–505

Olson, J.L., Rennke, H.G. and Venkatachalam, M.A. (1981) 'Alteration in Charge and Size Selectivity Barrier of Glomerular Filter in Aminonucleoside Nephrosis', *Lab. Invest.*, *44*, 271–9

Olson, J.L., Hostetter, T.H., Rennke, H.G., Brenner, B.M. and Venkatachalam, M. A. (1982) 'Altered Glomerular Permselectivity and Progressive Sclerosis Following Extreme Ablation of Renal Mass', *Kidney Int.*, *22*, 112–6

Pappenheimer, J.R. (1953) 'Passage of Molecules through Capillary Walls', *Physiol. Rev.*, *33*, 387–423

Poortmans, J.R. (1970) 'Proteinuria after Muscular Work', in Y. Manuel, J.P. Revillard and H. Betuel, (eds), *Proteins in Normal and Pathological Urine*, Karger, Basel, pp. 229–34

Purtell, J.N., Pesce, A.J., Clyne, D.H., Miller, W.C. and Pollack, V.E. (1979) Isoelectric Point of Albumin: Effect on Renal Handling of Albumin', *Kidney Int.*, *16*, 366–76

Renkin, E.M. and Gilmore, J.P. (1973) 'Glomerular Filtration', in J. Orloff and R.W. Berliner (eds), *Handbook of Physiology, section 8, Renal Physiology*,American Physiological Society Washington, DC, pp. 185–248

Rennke, H.G. and Venkatachalam, M.A. (1977) 'Glomerular Permeability: *in vivo* Tracer Studies with Polyanionic and Polycationic Ferritins', *Kidney Int.*, *11*, 44–53

Rennke, H.G. and Venkatachalam, M.A. (1979) 'Glomerular Permeability of Macromolecules: Effect of Molecular Configuration on the Fractional Clearance of Uncharged Dextran and

Neutral Horseradish Peroxidase in the Rat', *J. Clin. Invest.*, *63*, 713–17

Rennke, H.G., Cotran, R.S. and Venkatachalam, M.A. (1975) 'Role of Molecular Charge in Glomerular Permeability: Tracer Studies with Cationized Ferritins', *J. Cell Biol.*, *67*, 638–46

Rennke, H.G., Patel, Y. and Venkatachalam, M.A. (1978) 'Glomerular Filtration of Proteins: Clearance of Anionic, Neutral and Cationic Horseradish Peroxidase in the Rat', *Kidney Int.*, *13*, 324–8

Rhodin, J.A.G. (1962) 'The Diaphragm of Capillary Endothelial Fenestrations', *J. Ultrastruct. Res.*, *6*, 171–85

Robinson, G.B. and Cotter, T.G. (1980) 'Concentration Polarization: a Determining Factor in Filtration across Basement Membranes?', in A.B. Maunsbach, T.S. Olsen and E.I. Christensen (eds), *Functional Ultrastructure of the Kidney*, Academic Press, London, pp.75–89

Robinson, R.R. (1970) 'Postural Proteinuria', in Y. Manuel, J.P. Revillard and H. Betuel (eds), *Proteins in Normal and Pathological Urine*, Karger, Basel, pp. 224–8

Rodewald, R. and Karnovsky, M.J. (1974) 'Porous Substructure of the Glomerular Slit Diaphragm in the Rat and Mouse', *J.Cell Biol.*, *60*, 423–33

Rosenzweig, L.J. and Kanwar, Y.S. (1982) 'Removal of Sulfated (Heparan Sulfate) or Unsulfated (Hyaluronic Acid) Glycosaminoglycans Results in Increased Permeability of the Glomerular Basement Membrane to ^{125}I-Bovine Serum Albumin', *Lab. Invest.*, *47* 177–84

Roy, L.P., Vernier, R.L. and Michael, A.F. (1972) 'Effect of Protein-Load Proteinuria on Glomerular Polyanion', *Proc. Soc. Exp. Biol. Med.*, *141*, 870–4

Ryan, G.B. (1979) 'Ultrastructural Studies of the Mechanisms of Proteinuria in Glomerular Disease', in P. Kincaid-Smith, A.J.F. d'Apice and R.C. Atkins (eds), *Progress in Glomerulonephritis*, Wiley Medical, New York pp.145–56

Ryan, G.B. and Karnovsky, M.J. (1975) 'An Ultrastructural Study of the Mechanics of Proteinuria in Aminonucleoside Nephrosis', *Kidney Int.*, *8*, 219–32

Ryan, G.B. and Karnovsky, M.J. (1976) 'Distribution of Endogenous Albumin in the Rat Glomerulus: Role of Hemodynamic Factors in Glomerular Barrier', *Kidney Int.*, *9*, 36–45

Ryan, G.B., Leventhal, M. and Karnovsky, M.J. (1975a) 'A Freeze-fracture Study of the Junctions between Glomerular Epithelial Cells in Aminonucleoside Nephrosis', *Lab. Invest.*, *32*, 397–403

Ryan, G.B.,Rodewald, R. and Karnovsky, M.J. (1975b) 'An Ultrastructural Study of the Glomerular Slit Diaphragm in Aminonucleoside Nephrosis', *Lab. Invest.*, *33*, 461–8

Ryan, G.B., Hein, S.J. and Karnovsky, M.J. (1976) 'Glomerular Permeability to Proteins: Effects of Hemodynamic Factors on the Distribution of Endogenous Immunoglobulin G and Exogenous Catalase in the Rat Glomerulus', *Lab. Invest.*, *34*, 415–27

Ryan, G.B., Hein, S.J. and, Karnovsky, M.J. (1978a) 'The Distribution of Albumin and Immunoglobulin G in the Glomerular Capillary Wall in Aminonucleoside Nephrosis', *Pathology*, *10*, 335–41

Ryan, G.B., Hein, S.J., Kreisberg, J.I. and Karnovsky, M.J. (1978b) 'Effect of Hemodynamic Factors on the Distribution of Anionic Groups in the Glomerular Capillary Wall', *J. Ultrastruct. Res.*, *65*, 227–33

Schneeberger, E.E., O'Brien, A. and Grupe, W.E. (1979) 'Altered Glomerular Permeability in Munich-Wistar Rats with Autologous Immune Complex Nephritis', *Lab. Invest.*, *40*, 227–35

Schurer, J.W., Fleuren, G-J., Hoedemaeker, P.J. and Molenaar, I. (1980) 'A Macromolecular Model of the Glomerular Basement Membrane', in A.B. Maunsbach, T.S. Olsen and E.I. Christensen (eds), *Functional Ultrastructure of the Kidney*, Academic Press, London, pp. 105–17

Seiler, M.W., Venkatachalam, M.A. and Cotran, R.S. (1975) 'Glomerular Epithelium: Structural Alterations Induced by Polycations', *Science*, *189*, 390–3

Seiler, M.W., Rennke, H.G., Venkatachalam, M.A. and Cotran, R.S. (1977) 'Pathogenesis of Polycation-induced Alterations ('Fusion') of Glomerular Epithelium', *Lab. Invest.*, *36*, 48–61

Shea, S.M. and Morrison, A.B. (1975) 'A Stereological Study of the Glomerular Filter in the Rat. Morphometry of the Slit Diaphragm and Basement Membrane', *J. Cell Biol.*, *67*, 436–43

Shea, S.M., Raskova, J. and Morrison, A.B. (1980) 'Ultrastructure of the Glomerular Basement Membrane of Rats with Proteinuria due to Subtotal Nephrectomy', *Am. J. Pathol.*,

100, 513–28

Smith, H.W. (1951) *The Kidney. Structure and Function in Health and Disease*, Oxford University Press, New York

Stolte, H., Schurek, H-J. and Alt, J.M. (1979) 'Glomerular Albumin Filtration: Comparison of Micropuncture Studies in the Isolated Perfused Rat Kidney with *in vivo* Experimental Conditions', *Kidney Int.*, *16*, 377–84

Swanson, J.W., Besarab, A., Pomerantz, P.P. and DeGuzman, A. (1981) 'Effect of Erythrocytes and Globulin on Renal Functions of the Isolated Rat Kidney', *Am. J. Physiol.*, *241*, F139–50

Vehaskari, V.M., Root, E.R., Germuth, F.G. and Robson, A.M. (1982) 'Glomerular Charge and Urinary Excretion: Effect of Systemic and Intrarenal Polycation Infusion in the Rat', *Kidney Int.*, *22*, 127–35

Venkatachalam, M.A., Karnovsky, M.J. and Cotran, R.S. (1969) 'Glomerular Permeability. Ultrastructural Studies in Experimental Nephrosis Using Horseradish Peroxidase as a Tracer', *J. Exp. Med.*, *130*, 381–9

Venkatachalam, M.A., Cotran, R.S. and Karnovsky, M.J. (1970b) 'An Ultrastructural Study of Glomerular Permeability in Aminonucleoside Nephrosis Using Catalase as a Tracer Protein', *J. Exp. Med.*, *132*, 1168–80

Venkatachalam, M.A., Karnovsky, M.J., Fahimi, H.D. and Cotran, R.S. (1970a) 'An Ultrastructural Study of Glomerular Permeability Using Catalase and Peroxidase as Tracer Proteins', *J. Exp. Med.*, *132*, 1153–67

Vernier, R.L., Papermaster, B.W. and Good, R.A. (1959) 'Aminonucleoside Nephrosis: I Electron Microscopic Study of the Renal Lesion in Rats', *J. Exp. Med.*, *109*, 115–26

Weening, J.J. and Rennke, H.G. (1983) 'Glomerular Permeability and Polyanion in Adriamycin Nephrosis in the Rat', *Kidney Int.*, *24*, 152–9

Weinberg, J.M., Simmons, C.F. and Humes, H.D. (1979) 'The Molecular Basis of Aminoglycoside (A) and Diethylaminoethyl (DEAE) Dextran Nephrotoxicity', *Kidney Int.*, *16*, 778 (abstract)

2 GLOMERULAR FILTRATION DYNAMICS

Christine Baylis

Introduction

This chapter will focus on information obtained over the last 12 to 15 years from studies using *in vivo* micropuncture and certain *in vitro* techniques which have recently become available for the study of glomerular function. These techniques have permitted a detailed evaluation of the different determinants of glomerular ultrafiltration. *In vivo* micropuncture studies have been greatly advanced by the discovery of the Munich-Wistar rat strain. These rats possess glomerular capillaries on the surface of the renal cortex which permit direct measurement of the hydraulic pressures in the glomerular capillaries and Bowman's space, thus allowing direct measurement (or calculation) of all the dynamic determinants of glomerular ultrafiltration. Information derived from whole kidney studies in anaesthetised and awake animals has been considered by others (Renkin and Gilmore, 1973; O'Connor, 1982) and will not be described in great detail here.

Anatomy and Morphology

The glomerulus is unique in the microcirculation in that arteriolar resistance vessels are arranged, in series, both before and *after* the glomerular capillary, and a second capillary system, the peritubular capillary network, is located between the efferent (postglomerular) arterioles and the venules (Fourman and Moffat, 1971). The cortical glomeruli give rise to the efferent arterioles which break up to form the peritubular capillaries surrounding the tubules of cortical nephrons (Fourman and Moffat, 1971). The branching patterns of efferent arterioles which originate from cortical glomeruli have been described for the human, dog and rat kidney, and are highly variable (Beeuwkes, 1971; Evan and Dail, 1977; Moffat, 1981). In the outer (superficial) cortex some efferent arterioles are relatively long and run to the surface of the kidney to form the star vessels or welling points before they branch; in the rat 40 per cent or more of superficial efferent arterioles have this structure (Evan and Dail, 1977; Weinstein and Szyjewicz, 1978). Microinjection studies in the rat by Briggs and Wright (1979) have shown that the majority of superficial efferent arterioles are surrounded by tubules from at least two and up to four different nephrons. However, in approximately 30 per cent of cases the efferent arteriole was completely surrounded by tubules that belonged to the same nephron and had originated from the same parent glomerulus as the efferent arteriole. The afferent or preglomerular arterioles arise from the interlobular arteries and are extremely variable in length. The vascular smooth-muscle cells diminish in number as the afferent arteriole approaches the glomerulus and are replaced by the specialised cells of the juxtaglomerular apparatus, which lies in close proximity to the glomerulus. The juxtaglomerular apparatus is a specialised structure located in the wall of the afferent and to a lesser extent the efferent arterioles at the point where these vessels come into close apposition at the hilus of the glomerulus (Latta, 1973). The juxtaglomerular apparatus contains specialised cells, some of which are granular (the myoepithelioid cells), and secrete renin, an enzyme that acts on renin substrate to produce the potent renal and systemic vasoconstrictor, angiotensin II (AII). Renin release from the myoepithelioid cells occurs both in the direction of the arteriolar lumen and the interstitium, and much of the interstitial renin reaches the systemic circulation via the lymph (Ryan *et al.*, 1982). In addition to the systemic formation of AII, intrarenal AII generation also occurs where it may function as a 'local' hormone (Burghardt et al., 1982; Mendelsohn, 1982, Morgan *et al.*, 1982;). A part of the distal tubule also comes into close contact with the juxtaglomerular apparatus and here the distal tubular cells are highly specialised and form the macula densa (Latta, 1973). This system is believed to provide a mechanism by which the release of renin is controlled by a signal in the distal tubular fluid (Thurau *et al.*, 1982), and to be involved in the tubuloglomerular feedback control system, discussed in Chapter 4 of this volume.

In the outermost (superficial) cortical glomeruli, the afferent arteriole always enters the glomerulus from below; thus afferent arterioles never appear on the subcapsular surface of the kidney (Fourman and Moffat, 1971; Barger and Herd, 1973). The individual deep or juxtamedullary glomeruli are only about 20 per cent of the total glomeruli per kidney. In contrast to the cortical glomeruli, juxtamedullary glomeruli give rise to longer efferent arterioles. Some of the these arterioles form the corticomedullary capillary plexus and others divide into multiple vasa recta, which run in close proximity to the loops of Henle and the collecting ducts (Fourman and Moffat, 1971; Barger and Herd, 1973).

The glomerulus itself is a complex knot of capillaries occupying a roughly spherical area. As shown in Figure 2.1, large capillary loops arise at the afferent arteriole and terminate at the efferent arteriole (Latta, 1973). In addition, smaller anastomotic channels are also apparent, which branch off at about 90° angles from the large loops. As described by Hall (1957), the patency of these small anastomotic loops will be determined by the pressure and rate of blood flow through the larger loops; thus redistribution of blood flow may occur within a glomerulus. The kidney receives a rich supply of sympathetic nerves, many of which innervate the blood vessels up to, but not including, the glomerulus. The cortical efferent arteriole receives relatively little nerve supply although the juxtaglomerular region is innervated, and efferent arterioles and the vasa recta arising from juxtamedullary glomeruli receive a richer innervation (Barger and Herd, 1973; Moss, 1982). The renal sympathetic supply consists of both adrenergic and dopaminergic neurones (Moss, 1982).

Figure 2.1: Diagram of a Human Glomerulus Showing the Afferent Arteriole, Indicated by the Solid Arrow Entering the Glomerulus, Breaking up to Form Long Capillary Loops which are Joined by Lateral, Anastomotic Channels. Each lobule is enveloped by basement membrane. The long, glomerular, capillary channels reconnect on the efferent side of the glomerulus and the blood exists through the efferent arteriole, given by the solid arrow leaving the glomerulus. The broken arrow shows direct connections between the afferent and efferent arterioles.

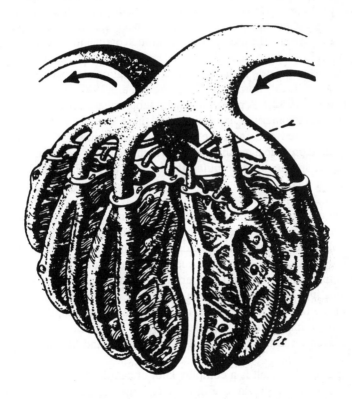

Reproduced with permission from Barger and Herd (1973).

The ultrastructure of the wall of the glomerular capillary has been well described. On the blood side of the capillary lies a discontinuous layer of endothelial cells, separated by large fenestrations or gaps which may exceed 1000 Å in diameter in some species (Latta, 1973). The consensus of opinion holds that these fenestrae are *not* covered with a diaphragm, or at least do not provide a physical barrier to the passage of large molecules (Moffat, 1981).

The endothelial cells rest on the glomerular basement membrane (GBM), an acellular gel composed of acidic glycosaminoglycans and a supporting matrix of collagen fibres (Farquhar *et al.*, 1981). The epithelial cells lie on the urinary side of the GBM with the cell bodies projecting into Bowman's space. The epithelial surface in close contact with the GBM is characterised by the foot processes arranged in an interdigitating fashion, which gives rise to the epithelial slit pores: narrow channels lying between adjacent foot processes. These slit pores are invested with a fine diaphragm which lies close to the subepithelial surface of the GBM (Moffat, 1981). The morphology of these components of the glomerulus is described in detail in Chapter 1 of this volume.

The glomerulus also contains a fourth type of highly differentiated area, the mesangial cells. These cells are not distributed freely throughout the wall of the glomerulus but are located at the hilus of the glomerulus from whence they send out 'branch-like' processes (Latta, 1973; Moffat, 1981). Mesangial cells possess contractile elements and are enclosed in a matrix which is contiguous with cells of the juxtaglomerular apparatus (Latta, 1973; Moffat, 1981).

Determinants of Glomerular Ultrafiltration

The glomerular filtration rate (GFR) is determined by the 'Starling forces' acting across the wall of the glomerular capillary. The glomerular capillary bed is unique in the microcirculation in that the net fluid flux across the wall of the capillary passes into a discrete area (Bowman's space) and this flux (the single nephron GFR, SNGFR) may be directly measured by micropuncture techniques. Micropuncture measurements have also permitted an evaluation of the pressures and flows that determine the SNGFR.

The local rate of fluid flux across a capillary wall (J_v) and the direction of fluid movement is determined by the imbalance between the transcapillary hydraulic pressure gradient (ΔP) and the corresponding oncotic pressure gradient ($\Delta \pi$). At the glomerulus, only filtration is believed to occur, thus the transcapillary hydraulic pressure gradient (ΔP) always exceeds or equals the oncotic pressure gradient ($\Delta \pi$) and the difference is the ultrafiltration pressure, P_{UF}. At any point along the glomerular capillary wall the local rate of ultrafiltration (J_v) is equal to the product of the local net ultrafiltration pressure (P_{UF}) and the local effective hydraulic permeability of the glomerular capillary wall (k), as given by the Starling equation:

$$J_v = (\Delta P - \Delta \pi)\, k \qquad (1)$$

The rate of ultrafiltration across an entire glomerulus, the SNGFR, is given by equation 2:

$$\text{SNGFR} = \overline{(P_{\text{UF}})} \, kS$$

$$= [\,(P_{\text{GC}} - P_{\text{BS}}) - (\pi_{\text{GC}} - \pi_{\text{BS}})\,]\,K_{\text{f}} \tag{2}$$

where the SNGFR is the product of the net ultrafiltration pressure averaged over the length of the glomerular capillary ($\overline{P_{\text{UF}}}$), the capillary wall hydraulic permeability (k) and the surface area over which filtration occurs (S). In terms specific to the glomerulus, the value of P_{UF} is determined by the difference between hydraulic pressure in the glomerulus (P_{GC}) and that in Bowman's space (P_{BS}) minus the difference between the corresponding oncotic pressures (π_{GC} and π_{BS}). Since the hydraulic pressures measured in Bowman's space and in superficial proximal-tubule segments of the same nephron (P_{T}) are similar, P_{BS} and P_{T} are used interchangeably and P_{T} is routinely measured and its value employed in equation 2 (Brenner *et al.*, 1971). Because the glomerular filtrate is an almost ideal plasma ultrafiltrate, the total protein concentration of the fluid in Bowman's space is extremely low (Eisenbach *et al.*, 1975). Thus π_{BS} is negligible and may be ignored, and the transglomerular oncotic pressure gradient ($\Delta\pi$) is exclusively determined by the glomerular capillary oncotic pressure, π_{GC}. The product of the intrinsic characteristics of the glomerulus, which also determine the magnitude of SNGFR, the hydraulic permeability and the filtration surface area (k and S), is termed the glomerular capillary ultrafiltration coefficient, usually abbreviated as K_{f} but also $L_{\text{P}}A$.

Measured Values of the Determinants of SNGFR under Control Conditions

The majority of the data to be described here and in subsequent sections has derived from studies that have been performed in the Munich–Wistar rat. The kidneys of rats of this inbred strain possess glomerular capillaries on the subcapsular surface which are accessible to direct micropuncture measurement of the hydraulic pressure of the blood within the glomerulus. Direct measurements of the hydraulic pressures in superficial proximal tubules, efferent arterioles and terminal peritubular capillaries are also possible. Further, by collection of fluid from superficial nephron tubules and comparison of tubule fluid with plasma inulin concentrations, as well as collection of blood from superficial efferent arterioles and comparison of efferent and afferent (systemic) plasma protein concentrations, it is possible to calculate SNGFR, single nephron filtration fraction (SNFF), glomerular plasma flow rate (Q_{A}), afferent and efferent arteriolar oncotic pressures (π_{A} and π_{E}) as well as afferent and efferent arteriolar resistances (R_{A} and R_{E}, respectively) and the glomerular capillary ultrafiltration coefficient K_{f}. The methods by which these variables are calculated, as well as more precise details about the methods of measurement and collection employed in this technique, are given elsewhere (Deen *et al.*, 1972; Baylis *et al.*, 1976; Blantz and Tucker, 1978).

Glomerular Capillary Hydraulic Pressure

Direct pressure measurements of glomerular capillary hydraulic pressure (P_{GC}) under conditions of control hydropenia have now been reported by many workers and some of these data are summarised in Table 2.1a. This is not intended to represent an inclusive survey of the literature but does give representative data from most of the laboratories that have made these measurements. It is evident that the average value of P_{GC} of about 34–50 mmHg is higher than the hydraulic pressure seen in peripheral capillary beds (Landis and Pappenheimer, 1963; Intaglietta *et al.*, 1970). It is now recognised that hydropenia represents a state of moderate acute volume contraction due to the unreplaced fluid losses occasioned by anaesthesia and the extensive surgical preparation necessary for micropuncture (Maddox *et al.*, 1977). Recently the 'euvolaemic' protocol has been adopted as more truly representative of a 'control' baseline state. This protocol was first described by Ichikawa *et al.* (1978b), who showed that with a carefully controlled infusion of donor rat plasma, the plasma volume could be successfully maintained at the awake, pre-anaesthesia value throughout the micropuncture experiment. Representative values of P_{GC} measured in euvolaemia are given in Table 2.1b. P_{GC} in the euvolaemic preparation is only slightly higher, averaging $\sim$ 48–56 mmHg, compared with the value seen in hydropenia. Surface glomeruli are also present in the squirrel monkey, and the directly measured P_{GC} in this species averages $\sim$ 48 mmHg in control hydropenia conditions (Maddox *et al.*, 1974a).

Because of the anatomy of the glomerulus, it is not possible to ascertain whether the pressure pipette is placed close to the afferent or efferent end of the glomerulus during a glomerular puncture; however, repeat measurements of P_{GC} from different sites in the same glomerulus, or values of P_{GC} measured in different glomeruli in the same kidney, have yielded values within a remarkably narrow range (Baylis and Brenner, 1978b, Blantz, 1980). These findings suggest that the axial pressure drop along the glomerulus is small, i.e. that glomerular capillary resistance is low and that P_{GC} values derived from randomly punctured sites along the glomerular capillary network are representative of the average value of P_{GC}. The value of P_{GC} is determined by both the afferent and efferent arteriolar resistances, R_A and R_E, respectively, and micropuncture studies in the Munich–Wistar rat have indicated that about 60 per cent of the total renal vascular resistance is provided by R_A (this estimate includes the resistance contributed by preafferent arteriolar vessels; the contribution of the glomerulus as a resistance site is negligible; R_E contributes about 30 per cent and the remaining 10 per cent of the renal vascular resistance resides beyond the efferent arteriole (Baylis and Brenner, 1978b; Blantz, 1980). Increases in R_A will tend to reduce P_{GC} whereas increases in R_E will tend to elevate P_{GC}; thus the unique anatomical arrangement of these pre- and post-glomerular resistances permits P_{GC} to be

Table 2.1: Summary of Glomerular Pressure Measurements in Munich–Wistar (M–W) Rats by Several Groups of Workers. Where more than one reference is cited by a particular group, values have been averaged. Where more than one group of data is given for one reference, data are derived from different populations of M–W rats

	$\overline{AP}$	P_{GC}	$P_{T/BS}$	$\overline{\Delta P}$	π_A	π_E	$\pi_E/\overline{\Delta P}$
(a) *Hydropenia*				mmHg			
Reference							
Andreucci *et al.*, 1976 (♂)	122	49	—	—	—	—	—
Baylis and Brenner, 1978a (♂)	119	46	11	35	15	33	0.98
Baylis *et al.*, 1976 (♂)	114	47	11	36	16	35	0.99
Blantz, 1974, 1975 (♂)	134	44	13	31	18	35	1.13
Blantz *et al.*, 1972 (♂)	120	47	14	33	16	—	—
Blantz *et al.*, 1974 (♂)	—	45	12	34	16	33	0.97
	119	48	16	32	16	28	0.86
Brenner *et al.*, 1971, 1972a (♂)	120	45	9	36	19	35	0.99
Dal Canton *et al.*, 1982 (♀)	102	45	14	31	15	29	0.95
Myers *et al.*, 1975a (♂)	120	46	11	35	17	35	1.01
Ott *et al.*, 1976 (♂)	117	47	—	—	12	—	—
Sakai *et al.*, 1984 (♂)	110	43	13	30	21	34	1.15
Tucker and Blantz, 1983 (♂)	110	49	15	34	20	33	0.96
(b) *Euvolaemia*							
Arendshorst and Gottschalk, 1980 (♂)	122	55	13	42	18	35	0.82
	126	56	13	43	19	38	0.89
Baylis, 1979/80a (♂)	113	49	14	35	20	35	1.00
Baylis, 1979/80b, 1980, 1982 (♀)	116	53	14	39	21	39	0.99
Ichikawa *et al.*, 1978b (♂)	113	48	14	34	19	34	1.00
Schor, 1981a, b (♂)	111	49	12	37	19	36	0.93
Tucker *et al.*, 1982 (♂)	114	48	14	34	17	33	0.96

controlled independently of the arterial blood pressure, a point which is discussed in more detail in the later section dealing with autoregulation.

Glomerular pressures have also been measured by the 'stop-flow' technique in rat strains that do not regularly exhibit superficial glomerular capillaries and in the dog. This technique utilises the following principle: when tubular fluid flow rate is obstructed by the introduction of an oil or wax block into an early proximal tubule, pressure within the tubule rises rapidly to a stable value, the 'stop-flow' pressure, P_{SF}. P_{SF} plus the oncotic pressure of the blood arriving at the glomerulus (π_A) is equal to the pressure required to prevent further formation of glomerular filtrate, which must therefore equal the value of P_{GC} at that moment. The validity of this technique has been questioned since the cessation of filtration must imply that the volume of fluid normally exiting from the glomerulus is diverted back and augments the glomerular blood flow rate (by about one-third of the plasma flow entering the glomerulus). However, directly measured P_{GC} has been continually monitored before, during and after the introduction of an obstructing oil block in the proximal tubule, and has been found to rise transiently following cessation of filtration but then to return to control values within about half a minute (Blantz *et al.*, 1972). These workers suggest this must imply alteration in pre- and post-glomerular arteriolar resistances, and probably reflects efferent arteriolar dilatation. This perfect maintenance of P_{GC} due to compensatory resistance changes was noted in rats studied under conditions of control hydropenia, but acute volume expansion led to sustained elevations in the directly measured P_{GC} (by about 6 mmHg) under conditions of stopped flow, unless tubular fluid was aspirated proximal to the block (Blantz *et al.*, 1972). Thus, estimation of P_{GC} by the use of P_{SF} when the kidney is already vasodilated (e.g. during acute volume expansion) may lead to an overestimation of the true values of P_{GC} in the absence of cessation of SNGFR, since further compensatory alterations in renal resistances may not be possible. This question has more recently been directly addressed by Ichikawa, who found that in the hydropenic Munich–Wistar rat, cessation of SNGFR caused by proximal-tubule obstruction led to a significant overestimation of P_{GC} whether measured directly or as P_{SF} (Ichikawa, 1982). Care was taken in the design of this experiment to prevent the possibility of the introduction of a vent in Bowman's capsule, which Ichikawa believes must normally occur during the localisation procedure employed to define the surface convolutions belonging to a given superficial glomerulus. It was demonstrated in this study that the P_{GC} estimated as P_{SF} was significantly lower when Bowman's space had previously been vented by the introduction of a small localising pipette for injection of dye, in order to define the pattern of superficial tubules belonging to a given parent superficial glomerulus. Thus, Ichikawa believes that even under the relatively vasoconstricted condition of hydropenia, P_{SF} overestimates the true P_{GC} in the absence of a hole in Bowman's capsule, and that when such a hole is present (as in the study previously described by Blantz *et al.*, 1972), true P_{GC} measured at the moment of 'stopped-flow' is underestimated as a result of leakage of fluid from Bowman's space and thus incomplete cessation of SNGFR. Thus, although mention will be made of studies in which P_{GC} is estimated from the P_{SF} in rat strains and in the dog where surface glomeruli are not evident, some caution should be exercised in the interpretation of these data, for the reasons outlined above.

Values of P_{GC} have been estimated from P_{SF} in several rat strains and are generally higher than the directly measured value obtained in the Munich–Wistar, often being close to 60 mmHg (Kallskog *et al.*, 1975a; Arendshorst and Beierwaltes, 1979; Azar *et al.*, 1979; Schweitzer and Gertz, 1979). Directly measured values of P_{GC} have also been reported to exceed 60 mmHg in the Sprague-Dawley rat (Kallskog *et al.*, 1975a). In the immature Sprague-Dawley rat, low values of P_{GC}, estimated for P_{SF}, were reported in superficial glomeruli, whereas juxtamedullary P_{GC} was found to be much higher, around 52 mmHg (Ericson *et al.*, 1982). Measurement of P_{GC} from P_{SF} in the dog yielded values for control hydropenic conditions which are greater than those observed by direct measurement in the Munich–Wistar rat, and average 55–70 mmHg (Navar, 1970; Ott *et al.*, 1976; Navar *et al.*, 1977b, 1979; Osswald *et al.*, 1979; Heller and Horacek, 1984). In some of these same studies in the dog a direct estimate of P_{GC} has also been obtained in subsurface glomeruli by utilisation of the corticotomy technique, and values obtained by this method have averaged 60 mmHg. The corticotomy technique was first described for the rat kidney and involves cutting out a 'lens'-shaped slice from the dorsal kidney surface and directly measuring the hydrostatic pressure in the glomeruli exposed by this technique (Aukland *et al.*, 1977). When pressures are measured by this method, P_{GC} in outer cortical glomeruli of both Wistar and Sprague-Dawley rats averaged 60 mmHg and was lower in inner cortical glomeruli, around 54 mmHg. In later studies by this same group, however, using the same technique, pressure of approximately 50 mmHg were reported for outer cortical glomeruli of both Wistar and Munich–Wistar rats (Tonder and Aukland, 1979). Until recently it has not been possible to directly and atraumatically measure P_{GC} in deep nephrons, although indirect estimates (from P_{SF}) have suggested that P_{GC} may be higher in juxtamedullary compared with superficial cortical glomeruli in immature Sprague-Dawley rats (Müller-Suur *et al.*, 1982). A unique population of juxtamedullary nephrons has recently been described which lies on the inner cortical surface of the pelvis. When the vessels supplying these glomeruli are perfused with blood, *in situ* at a perfusion pressure of 100 mmHg, their P_{GC} averages about 50 mmHg (Casellas and Navar, 1984). Thus, as with superficial cortical glomeruli, the afferent arterioles probably provide 50–60 per cent of the resistance to blood flow.

In summary, a wide range of values of P_{GC} have been reported for the rat. Values of P_{GC} in the dog are also thought to be high compared with that seen in the Munich–Wistar rat. However, in view of the concerns described above for the stop-flow pressure-measuring method of estimating P_{GC}, and the obvious questions regarding the validity of the corticotomy technique, most of the experimental evidence discussed below will be derived from studies in the Munich–Wistar rat in which direct pressure measurements are made. It is true that information derived from these studies applies directly only to the small population of nephrons located on the kidney surface of this particular rat strain, and it is also true that these nephrons (a) may not be representative of deeper nephrons in the same kidney, and (b) may differ from those of other rat strains. However, the great advantage of this preparation is that it permits an evaluation, based on direct measurements, of the mechanisms by which SNGFR is controlled in response to a variety of acute and chronic interventions. Presumably, also, information derived from these studies will be qualitatively applicable to the control of glomerular filtration in other species.

The hydraulic pressure in Bowman's space opposes the formation of glomerular ultrafiltrate. Values representative of hydropenia and euvolaemia are summarised in Table 2.1. It is evident that P_T ($\simeq P_{BS}$) is fairly uniform and tends to average 10–15 mmHg, thus the normal transglomerular hydraulic pressure gradient ($\overline{\Delta P}$) averages 35–40 mmHg. Tubule pressure rises to 20–25 mmHg during the following: volume expansion with hypotonic solutions (Ichikawa and Brenner, 1977) or isotonic solutions (Baylis *et al.*, 1977a); diuresis induced by hyperglycaemia (Blantz *et al.*, 1983); diuretic administration (Tucker and Blantz, 1984); carbonic anhydrase inhibition (Tucker *et al.*, 1978); in a homogeneous model of polyuric acute renal failure (Baylis *et al.*, 1977b); and in conditions of acute ureteral obstruction (Blantz *et al.*, 1975). However, unless urine flow rate is disproportionately high for the prevailing GFR, variations in $\overline{\Delta P}$ are usually achieved by changes in P_{GC}.

Transcapillary Oncotic Pressure Difference ($\Delta\pi$)

As mentioned earlier, the glomerular ultrafiltrate is essentially protein-free and thus the intraglomerular protein concentration rises as blood flows along the glomerular network, due to the loss of about a third of (the colloid-free fraction of) the plasma. Because of the inaccessibility of the afferent arteriole, afferent arteriolar protein concentration (C_A) cannot be measured directly but is taken to be equal to the value of the systemic (usually femoral) arterial plasma-protein concentration (C_A). The value of efferent arteriolar plasma-protein concentration (C_E) can be determined directly from measurements made on plasma collected from superficial efferent arterioles (or star vessels) (Brenner *et al.*, 1972b). Values for C_A and C_E in control hydropenia and euvolaemia generally tend to range between 5–6.5 g dl^{-1} and 7.5–9.0 g dl^{-1} respectively, and, as shown in Table 2.1, the oncotic pressure (π) calculated from these measured values of C_A and C_E increases from 15–20 mmHg at the beginning (π_A) to 35–40 mmHg at the end (π_E) of the glomerulus. In view of the relative constancy of P_{GC} and thence $\overline{\Delta P}$ along the length of the glomerulus, the local net ultrafiltration pressure (P_{UF}; $\Delta P - \Delta\pi$) therefore declines from a value of 13–24 mmHG (mean $\simeq$ 18) at the beginning of the glomerular capillary network to zero at the end of the glomerulus, as shown in Figure 2.2, curves A and B. Therefore, in most laboratories under conditions of control hydropenia or euvolaemia, the transglomerular oncotic pressure difference ($\Delta\pi$) has risen to a value, by the end of the glomerulus, which on average equals and opposes ΔP and thus prevents further net filtration (Table 2.1). This equality of ΔP and $\Delta\pi$ at the end of the glomerulus is referred to as filtration pressure equilibrium.

As shown in Figure 2.2, the profile of $\Delta\pi$ along the glomerular capillary is non-linear. This non-linearity occurs because the *local* rate of ultrafiltration is proportional to the *local* net driving pressure ($\Delta P - \Delta\pi$) so that the formation of ultrafiltrate will occur most rapidly at the beginning of the glomerulus where *local* P_{UF} is at a maximum. This high rate of filtrate formation at the afferent side of the glomerulus will lead to a rapid initial rate of concentration of

Figure 2.2: Graph to Show Several Possible Profiles of the Transcapillary Oncotic Pressure Difference ($\Delta\pi$) under Conditions of Filtration Pressure Equilibrium (curves A, B and C) and Filtration Pressure *Dis*equilibrium (curve D), for a Given Transcapillary Hydraulic Pressure Difference, ΔP, along an Idealised Glomerular Capillary. The area between the ΔP and a given $\Delta\pi$ curve gives the net ultrafiltration pressure, P_{UF}

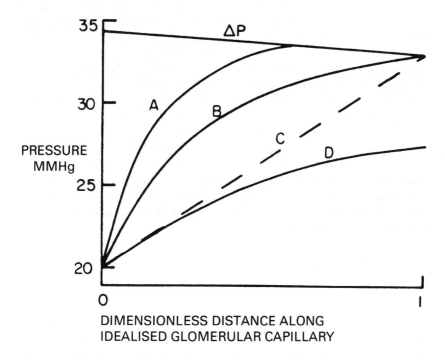

Reproduced with permission from Baylis and Brenner, (1978b)

intraglomerular protein, a rapid initial rise in the local value of $\Delta\pi$ and hence a rapid initial reduction in the *local* P_{UF}. This will have the effect of limiting the rate of ultrafiltration in further downstream sites, which in turn will further limit the rate of rise of $\Delta\pi$. Thus the $\Delta\pi$ profile along the glomerulus will take an exponential shape with the most rapid rise occurring at the beginning of the glomerulus. An additional effect contributing to the exponential rise in $\Delta\pi$ with distance along the glomerulus is that π increases in a non-linear manner with increases in protein concentration (Landis and Pappenheimer, 1963; Deen *et al.*, 1972).

Measurements of π can only be performed on samples of systemic ($\equiv$ afferent arteriolar) blood, and blood from efferent arterioles, since it is impossible, under *in vivo* micropuncture conditions, to determine a given location along the glomerular capillary network. The $\Delta\pi$ curves A and B in Figure 2.2 are only two of an infinite number of possible $\Delta\pi$ profiles consistent with the measurements of π_A and π_E obtained under conditions of filtration pressure equilibrium, i.e. when $\pi_E \simeq \overline{\Delta P}$. However, a knowledge of the exact $\Delta\pi$ profile is necessary in order to calculate an exact value of the mean net ultrafiltration pressure, P_{UF}, which is equal to the area between the ΔP and any of the $\Delta\pi$ curves in Figure 2.2. In view of the uncertainty in determining the exact $\Delta\pi$ profile in an animal at filtration pressure equilibrium, it is therefore not possible to calculate an exact value of $\overline{P_{UF}}$ under the control conditions of hydropenia or euvolaemia. Only a maximum value of $\overline{P_{UF}}$ may be calculated, and only then by assuming (1) a linear rate of rise of $\Delta\pi$ along the glomerular capillary, and (2) that $\Delta\pi$ becomes equal to ΔP at the efferent-most point of the glomerular network, as shown by curve C in Figure 2.2. The extent to which these assumptions overestimate the true value of $\overline{P_{UF}}$ will always be unknown, and will depend on (1) the degree of departure from linearity of the true $\Delta\pi$ curve, and (2) the exact site along the glomerulus at which $\Delta\pi$ comes to be equal to $\overline{\Delta P}$, i.e. the point at which filtration pressure equilibrium is reached and filtration therefore stops. In view of these uncertainties in calculating an exact value of $\overline{P_{UF}}$ under conditions of filtration pressure equilibrium, it is also impossible to calculate an exact value of the glomerular capillary ultrafiltration coefficient, K_f, as shown below in equation 3, which is a rearrangement of equation 2:

$$K_f = \frac{SNGFR}{\overline{P_{UF}}} \tag{3}$$

The best that is possible under these circumstances is that, for a given measured value of SNGFR and a given MAXIMUM estimate of P_{UF}, a minimum value of K_f may be calculated using equation 3 and employing the assumptions already described in the computation of curve C in Figure 2.2.

Although not described explicitly in equation 2, the rate of plasma flow to a glomerulus, Q_A, will also influence the magnitude of SNGFR by affecting the $\Delta\pi$ profile, and thence $\overline{P_{UF}}$. For example, an increase in Q_A will reduce the rate of rise of $\Delta\pi$ and thus increase both the local and net P_{UF}, thereby increasing SNGFR. Conversely, a reduction in Q_A will have the opposite effect of increasing the local rate of rise of $\Delta\pi$ and thus reducing P_{UF} and SNGFR (Brenner *et al.*, 1972a). Development of a mathematical model of glomerular ultrafiltration by Deen *et al.* (1972) led to the prediction that, with significant increases in the value of Q_A and without significant changes in the other determinants of glomerular ultrafiltration, the rate of rise of intraglomerular protein concentration and thence in $\Delta\pi$ would be sufficiently attenuated to prevent the achievement of filtration pressure equilibrium. In other words, with sufficient elevation in Q_A, the value of $\Delta\pi$ attained by the end of the glomerulus (π_E) would be significantly less than the corresponding value of $\overline{\Delta P}$, as depicted by curve D in Figure 2.2. The advantage of situations in which filtration pressure equilibrium is not obtained, i.e. when filtration pressure *dis*equilibrium exists ($\pi_E < \overline{\Delta P}$) is that, using the mathematical model of Deen *et al.* (1972), an exact $\Delta\pi$ curve can be computed which connects the measured values of π_A and π_E. Thus, when filtration pressure *dis*equilibrium exists, an exact value of P_{UF} and also K_f can be calculated from measured values of SNGFR, $\overline{\Delta P}$, π_A and π_E.

The Glomerular Capillary Ultrafiltration Coefficient, K_f

An exact estimate of the ultrafiltration coefficient, K_f, has been obtained in the normal rat during the i.v. infusion of 5 per cent body weight of donor-rat plasma. This degree of plasma volume expansion increases glomerular plasma flow rate (Q_A) to sufficiently high values to produce filtration pressure *dis*equilibrium (Deen *et al.*, 1973). Calculated values of K_f in this study were found to average 0.08 nl/(s.mmHg), and it was also shown that with further large increases in Q_A (over a twofold range of *dis*equilibrium-producing Q_A values) K_f remained unchanged. It therefore seems unlikely that the experimental manoeuvre of increasing Q_A would of itself alter the values of K_f. This assumption is further supported by data from studies in which K_f was reduced due to glomerular injury, and variation of Q_A over a lower range of values was still found to have no effect on the calculated (low) value of K_f (Chang *et al.*, 1976). In addition, in studies in which Q_A was increased during isovolaemic reduction in the hematocrit, i.e. without plasma volume expansion, filtration pressure *dis*equilibrium was again produced and the exactly calculated value of K_f was found to be similar to the value observed during conditions of plasma volume expansion (Deen *et al.*, 1973; Myers *et al.*, 1975b).

Although only minimum estimates of K_f are possible under control conditions of hydropenia and euvolaemia (because filtration pressure equilibrium exists in these conditions), these minimum estimates fall in the range 0.06–0.10 nl/(s.mmHg) in most of the studies summarised in Table 2.1. Given that the normal true value of K_f, at least for the superficial glomeruli in the Munich–Wistar rat kidney, averages about 0.08 nl/(s.mmHg), this gives values for the mean, net ultrafiltration pressure, P_{UF}, of 4–6 mmHg in hydropenia and 6–8 mmHg in euvolaemia, using the measured values of SNGFR reported in the studies summarised in Table 2.1 and by rearranging equation 3. In a few of the groups of Munich–Wistar rats summarised in Table 2.1, however, filtration pressure *dis*equilibrium was observed even under the relatively low plasma flow rate conditions of hydropenia and euvolaemia (Blantz *et al.*, 1974; Arendshorst and Gottschalk, 1980). For some unknown reason Munich–Wistar rats from substrains developed in Dallas and North Carolina exhibited an unusually low value of K_f, and this was responsible for the development of filtration pressure *dis*equilibrium at normal plasma flow rates.

Studies in other rat strains in which K_f is calculated from indirectly estimated values of P_{GC} have generally reported lower values of K_f, which causes filtration pressure *dis*equilibrium under control conditions; these include observations in the Sprague-Dawley rat (Arendshorst and Gottschalk, 1974; Michels *et al.*, 1981; Larson *et al.*, 1983); in Wistar–Kyoto normotensive and Wistar spontaneously hypertensive rats (DiBona and Rios, 1978; Arendshorst and Beierwaltes, 1979; Azar *et al.*, 1979) and in Holtzman rats (Azar *et al.*, 1977). In the dog, estimated values of K_f are high and are generally comparable with the directly measured values reported for the Munich–Wistar rat; however, despite the high K_f, filtration pressure *dis*equilibrium apparently exists in the dog, presumably due to the higher rate of glomerular plasma flow under control conditions (Ott *et al.*, 1976; Navar *et al.*, 1977b, 1979; Osswald *et al.*, 1979; Thomas *et al.*, 1979; Heller and Horacek, 1984). The implications of the presence of filtration pressure equilibrium or *dis*equilibrium will be made apparent in the section dealing with selective effects of alterations of the individual determinants of SNGFR.

As shown in equation 2, the glomerular capillary ultrafiltration coefficient, K_f, is the product of filtration surface (S) and the water permeability of the glomerular capillary wall (k). Using the micropuncture measurements obtained in the Munich–Wistar rat, it is possible only to arrive at a calculated value of the product K_f but not to determine separately either of the intrinsic characteristics of the glomerular capillary wall, i.e. k and S. Estimates of surface area (S) of the glomerulus in an adult rat have, however, been obtained using morphometric techniques, and values of 0.0019 and 0.0028 cm^2 per glomerulus have been reported (Kirkman and Stowell, 1942; Shea and Morrison, 1975). Also, studies by Knutson *et al.* (1978) used the binding of antiglomerular basement–membrane antibodies as a measure of the relative glomerular capillary surface area during growth in the rat. These workers observed that in the immature rat, glomerular capillary surface area (S) increased in proportion to increases in body weight, but that in the mature rat, when body weight exceeded 200 g, S remained constant and no longer increased with further increases in body weight. This independence of S and body weight allows one to employ the absolute values of S estimated from morphometric studies (in adult rats) to calculate a value for glomerular capillary water permeability, k, using the average value of K_f of 0.08nl/(s.mmHg) derived from micropuncture studies in mature rats over a wide range of body weights. This approach yields calculated values of k of 28.6 and 42.1 nl/(s.mmHg)/cm^2 (using the two available surface-area measurements). Taking either of these values for k, it is apparent that the water permeability of the rat glomerulus is one or two orders of magnitude greater than that reported for a variety of other, peripheral capillaries (Renkin, 1979). This very high hydraulic permeability in the superficial glomeruli of the Munich-Wistar rat therefore allows glomerular filtration to proceed rapidly with mean driving pressures that average only 4–8 mmHg in the normal rat.

A novel *in vitro* technique, recently described by Savin and Terreros (1981), has permitted a direct estimation of K_f and both of its component terms (filtration surface area and hydraulic permeability) in a number of species. Briefly, this technique involves the isolation of glomeruli which are observed by high-magnification video recording during their subjection to an osmotic gradient. The osmotic pressure of the bathing solution is abruptly reduced, which causes fluid movement into the glomerulus (i.e. in the opposite direction to that which occurs *in vivo*). The increase in glomerular diameter that occurs during this procedure is used to estimate the rate of fluid flux across the glomerulus. This measurement, together with the magnitude of the oncotic gradient applied and morphometric measurements of the glomerular geometry, allow a calculation of K_f. Using this technique, values for K_f in the rat have been reported which are similar to those seen in the Munich-Wistar rat under conditions of *in vivo* micropuncture, whereas values in the dog are considerably higher than those calculated from indirectly estimated values of P_{GC} (Savin and Terreros, 1981; Savin and Patak, 1982). Measurements using this technique have also been made in glomeruli obtained from human cadaveric kidneys, and the calculated mean water permeability of the glomerular capillary wall was similar to that calculated in the Munich-Wistar rat *in vivo*, although K_f was greater due to the greater surface area of the human glomerulus (Savin, 1983). Savin and co-workers have concluded that variations in K_f between and within species relate mainly to differences in glomerular surface area, with water permeability being fairly similar.

The Single Nephron Filtration Fraction

SNGFR may also be described as the product of the glomerular plasma flow rate (Q_A) and the single nephron filtration fraction (SNFF) as shown in equation 4.

$$SNGFR = Q_A \cdot SNFF \tag{4}$$

Thus SNFF may be expressed as:

$$SNFF = \frac{SNGFR}{Q_A} \tag{5}$$

The value of SNFF may be calculated from the measured values of the afferent and efferent arteriolar protein concentrations (C_A and C_E, respectively), thus:

$$SNFF = 1 - \frac{C_A}{C_E} \tag{6}$$

$$\simeq 1 - \frac{\pi_A}{\pi_E} \tag{7}$$

In rats at filtration pressure equilibrium ($\pi_E \simeq \overline{\Delta P}$) equation 7 may be rewritten as

$$\text{SNFF} \simeq 1 - \frac{\pi_A}{\overline{\Delta P}} \qquad (8)$$

Thus, at filtration pressure equilibrium, the value of SNFF is determined exclusively by π_A and thence the value of afferent arteriolar protein concentration (C_A) and the value of $\overline{\Delta P}$. The value of $\overline{\Delta P}$ limits the final value to which C_E and thence π_E can rise by the efferent end of the glomerulus. The dependence of SNFF on C_A has been described in greater detail previously (Baylis and Brenner, 1978b).

Effects of Selective Variations in the Determinants of SNGFR

A. Variations of $\Delta\pi$ Evoked by Variations in Glomerular Plasma Flow Rate, Q_A. It is evident from Figure 2.2, curves A and B, and equations 4, 6 and 8 that, in an animal at filtration pressure equilibrium, changes in Q_A in the absence of changes in C_A and $\overline{\Delta P}$ will not influence the value of π_E, since at equilibrium the value to which π_E can rise will be determined solely by the value of $\overline{\Delta P}$. Under these (equilibrium) conditions, SNFF will remain constant with alterations in Q_A, and SNGFR will vary in direct proportion to the changes in Q_A, i.e. glomerular filtration rate will be highly 'plasma-flow' dependent. When a sufficiently large increase in Q_A occurs to produce filtration pressure *dis*equilibrium, however, the resultant attenuation of the rate of rise to $\Delta\pi$ will cause π_E to fall (curve D, Figure 2.2). Thus, at *dis*equilibrium and with values of K_f, C_A and $\overline{\Delta P}$ remaining constant, SNFF must fall with further increases in Q_A.

The theoretical relationship between SNFF and Q_A is presented graphically in Figure 2.3A, calculated assuming values of K_f, C_A and $\overline{\Delta P}$ that are representative of the normal, hydropenic Munich-Wistar rat (Baylis and Brenner, 1978b). As shown, SNFF is predicted to remain constant (at about 0.33, the value observed in the normal rat under control conditions) with values of Q_A up to about 110 nl min.$^{-1}$. Further increases in Q_A, however, lead to progressively lower values of SNFF once filtration pressure *dis*equilibrium has been reached.

The theoretical dependence of SNGFR on Q_A is shown in Figure 2.4A. It follows from equation 4 that as long as SNFF remains constant, i.e. as long as filtration pressure equilibrium persists, SNGFR will vary linearly with Q_A. For values of Q_A above about 110 nl min^{-1}, where *dis*equilibrium occurs and SNFF begins to decline, SNGFR is predicted to increase less than in proportion to the rise in Q_A. This is indicated in Figure 2.4A by the divergence of the solid line and the broken line, the latter denoting a constant filtration fraction of 0.33. Thus, even at filtration pressure *dis*equilibrium, SNGFR will be predicted to vary directly with Q_A but to a lesser extent than when

Figure 2.3A–D: Graph Showing the Predicted Effects on Single Nephron Filtration Fraction SNFF, of Selective Alterations in (A) Glomerular Plasma Flow Rate, Q_A; (B) the Mean Transglomerular Hydraulic Pressure Gradient, $\overline{\Delta P}$; (C) the Glomerular Capillary Ultrafiltration Coefficient, K_f; and (D) the Protein Concentration of Systemic Plasma, C_A, or the Oncotic Pressure Due to the Plasma Proteins, π_A. These graphs are computed from data obtained in the normal hydropenic Munich–Wistar rat, and, unless specified otherwise, $Q_A = 75$ nl min^{-1}; $\overline{\Delta P} = 35$ mmHg; $K_f = 0.08$ nl/(s.mmHg) and $C_A = 5.7$ g dl^{-1} ($\equiv \pi_A = 19$ mmHg)

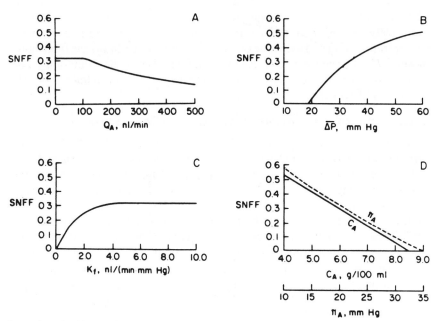

Reproduced with permission from Baylis and Brenner, (1978b)

equilibrium exists. It is worthy of note that it is only at extremely high values of Q_A (at least three to five times greater than seen under conditions of control hydropenia or euvolaemia) that SNGFR becomes almost independent of the effect of further alterations in Q_A.

Numerous experimental observations have supported these predictions. For example, when Q_A was elevated within the equilibrium range in normal rats and without producing major alterations in the other determinants of glomerular ultrafiltration, by mildly plasma-volume-expanding previously hydropenic rats by the chronic administration of the glucocorticoid, methylprednisolone, or by comparing euvolaemic and hydropenic conditions, SNGFR rose in near proportion to the rise in Q_A with relatively little change in SNFF (Brenner *et al.*, 1972a; Baylis and Brenner, 1978a; Ichikawa *et al.*, 1978b; Tucker and Blantz, 1983). Elevation of Q_A to supernormal (*dis*equilibrium-producing) levels, either by various degrees of plasma volume expansion with or without concomitant carotid occlusion or aortic constriction or by isovolaemic reduction in haematocrit, led to less than proportional rises

Figure 2.4A–D: Graph Showing the Predicted Effects on SNGFR of Selective Alterations in (A) Glomerular Plasma Flow Rate, Q_A; (B) the mean transglomerular hydraulic pressure gradient, $\overline{\Delta P}$; (C) the glomerular capillary ultrafiltration coefficient, K_f; and (D) the protein concentration of systemic plasma, C_A, or the oncotic pressure due to the plasma proteins, π_A. The conditions are the same as those described for Figure 2.3. The broken lines in Figures 2.4A and 2.4B are explained in the text

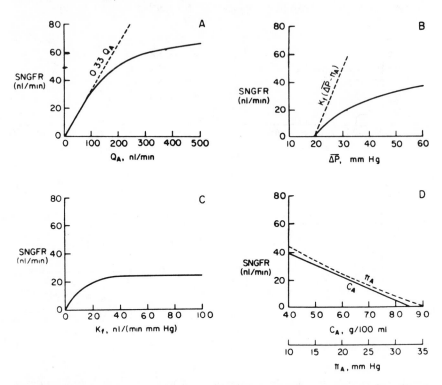

Reproduced with permission from Baylis and Brenner (1978b)

in SNGFR together with falls in SNFF (Deen *et al.*, 1973; Myers *et al.*, 1975b; Baylis *et al.*, 1977a). In uninephrectomised rats, plasma loading produced filtration *dis*equilibrium without significantly altering π_A, $\overline{\Delta P}$ or K_f, and SNGFR rose but less than in proportion to the increase in Q_A due to a reduction in SNFF (Deen *et al.*, 1974a).

Studies on glomerular haemodynamics in spontaneously hypertensive rats (SHR) have also yielded interesting insights into the control of glomerular filtration. In the adult (hypertensive) SHR, values for SNGFR are comparable to those considered normal in normotensive rat strains, and although, unfortunately, surface glomeruli are not present in this strain, estimates of glomerular capillary hydraulic pressure have been obtained from 'stop-flow' pressure measurements and are not elevated above values considered normal for this strain. This must imply preferential afferent arteriolar constriction (DiBona and Rios, 1978; Arendshorst and Beierwaltes, 1979; Azar *et al.*, 1979). Under control conditions, rats of the SHR strain always seem to be at filtration pressure *dis*equilibrium (Rios, 1978; DiBona and Rios, 1978; Azar *et al.*, 1979). In these animals, Q_A is low (because of the presumed afferent arteriolar constriction) but SNFF is elevated compared with normotensive controls, thus accounting for the near normal values of SNGFR (Feld *et al.*, 1977; DiBona and Rios, 1978; Azar *et al.*, 1979). This is exactly what would be predicted in an animal at filtration pressure *dis*equilibrium since a reduction in Q_A would lead to an increase in SNFF (Figure 2.3A) and SNGFR would be reduced by proportionally less than the fall in Q_A (Figure 2.4A). In human essential hypertension it is also observed that kidney filtration fraction rises when a fall in renal plasma flow rate occurs, thus GFR is relatively protected (Hollenberg *et al.*, 1969; Reubi *et al.*, 1978) and this may well be due to the same mechanism as occurs in the SHR.

Studies by Arendshorst and Gottschalk have described a substrain of Munich–Wistar rats that exhibits a low value of K_f under control, euvolaemic conditions. Because of their low K_f these rats are at filtration pressure *dis*equilibrium under control conditions, and plasma loading produces large increases in Q_A, marked falls in SNFF and little increase in SNGFR as predicted by Figure 2.4A (Arendshorst and Gottschalk, 1980). Thus, whether an animal is at filtration pressure equilibrium or *dis*equilibrium under control conditions will influence the magnitude of the response of SNGFR to changes in plasma flow rate, and the degree of dependency of GFR on renal plasma flow rate has been used as an index of whether a particular species is normally at filtration pressure equilibrium or *dis*equilibrium. At present it is not known which of these conditions is normal for the human, although Oken has suggested, using a mathematical modelling approach, that man is normally at filtration pressure *dis*equilibrium (Oken, 1982). However, it should be noted that under the physiological conditions of variations in protein intake and pregnancy, GFR and renal plasma flow rate rise in near proportion, which is indicative of the fact that the normal set-point for the human is close to, or at, filtration pressure equilibrium (Pullman *et al.*, 1954; Davison and Dunlop, 1980).

B. Variations in the Glomerular Transcapillary Hydraulic Pressure Difference ($\overline{\Delta P}$). The predicted effects of selective variations in $\overline{\Delta P}$ on both SNFF and SNGFR in rats at filtration pressure equilibrium are shown in Figures 2.3B and 2.4B. Glomerular filtration will only occur when there is a net positive driving pressure (P_{UF}), and thus $\overline{\Delta P}$ must exceed the value of afferent arteriolar oncotic pressure (π_A, about 20 mmHg) for SNFF and SNGFR to rise above zero. Both SNGFR and SNFF are predicted to increase in a non-linear fashion with increasing $\overline{\Delta P}$, with the rate of rise of SNFF and SNGFR being less for larger values of $\overline{\Delta P}$. These non-linear relationships result from the fact that as $\overline{\Delta P}$ is increased, the resulting increase in the rate of filtration leads to (smaller) increases in $\Delta\pi$. The rise in $\Delta\pi$ tends to partially offset the increment in $\overline{\Delta P}$, thus diminishing the increase in $\overline{P_{UF}}$. Were this increase in $\Delta\pi$ not to occur, $\overline{P_{UF}}$ and SNGFR would rise in a linear fashion with $\overline{\Delta P}$, as shown by the broken line in Figure 2.4B. It has proved particularly difficult to evaluate experimentally the selective effects of alterations in $\overline{\Delta P}$ on SNGFR since manoeuvres designed to alter $\overline{\Delta P}$, such as aortic constriction or carotid occlusion, also produce marked variations in Q_A (Robertson *et al.*, 1972; Deen *et al.*, 1973). However, comparison of data from several groups of rats which fortuitously exhibited quite similar values of Q_A but a range of values of $\overline{\Delta P}$ reveal a similar relationship to that predicted by Figure 2.4B (Baylis and Brenner, 1978b).

Under conditions of filtration pressure *dis*equilibrium, increased in $\overline{\Delta P}$ will be predicted to have a greater influence on SNGFR than in equilibrium states, as shown in Figure 2.5. Here, the curve for a rat at equilibrium is redrawn from Figure 2.3B, connecting the open circles; and the upper curve, connecting the solid circles, has been computed from data obtained during infusion of a pressor dose of angiotensin II. This manoeuvre acutely lowers K_f to *dis*equilibrium values, an effect discussed in more detail later (Baylis and Brenner, 1978c). The reason for the greater predicted influence of $\overline{\Delta P}$ on SNGFR at *dis*equilibrium is that the rate of rise of the intraglomerular oncotic pressure (and then $\Delta\pi$) will automatically be attenuated under *dis*equilibrium conditions, whether due to a low K_f or to increases in Q_A. Thus, the factor that limits the influence of a rise in $\overline{\Delta P}$ on the net ultrafiltration pressure, $\overline{P_{UF}}$, under equilibrium conditions, i.e. the rise in $\Delta\pi$, will be diminished, and at *dis*equilibrium, increases in $\overline{\Delta P}$ will be predicted to produce a greater rise in $\overline{P_{UF}}$ and then in SNGFR. This prediction has not been critically examined experimentally; however, with acute infusions of angiotensin II, and in chronic, immune-mediated glomerulonephritis, filtration pressure *dis*equilibrium exists and both K_f and Q_A are low but values of SNGFR remain normal (Baylis and Brenner, 1978c; Wilson and Blantz, 1984). The only determinant of filtration that is acting to offset the anticipated fall in SNGFR (due to reductions in K_f and Q_A) is a rise in $\overline{\Delta P}$, which suggests that the dependence of SNGFR on $\overline{\Delta P}$ is enhanced under conditions of filtration pressure *dis*equilibrium. Tucker and Blantz (1981) have employed multiple regression analysis to examine possible relationships between some of the determinants of glomerular ultrafiltration and the glomerular capillary ultrafiltration coefficient (K_f). This statistical approach has the advantage that correlations between two given variables may be described, although such correlations may apparently be obscured by simultaneous alterations in the other determinants of SNGFR. Three different protocols were employed, namely hydropenia to saline expansion, saline expansion to acute restoration of systemic plasma protein concentration with persistent expansion, and saline expansion to acute restoration in systemic plasma protein concentration and partial restoration of haematocrit. In these experimental situations a

Figure 2.5: Graph to Show the Predicted Effects on SNGFR of $\overline{\Delta P}$ under Conditions of Filtration Pressure *Dis*equilibrium (Solid Circles) and Compared with Conditions of Filtration Pressure Equilibrium (open circles), redrawn from Figure 2.4B. The graph for filtration pressure *dis*equilibrium was constructed from data derived during infusion of angiotensin II (Baylis and Brenner, 1978c) where $Q_A = 100$ nl min^{-1}; $K_f = 0.037$ nl/(s.mmHg) and $C_A = 5.1$ g dl^{-1}. The equilibrium curve was constructed from data obtained in normal hydropenic rats where $Q_A = 75$ nl min^{-1}; $K_f = 0.08$ nl min^{-1} and $C_A = 5.7$ g dl^{-1}

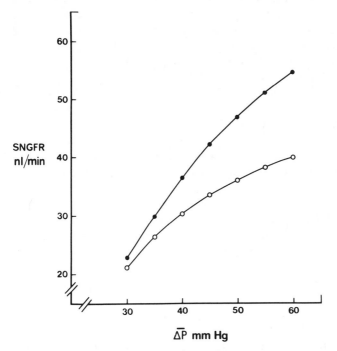

significant inverse relationship between $\overline{\Delta P}$ and K_f was detected, and a similar relationship was also observed when this same statistical test was applied to data derived from earlier studies by Baylis *et al.* (1977a). If this inverse relationship between $\overline{\Delta P}$ and K_f holds true under all conditions, then the dependence of SNGFR on $\overline{\Delta P}$ under *dis*equilibrium conditions, described in Figure 2.5, may not be as great as postulated.

C. Variations in Ultrafiltration Coefficient. The theoretical relationships between K_f and both SNFF and SNGFR are shown in Figures 2.3C and 2.4C, and assume values of Q_A, C_A and $\overline{\Delta P}$ which are representative of the normal hydropenic rat. When K_f is greater than about 0.06 nl/(s.mmHg) ($\simeq$ 3.6 nl/(min. mmHg), filtration pressure equilibrium is achieved and SNFF remains constant at 0.33; SNGFR is also independent of the value of K_f, but varies directly with P_{UF}. Thus, as indicated by equations 4 and 8, under conditions of filtration pressure equilibrium, SNGFR is determined solely by the values of Q_A, π_A and $\overline{\Delta P}$. Therefore, so long as the value of K_f is sufficiently high for filtration pressure equilibrium to be achieved, variations in K_f will have no influence on either SNFF or SNGFR. At the pressures and flows that are representative of hydropenia, a reduction in K_f to below about 0.05 nl/(s.mmHg) i.e. 3.0 nl/(min.mmHg) will lead to filtration pressure *dis*equilibrium, causing SNFF to fall. In the absence of any compensating changes in the other determinants of ultrafiltration, SNGFR will also fall in proportion to the reduction in K_f. It is important to make the point that the closer the animal is to filtration pressure *dis*equilibrium, i.e. when Q_A is relatively high, the smaller the fall in K_f that will be required to produce *dis*equilibrium and then dependency of SNGFR on the absolute magnitude of K_f. Thus, in the euvolaemic rat, where plasma flow rates are elevated compared with hydropenia (averaging 90–100 nl/min^{-1} as opposed to 60–100 nl/min^{-1}), the rat is close to the inflection point where the magnitude of K_f will begin to influence SNGFR. It should also be stated explicitly that if an *increase* in K_f occurs, the rat will immediately move back to the condition of filtration pressure equilibrium where further rises in K_f will have no additional effect on SNGFR. In recent studies in euvolaemic female virgin and retired breeder Munich–Wistar rats, rather low values of K_f have been observed of around 0.05 nl/(s.mmHg) and all rats in both groups were at filtration pressure *dis*equilibrium. Values of GFR and SNGFR were not low, however, since Q_A in these animals was higher than is normally observed in the euvolaemic preparation (Baylis and Rennke, 1984). These rats were approximately 1 year old at the time of study, much older than the usual age at which Munich–Wistar rats have been studied in the past (3–5 months), and this decline in K_f may reflect an age-dependent defect, possibly associated with the thickening of the glomerular basement membrane that is known to occur during ageing (Asworth *et al.*, 1960; Schurek *et al.*, 1982). It is interesting to note that in the ageing Munich–Wistar female a reduction in K_f to just around the value at which filtration pressure *dis*equilibrium is predicted to occur and SNGFR is predicted to become dependent on K_f (Figure 2.4C) does not result in subnormal values of SNGFR because the increase in Q_A compensates. It is possible that later age-dependent declines in GFR, which in the human do not become evident until after the sixth decade (Thomson *et al.*, 1983), may reflect a further age-dependent decline in K_f to a value where the other determinants of glomerular ultrafiltration can no longer compensate.

Marked reductions in K_f have been produced in a number of models of experimentally induced renal injury, including toxic injury following the administration of gentamicin, uranyl nitrate and puromycin aminonucleotide (Blantz, 1975; Baylis *et al.*, 1977b; Bohrer *et al.*, 1977; Hostetter *et al.*, 1980), various forms of glomerulonephritis (Maddox *et al.*, 1975; Bohrer *et al.*, 1978; Wilson and Blantz, 1984) ischaemia-induced damage (Cox *et al.*, 1974; Hostetter *et al.*, 1980) and untreated diabetes (Hostetter *et al.*, 1981). In some situations SNGFR fell with the reduction of K_f when no compensatory changes occurred in the other determinants of SNGFR, e.g. with gentamicin, uranyl nitrate and puromycin administration and in untreated diabetes (Blantz, 1975; Baylis *et al.*, 1977b; Bohrer *et al.*, 1977; Hostetter *et al.*, 1981) whereas in glomerulonephritis, compensatory increases in Q_A and $\overline{\Delta P}$ occur which serve to maintain the SNGFR at close to the normal value (Maddox *et al.*, 1975; Bohrer *et al.*, 1978; Wilson and Blantz, 1984). Thus, although it has not always proved possible to isolate experimentally the relationship between SNGFR and K_f, in those situations (described above) where K_f falls markedly to *dis*equilibrium-producing values, SNGFR generally behaves as predicted by equations 2 and 4 and Figures 2.3C and 2.4C.

D. Variations in Afferent Arteriolar Protein Concentration (and π_A). The theoretical relationships between afferent protein concentration (C_A) and also π_A and SNFF and SNGFR are shown in Figures 2.3D and 2.4D, again assuming values of K_f, $\overline{\Delta P}$ and Q_A representative of the normal, hydropenic rat. Both SNFF and SNGFR are predicted to vary inversely with C_A, since as C_A and thus π_A are reduced, the oncotic pressure opposing formation of ultrafiltrate is also reduced and, according to equation 2, in the absence of any other changes, the value of the net ultrafiltration pressure, P_{UF}, will be increased. As shown in Figures 2.3D and 2.4D, as the value of π_A approaches 35 mmHg ($\simeq$ the value of $\overline{\Delta P}$ in the rat), both SNFF and SNGFR will tend towards zero, since P_{UF} is also approaching zero.

Several studies have been designed which attempt to test directly the predictions made by the Starling equation (equation 2) of an inverse relationship between π_A and SNGFR. In experiments by Baylis *et al.* (1977a), C_A was reduced by a variety of manoeuvres and *SNGFR failed to rise* as predicted, despite large measured increases in P_{UF}, although SNGFR does rise when the extracellular fluid volume is expanded with colloid-free solutions. The reason that these large rises in P_{UF} did not evoke predictable increases in SNGFR was that a concomitant reduction in K_f also occurred. This reduction in K_f with falls in C_A was acutely reversible by infusion of hyperoncotic rat plasma and restoration of C_A to normal values. Studies by Blantz and co-workers have also demonstrated a direct relationship between C_A and K_f with both reduction and elevation in C_A (Blantz, 1974; Blantz *et al.*, 1974), as well as in more recent studies in which a marked direct correlation between C_A (and thus π_A) was revealed in data subjected to multiple regression analysis (Tucker and Blantz, 1981). A direct relationship between C_A and K_f has also been reported in studies in the dog, in which P_{GC} was estimated by 'stop-flow' pressure measurement, during acute elevation in C_A (Thomas *et al.*, 1979). In earlier studies in the dog, isovolaemic reduction in C_A, in the absence of changes in renal plasma flow rate, failed to invoke the predicted rise in GFR (Vereerstaten and Toussaint, 1969).

Studies in the isolated perfused kidney have also supported a direct relationship between C_A and K_f; in both the isolated perfused dog and rat kidney, reductions in the total protein concentration of the perfusate (and thus π_A) were not accompanied by the expected rise in GFR (Nizet, 1968; Bowman and Mack, 1974; Little and Cohen, 1974) although recent observations have suggested that technical reasons may have caused these results (Schurek and Alt, 1981). Even in this later study, however, variation in perfusate protein concentration between 4.7 and 5.7 g/dl^{-1} (approximating a physiologically normal range of values) shows constancy of both perfusate flow rate and GFR despite a large difference in the oncotic pressure opposing formation of glomerular ultrafiltrate, which suggests the operation of some offsetting action such as a direct effect of perfusate protein concentration on K_f. A recent *in vitro* preparation, the isolated perfused dog glomerulus, has been described (Osgood *et al.*, 1983), and this group has reported that K_f is *lower* at a perfusate protein concentration of 3.5–4.0 dl^{-1} than at zero, i.e. they see an *inverse* rather than a direct relationship between K_f and perfusate protein concentration (Osgood *et al.*, 1981). Although the physiologically relevant range of perfusate protein concentrations has not yet been tested in this preparation, this finding of an inverse rather than a direct relationship between C_A and K_f is in agreement with numerous observations made in peripheral capillaries (Landis and Pappenheimer, 1963; Mason *et al.*, 1977). The reason for this difference is unclear although the use of zero or trace quantities of protein in the intravascular perfusate may interfere with capillary integrity by some osmotic pressure effect. However, despite these discordant findings in the isolated perfused dog glomerulus and in peripheral capillaries, *in vivo* studies in the dog and rat kidney have all confirmed a direct relationship between C_A and K_f.

The functional significance of this direct relationship between C_A and K_f is that, for example, when C_A is reduced to subnormal values, the reduction in π_A and thus elevation in P_{UF} that occurs will be accompanied by a concomitant fall in K_f. Providing that the fall in K_f is sufficient to produce filtration pressure *dis*equilibrium, the reduction in K_f will at least partially offset the effect of the increase in P_{UF}, and thus little net increase in SNGFR will be predicted to occur. On the other hand, if the animal remains at filtration pressure equilibrium, any reduction in K_f which has occurred will have no influence on SNGFR, as described earlier (Figures 2.3C and 2.4C); thus the reduction in C_A will exert its full effect to increase SNGFR as predicted by equation 2 and Figures 2.3D and 2.4D. Increases in C_A and thus K_f will tend to maintain filtration pressure equilibrium, in which case the high K_f will exert no net effect on SNGFR and the increase in π_A, and thus decline in P_{UF} will be anticipated to cause a fall in SNGFR as predicted by equation 2 and Figures 2.3D and 2.4D.

The previous sections have been intended to provide a background knowledge of the qualitative and quantitative importance of the determinants of glomerular ultrafiltration and of the complex interactions that occur between individual determinants of SNGFR. The remainder of this chapter will be devoted to a consideration of the way in which SNGFR is actively controlled in several situations.

Renal Autoregulation

The ability of the kidney to somehow protect and maintain GFR relatively constant over a wide range of arterial blood pressures represents one of the important GFR control mechanisms that operate during normal life. GFR remains almost unchanged over a range of mean arterial blood pressures between 80 and 180 mmHg. The absolute value of the lower limits of the renal autoregulatory range are somewhat variable according to the preparation under study; for example, in the conscious, chronically catheterised rat, near perfect autoregulation of GFR occurs at arterial blood pressures above 80 mmHg (Conrad *et al.*, 1984). In studies under anaesthesia and following surgery, autoregulation of GFR in the rat is generally less efficient, the best autoregulation of GFR being evident at values above 100 mmHg (Arendshorst *et al.*, 1975; Conger and Burke, 1976; Arendshorst and Finn, 1977; Chevalier and Kaiser, 1983). These differences presumably relate to the experimental condition in which the animal is studied, since observations by Gellai and Valtin (1981) have demonstrated that the lower limit at which renal autoregulation of GFR occurs is elevated in rats studied after anaesthesia and minor surgery. Thus, studies performed under anaesthesia may obscure the true value of the lower autoregulatory threshold of arterial blood pressures. Nevertheless, renal autoregulation of GFR does occur in the anaesthetised animal, and since studies under anesthesia have illuminated our understanding of the intrarenal mechanisms involved, such studies will be discussed in some detail.

In addition to renal autoregulation of GFR, renal blood flow rate (RBF) is also maintained nearly constant over a wide range of arterial blood pressures in the rat, man, dog and rabbit (Forster and Maes, 1947; Selkurt *et al.*, 1949; Shipley and Study, 1951; Thurau, 1964; Arendshorst *et al.*, 1975; Chevalier and Kaiser, 1983; Conrad *et al.*, 1984). Autoregulation of RBF has been demonstrated in both denervated and some isolated perfused kidney preparations, and therefore appears to be a property intrinsic to the renal vasculature and independent of neural or extrarenal signals (Forster and Maes, 1947; Waugh, 1964). The intrinsic renal sensing mechanism that controls the autoregulatory response is not known but there are two major hypotheses. One is that the renal vessels respond to some index of transmural pressure, i.e. that an increase in transmural pressure (due to increased arterial blood pressure) will cause a myogenic reflex vasoconstriction, thus reducing blood flow: this is the myogenic theory of autoregulation. Alternatively, or additionally, it has been suggested that some signal created by a change in blood pressure is sensed by a tubuloglomerular feedback system which controls the level of angiotensin II by modulating renin release by the juxtaglomerular apparatus. The evidence in favour of these theories is described elsewhere (Renkin and Gillmore, 1973; Kiil, 1974; Knox *et al.*, 1974; Navar, 1978; see also chapter 4 of this volume).

A number of micropuncture studies have attempted to describe the alterations in renal vascular resistances and in the determinants of glomerular ultrafiltration by which renal autoregulation of the RBF and GFR is achieved. In one study in the Munich–Wistar rat, reductions in mean femoral arterial blood pressure from the resting value of 120 to 80 mmHg (by constriction of the aorta above the level of the renal arteries) in the hydropenic rat led to only slight declines in Q_A and SNGFR: Figure 2.6A (Robertson *et al.*, 1972). Further reductions in femoral arterial blood pressure (to 60 mmHg) led to steep declines in both Q_A and SNGFR. Over the entire range of femoral arterial blood pressures studied, the rats remained at filtration pressure equilibrium, i.e. $\pi_E \simeq \overline{\Delta P}$ (Figure 2.6A, middle panel); thus, in the absence of other changes in the determinants of glomerular ultrafiltration, SNGFR would be determined by the value of Q_A, and single nephron filtration fraction, SNFF, would remain constant. However, SNFF also fell slightly within the renal autoregulatory range (above renal perfusion pressures of 80 mmHg) and markedly when renal perfusion pressure was lowered to 60 mmHg (upper panel). The observed falls in SNFF were the results of falls in P_{GC} and thence in $\overline{\Delta P}$ (middle panel, Figure 2.6A). It should be noted, however, that when renal perfusion pressure was reduced by 40 mmHg from 120 to 80 mmHg, $\overline{\Delta P}$ declined by only 6 mmHg, from 36 to 30 mmHg, and thus was also autoregulated to a large extent. A steeper fall in $\overline{\Delta P}$ occurred when renal perfusion pressure was further reduced to 60 mmHg (Figure 2.6A, middle panel). Since tubular hydraulic pressure (P_T) remained almost constant over the entire range of renal perfusion pressures studied, the observed reductions in $\overline{\Delta P}$ were entirely the result of falls in P_{GC}. The calculated resistances of afferent and efferent arteriolar vessels (R_A and R_E, respectively) are given in the lower panel (Figure 2.6A). During reduction in femoral arterial blood pressure to 80 mmHg, the effective autoregulation of glomerular plasma flow rate, Q_A, was due to graded reductions in R_A; the relative constancy of P_{GC} and thence $\overline{\Delta P}$ was due also to the reductions in R_A while R_E remained constant. Autoregulation failed at femoral arterial blood pressures of below 80 mmHg because no further compensatory reductions in R_A occurred.

In Figure 2.6B, data are summarised from similar experiments carried out in plasma-expanded rats. Because of the plasma expansion, values of SNGFR and Q_A at normal mean blood pressures ($\simeq$ 120 mmHg in this preparation) were elevated compared with the hydropenic condition (upper panel). Also, autoregulation of both Q_A and SNGFR was better in the lower range of femoral arterial blood pressure, i.e. 60–80 mmHg and autoregulation of P_{GC}, and thence $\overline{\Delta P}$ was almost perfect over the range of femoral arterial blood pressures studied (middle panel). As shown in the lower panel, this improved

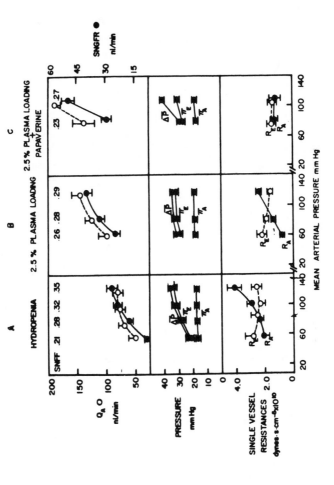

Figure 2.6A–C: Summary of the Effects of Variations in Mean Arterial Blood Pressure on Glomerular Plasma Flow Rate, Q_A (Open Circles), and SNGFR (Solid Circles), Upper Panel; Mean Transglomerular Hydraulic Pressure Gradient, $\overline{\Delta P}$, and Afferent and Efferent Arteriolar Oncotic Pressures π_A and π_E, Respectively, Middle Panel; Resistances of Single Afferent and Efferent Arterioles, R_A and R_E, Respectively. Lower Panel; Figure 2.6A describes data obtained in normal hydropenic Munich–Wistar rats; (B) in moderately (2.5% body weight) plasma-loaded rats; and (C) in plasma-loaded rats also receiving papaverine. Data are shown as mean ± SE

Reproduced with permission from Baylis and Brenner (1978b)

autoregulation at lower blood pressures during plasma loading was the result of an enhanced ability of the afferent arteriole to respond to low renal perfusion pressures by appropriate reductions in its resistance (lower panel). In addition, reciprocal changes in the value of the efferent arteriolar resistance were seen during plasma expansion, which accounted for the remarkable constancy of P_{GC} and thence $\overline{\Delta P}$ over a 60 mmHg range in femoral arterial blood pressure. As shown in the middle panel, values of afferent arteriolar plasma protein concentration and thence π_A were unaffected by changes in femoral arterial blood pressure, and values of π_E equalled $\overline{\Delta P}$ throughout the entire range of blood pressures investigated. Thus, rats remained at filtration pressure equilibrium (as in hydropenia) as shown by the near constancy of single nephron filtration fraction, SNFF; the small alterations in SNGFR which did occur were the result of changes in Q_A.

These studies in the Munich–Wistar rat indicate that autoregulation of SNGFR is the result of autoregulation of both Q_A and P_{GC}, and thence $\overline{\Delta P}$, due mainly to changes in afferent arteriolar resistance. When renal autoregulatory responses were investigated during plasma volume expansion and in the presence of a vascular smooth-muscle paralysing agent (such as papaverine), SNGFR, Q_A, P_{GC} (and thence $\overline{\Delta P}$) all fell precipitously with reductions in femoral arterial blood pressure from 110 to 80 mmHg, due to the inability of R_A and R_E to respond to the alteration in blood pressure (Figure 2.6C; Robertson *et al.*, 1972).

Micropuncture studies investigating the autoregulatory responses of superficial nephrons in the dog have also yielded essentially similar findings in that SNGFR (as well as whole kidney GFR and RPF) were efficiently autoregulated down to mean arterial blood pressures of 80 mmHg. Measurements of renal arterial blood pressure, and blood pressure in the peritubular capillaries (downstream from the glomerulus), together with measurements of renal blood flow rate, permitted calculation of total renal vascular resistance, which fell appropriately during graded reductions in renal arterial perfusion pressure (Navar *et al.*, 1977a).

Most workers have reported autoregulation of SNGFR and/or Q_A in superficial as well as in juxtamedullary nephrons (Aukland, 1966; Loyning, 1971; Bonvalet *et al.*, 1972; Grangsjo and Wolgast, 1972; Robertson *et al.*, 1972; Maddox *et al.*, 1974b; Navar *et al.*, 1977a); however, no autoregulation of outer cortical SNGFR was seen in a study by Kallskog *et al.* (1975b), despite pronounced autoregulation of whole kidney and inner medullary blood flow. Also, a lack of autoregulatory ability of juxtamedullary regions of the kidney has been reported (Thurau, 1964); the reasons for these disparate findings are not apparent but the consensus of opinion holds that both cortical and juxtamedullary glomeruli are capable of autoregulatory ability.

Humoral Control of SNGFR and its Determinants

Angiotensin II

Infusion of angiotensin II (AII) over a wide range of doses has been reported to produce either no change or a fall in whole kidney and/or SNGFR in the rat, dog and man (Zimmerman *et al.*, 1964; Regoli and Gauthier, 1971; Bonjour and Malvin, 1974; Myers *et al.*, 1975a; Blantz *et al.*, 1976; Steiner and Blantz, 1979). In these and other studies a marked reduction in renal plasma flow rate or glomerular plasma flow rate, Q_A, together with increases in whole kidney and single nephron filtration fraction, SNFF, are invariably seen during AII infusion. Studies in the hydropenic Munich–Wistar rat examined the effect of the intravenous infusion of pressor doses of AII on SNGFR and its determinants (Myers *et al.*, 1975a). All rats were at filtration pressure equilibrium during the control and AII infusion periods. A decline in Q_A occurred with AII, which was the result of increases in both afferent and efferent arteriolar resistances (R_A and R_E). SNGFR remained approximately constant due to concomitant increases in SNFF because of marked rises in P_{GC} and thence $\overline{\Delta P}$. In order to determine how much of the rise in P_{GC} was due to the large increase in arterial blood pressure, additional studies were performed, using the same dose of AII but with partial aortic occlusion (above the level of the renal artery) such that the AII-evoked rise in femoral arterial blood pressure (and renal artery perfusion pressure) were prevented. In this setting the changes in SNGFR, Q_A and P_{GC} that occurred during AII infusion were similar to those seen when the aorta was not clamped; however, the increase in R_A was partially prevented whereas the rise in R_E persisted. These observations suggest that the increases in R_A seen when arterial blood pressure was allowed to rise with AII were partly the result of an autoregulatory response to the increased blood pressure and not a direct action of AII on the afferent arteriole. This observation was confirmed by later studies in which a non-pressor dose of AII given directly into the renal artery *failed* to cause an increase in R_A but led to rises in R_E and thence $\overline{\Delta P}$, as well as to falls in Q_A and constancy of SNGFR (Ichikawa *et al.*, 1979). In both of these studies the persistence of the AII-evoked increase in R_E, despite constancy of renal perfusion pressure, suggests that AII exerts a direct, preferential action on the efferent arteriole. A selective rise in R_E would account for the AII-evoked rise in P_{GC} which was responsible for maintaining SNGFR despite the fall in Q_A. The suggestion that AII exerts a selective action on the efferent arteriole has received confirmation from recent *in vitro* studies by Edwards (1983) using isolated, cannulated interlobular arteries and afferent and efferent arterioles from the rabbit. No change in lumen diameter of interlobular arteries and afferent arterioles was seen over a contraluminal AII concentration range of 10^{-12} to 10^{-6} M, whereas efferent arterioles exhibited a significant vaso-constriction with 10^{-12} M AII and a maximal vasoconstriction (a 50 per cent reduction in resting lumen diameter) at 10^{-9} M AII. The physiological AII concentration range is 10^{-13} to 10^{-9} M (Burghardt *et al.*, 1982).

Under the conditions of the studies by Myers *et al.* (1975a), any AII-mediated effect on K_f would be undetectable and have no net influence on SNGFR because of the persistence of filtration pressure equilibrium. Studies by Blantz *et al.* (1976), however, revealed a significant AII-mediated reduction in K_f in rats which had been plasma loaded and were thus at filtration pressure *dis*equilibrium. In these studies K_f was reduced significantly by a low, non-pressor dose of AII and was further lowered when large (pharmacological) pressor doses were administered. SNGFR remained relatively stable during AII infusion, despite the fact that both Q_A and K_f declined with AII, and, in the setting of filtration pressure *dis*equilibrium that existed in these experiments, both of these variables would be expected to influence (i.e. reduce) SNGFR. Similar observations were also made in a later work by Baylis and Brenner (1978c) in which infusion of a pressor dose of AII led to marked falls in K_f and Q_A with relative constancy of SNGFR. In both of these studies the only factor that prevented a fall in SNGFR was the concomitant large rise in $\overline{\Delta P}$ (due to AII-evoked increases in P_{GC}). As described in an earlier section of this chapter, SNGFR would be far more sensitive to change in $\overline{\Delta P}$ under *dis*equilibrium conditions than in an animal at filtration pressure equilibrium (Figure 2.5).

Recent micropuncture studies have sought to describe more about the mechanism of the AII-evoked fall in K_f. Baylis and Brenner (1978c) demonstrated that the AII-mediated fall in K_f was unaffected by simultaneous prostaglandin (PG) synthesis inhibition with either indomethacin or meclofenamate. Inhibition of the PG system did, however, result in significant reductions in SNGFR during AII infusion due to large falls in Q_A, suggesting that endogenously formed PGs normally exert a protective, vasodilator action on the renal microcirculation under conditions in which AII levels are high. It has also been shown that PGs exert a modulating action on Q_A when endogenous AII concentrations are increased by partial ureteral obstruction (Ichikawa and Brenner, 1979a).

Despite the evidence of an interaction between the PG and AII systems on the renal resistance vessels, the AII-mediated decline in K_f is independent of the action of endogenously formed PGs (Baylis and Brenner, 1978c). However, as shown in Figure 2.7, studies have indicated that the actions of AII to increase the efferent arteriolar resistance and to lower K_f are mediated by a calcium-dependent effect (Ichikawa *et al.*, 1979). Rats were studied in an initial period of control euvolaemia, where only a minimum estimate of K_f was possible and then during an i.v. infusion of a pressor dose of AII which led to the usual pattern of change in the determinants of glomerular filtration. Namely, Q_A fell significantly but SNGFR was maintained at the control level (upper panel, Figure 2.7) due to a large increase in $\overline{\Delta P}$ (second panel) and despite a marked fall in K_f which was sufficient to produce filtration pressure *dis*equilibrium (third panel). The bottom panel shows the expected

Figure 2.7: Summary of Changes in Single Nephron Function during Intravenous Infusion of Angiotensin II (AII; 0.2 μg kg^{-1} body weight min^{-1}) and during Continued AII Infusion together with IV Verapamil (20 μg kg^{-1} body weight min^{-1}) in Euvolaemic Munich–Wistar Rats Compared with Controls. In the top panel, values of SNGFR (solid circles), and glomerular plasma flow rate, Q_A (open circles), are given. In the second panel the transglomerular hydraulic pressure gradient, $\overline{\Delta P}$ is given. In the third panel, the glomerular capillary ultrafiltration coefficient, K_f, is given; open circles denote minimum values obtained under conditions of filtration pressure equilibrium and the solid circle denotes exact values calculated under conditions of filtration pressure *dis*equilibrium. In the bottom panel, values are given for the afferent and efferent arteriolar resistances, R_A (solid circles), and R_E (open circles), respectively. Data are shown as mean $\pm$ SE

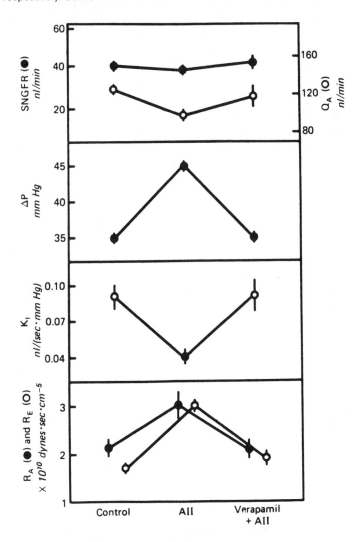

Reproduced with permission from Ichikawa *et al.* (1979)

AII-evoked increases in both afferent and efferent arteriolar resistances (R_A and R_E). In the third observation period the AII infusion was continued and an infusion of verapamil was also given. Verapamil inhibits calcium ion entry into smooth muscle cells (Golenhofen and Lammel, 1972; Langer *et al.*, 1975), and it has been shown that the contractile response to AII, in uterine smooth muscle, depends on the transcellular movement of calcium ion (Freer, 1975). As shown, verapamil, in the presence of AII, led to the complete restoration of SNGFR and all its determinants to control, pre-AII infusion values as well as to a reduction in arterial blood pressure. In another group of rats, the reduction in K_f seen during infusion of a non-pressor dose of AII directly into the renal artery was abolished by the concomitant infusion of manganese, also an inhibitor of calcium-ion entry into smooth-muscle cells (Langer *et al.*, 1975).

These observations suggest that AII exerts a direct action to lower K_f by a calcium-dependent mechanism, which in turn suggests that the fall in K_f is due to a contractile response causing loss of available filtering surface area at the glomerulus. Several types of *in vitro* studies have confirmed the observations from *in vivo* micropuncture studies, indicating that AII exerts a direct action on the glomerulus. For example, the presence of AII receptors in the isolated glomerulus has been demonstrated by receptor-binding studies (Beaufils *et al.*, 1976; Sraer *et al.*, 1977; Brown *et al.*, 1980; Skorecki *et al.*, 1981), and glomerular AII binding is known to be dependent on the external calcium concentration (Blanc *et al.*, 1978). Specific binding of AII has been reported in purified isolated fractions of rat glomerular basement membrane (Sraer *et al.*, 1977), and autoradiographic studies have demonstrated that mesangial cells possess AII receptors (Osborne *et al.*, 1975; Ausiello *et al.*, 1980; Foidart *et al.*, 1980; Mahieu *et al.*, 1980; Skorecki *et al.*, 1981). Scanning electron microscopy has demonstrated that AII infusion produces constriction of superficial glomerular capillary loops, although juxtamedullary glomeruli are reported to be unresponsive to administered AII (Hornych *et al.*, 1972; Hornych and Richet, 1977). Also, isolated glomeruli have been shown to contract in a dose-dependent manner, in response to administered AII (Caldicott *et al.*, 1981), although, in the *in vitro* preparation, a significant contractile response is only evident at pharmacological AII concentrations. It is interesting that the exposure of cultured glomerular mesangial cells to AII results in mesangial contraction (Ausiello *et al.*, 1980; Foidart *et al.*, 1980), which suggests that the reduction of K_f seen with AII in *in vivo* studies may result from a reduction in glomerular capillary surface area due to contraction of the mesangial cells. Using an *in vivo* video technique that allows a direct visual measurement of the glomerulus, it has recently been reported that with i.v. administration of AII, shunting of intraglomerular blood flow from long to short capillary loops occurs, although no reduction in glomerular diameter is evident in this preparation (Snoei *et al.*, 1984). This study provides direct evidence for an AII-evoked reduction in glomerular capillary surface area.

All the studies described so far have dealt with the renal actions of *administered* AII. However, as described in the introductory section, the renin-angiotensin system of the juxtaglomerular apparatus may provide high intrarenal concentrations of endogenously formed AII which function as a local renal hormone and never impinge on the systemic circulation (Burghardt *et al.*, 1982; Mendelsohn, 1982; Morgan *et al.*, 1982). Certainly the juxtaglomerular apparatus contains all the necessary enzymes to produce AII (Burghardt *et al.*, 1982), and the presence of AI as well as renin has been demonstrated, using immunohistochemical techniques, in the myoepithelial cells of the juxtaglomerular apparatus in rat and human kidney (Celio and Inagami, 1981; Celio, 1982). Studies have therefore been performed to evaluate the effects of endogenously formed AII on SNGFR and its determinants in a variety of conditions of different levels of activation of the renin-AII system. One experimental method that has been employed has involved the use of the AII-receptor antagonist saralasin, which is known to inhibit the renal vascular and glomerular AII receptors as well as AII receptors in the periphery (Taub *et al.*, 1977; Caldicott *et al.*, 1981). In *in vivo* micropuncture studies, saralasin infusion has been shown to reverse the reduction in K_f and the rise in efferent arteriolar resistance evoked by the i.v. infusion of a pressor dose of AII; however, for some unknown reason, the increase in afferent arteriolar resistance seen during AII infusion was not reversed by concomitant saralasin administration despite complete inhibition of the AII-evoked increase in arterial blood pressure (Steiner and Blantz, 1979).

Studies in which AII-receptor inhibition is achieved by i.v. saralasin infusion have demonstrated that in hydropenia and euvolaemia, little net effect is seen on either arterial blood pressure or the determinants of SNGFR, suggesting that in these experimental conditions, the AII system is not activated either peripherally or intrarenally (Steiner *et al.*, 1979; Schor *et al.*, 1981b). These observations are in agreement with studies in normotensive awake rats where saralasin infusion has little net effect on arterial blood pressure and/or renal blood flow and GFR, which presumably reflects a low level of activation of AII in these conditions also (Collins and Baylis, 1984). In a number of experimentally induced conditions, however, the renin-AII system is activated; for example, in chronic dietary restriction of sodium, arterial blood pressure and renal haemodynamics are under partial control of AII (Lohmeier *et al.*, 1977; Haber, 1979). Although circulating AII is inversely related to dietary sodium intake, intrarenal AII generation may be dissociated from sodium intake. For example, Mendelsohn (1980) has shown that whereas dietary sodium loading (for 3 weeks) leads to suppression of plasma renin activity, intrarenal AII levels are unchanged (Mendelsohn, 1980).

Micropuncture studies have been performed in sodium-deficient Munich–Wistar rats studied under hydropenic conditions, and K_f was found to be low compared with the values in rats maintained on a high sodium (AII-suppressed) diet (Schor *et al.*, 1980). In addition, AII infusion produced less of a pressor effect and an attenuated further fall in K_f in sodium-deplete vs. high-sodium-intake rats, suggesting prior receptor occupancy by endogenous AII in the sodium-restricted group. In studies by Steiner *et al.* (1979), values of whole kidney GFR and superficial SNGFR were significantly lower in sodium-deficient rats due to reductions that occurred in both Q_A and K_f in these animals compared with controls. Infusion of saralasin had no effect on SNGFR or any of its determinants in the normal sodium-intake group, but produced multiple effects in sodium-deplete animals. Mean arterial blood pressure fell with saralasin in sodium-deplete rats (but remained above the presumed autoregulatory range of the kidney), and SNGFR and Q_A rose significantly. Surprisingly, AII receptor inhibition did *not* reverse the fall in K_f due to sodium depletion, despite clear evidence of inhibition of the peripheral and renal arteriolar actions of the elevated endogenous AII system. The authors suggested that this might be due either to some glomerular structural changes brought about by the chronically raised AII levels or to activation of the antidiuretic hormone (consequent on the volume contraction) which is also known to reduce K_f (as discussed later). Alternatively, systemically administered saralasin may not readily gain access to intrarenal AII receptors.

In later studies by this same group of workers, an alternative method of AII inhibition was employed, namely, use of a converting enzyme inhibitor which prevents the conversion of the inactive angiotensin I to the vasoactive AII (Tucker and Blantz, 1983). Briefly, these experiments showed that with short-term converting enzyme inhibition (3–5 days) marked reductions in arterial blood pressure occurred, and SNGFR and Q_A but *not* K_f were restored to values similar to those observed in rats maintained on a normal sodium diet. Long-term converting enzyme inhibition (14 days) led to restoration of SNGFR, Q_A and K_f. Interestingly, in another group of rats in this same study, acute volume restoration, by i.v. infusion of donor rat plasma and Ringer solution during the micropuncture experiment, also led to complete restoration of SNGFR and all of its determinants, including K_f, to values not different from those seen in sodium-replete rats. Since the reduction in K_f seen with chronic sodium depletion is acutely reversible in this setting, this suggests that structural alterations are not responsible for the fall in K_f. It is possible, as the authors suggest, that local, intrarenally generated AII still mediates the fall in K_f of chronic sodium depletion but is not inhibited either by acute saralasin infusion or 3–5 days of converting enzyme inhibition because these AII inhibitors cannot gain ready access to the local synthesis/receptor sites. Also, it has been suggested that the intrarenal converting enzyme differs from that found in the periphery (Celio and Inagami, 1981) and may not therefore be sensitive to a 3- to 5-day course of the converting enzyme inhibitor (captopril) employed in the studies by Tucker and Blantz (1983). An alternative possibility raised by these observations is that the fall in K_f seen in chronic sodium-depleted states relates to some function of the volume contraction such as elevated antidiuretic hormone levels and/or differences in sympathetic nerve activity, to be discussed later.

An intrarenal role of endogenous AII has been strongly implicated in a number of other conditions in which K_f is found to be reduced; for example, chronic administration of the aminoglycoside antibiotic, gentamicin, has been shown to produce declines in SNGFR due, in large part, to reductions in K_f (Baylis *et al.*, 1977b). Later studies demonstrated that the declines in SNGFR and K_f with chronic gentamicin administration could be largely prevented by the concomitant administration of oral converting enzyme inhibitor (Schor *et al.*, 1981b). Experimentally induced two-kidney, one-clip Goldblatt hypertension is associated with elevations in plasma renin and AII levels (Leenen *et al.*, 1973; Gavras and Gavras, 1981), and reductions in K_f have also been reported in the contralateral kidney, exposed to the high arterial blood pressure (Schwietzer and Gertz, 1979; Steiner *et al.*, 1982). Ichikawa and colleagues have directly investigated the role of AII in the alteration in renal haemodynamics seen in Goldblatt hypertension, and, as with chronic sodium depletion, they found that acute administration of either saralasin or converting enzyme inhibitor led to reductions in renal vascular resistance and increases in SNGFR and Q_A, *but* that the K_f stayed *low* (Ichikawa *et al.*, 1983). However, when antidiuretic hormone was inhibited, the K_f was restored to a normal value (as discussed later).

One conclusion from these studies is that the glomerulus is not solely a passive filter whose function is determined exclusively by systemic factors and renal vascular resistances, but that it is also a site of synthesis and a target for the action of AII and is thus capable of modulating its own intrinsic characteristics to produce rapid and reversible changes in K_f. A second conclusion is that in states where endogenous levels of AII are chronically activated, the SNGFR and its determinants are controlled not only by the intrarenal actions of AII but also by other humoral (and possibly neural) systems. The actions of some of these other systems on glomerular dynamics will be discussed in the following sections.

Antidiuretic Hormone (Vasopressin)

The presence of specific receptors for vasopressin on glomerular mesangial cells has been described, and mesangial contraction in response to arginine-vasopressin (AVP) and AVP-induced cyclic AMP (cAMP) generation has been reported in isolated glomeruli and mesangial cells (Imbert *et al.*, 1974; Schlondorff *et al.*, 1978; Ausiello *et al.*, 1980; Mahieu *et al.*, 1980). Micropuncture studies have shown that in rats where AVP production is suppressed by water loading, the addition of exogenous AVP produced a significant reduction in K_f to *dis*equilibrium values (Ichikawa and Brenner, 1977). SNGFR remained relatively constant despite this fall in K_f since the transition from diuresis to antidiuresis, by the hydro-osmotic action of AVP, led to marked concomitant falls in Bowman's space hydraulic pressure and thence to rises in $\overline{\Delta P}$, which served to offset the effect of the reduction in K_f. Unlike AII, AVP produced no effect on either afferent or efferent arterioles, and thus did not change the value of Q_A. Administration of cAMP to water-diuretic animals also produced falls in K_f, and stimulation of endogenous AVP release (by acute haemorrhage) evoked a pattern of change similar to that seen with administered AVP (Ichikawa and Brenner, 1977).

It has been suggested that the maintenance of the high arterial blood pressure seen in Goldblatt hypertension is partly the result of the vaso-constrictor action of AVP (Mohring *et al.*, 1978) although others have reported that AVP is *antihypertensive* in Goldblatt hypertension (Leenen and de Jong, 1981). Recent studies by Ichikawa and colleagues addressed the question of whether AVP plays a role in the altered glomerular haemo-dynamics seen in this model of hypertension. Using a specific antagonist to the vascular AVP receptor (Lowbridge *et al.*, 1978), it was found that the saralasin-resistant reduction in K_f seen in two-kidney Goldblatt hypertension could be reversed by AVP-receptor blockade (Ichikawa *et al.*, 1983). Further evidence for an independent action of AVP on the glomerulus was provided by Schor *et al.* (1981a), who found that the fall in K_f seen with AVP infusion in euvolaemic rats was *not* reversible by concomitant saralasin, i.e. was not operating via a primary stimulus to AII production.

Thus AVP is another hormone which is apparently capable of exerting direct action on the superficial glomerulus to reduce K_f, and as with AII this effect is probably mediated by a mesangial contraction-induced reduction in surface area. However, the actions of AVP on the renal vasculature are multiple and complex; as discussed in the introductory section of this chapter, there is a marked degree of heterogeneity of both function and structure between superficial cortical and juxtamedullary glomeruli, with SNGFR and glomerular volume being considerably greater in deep compared with cortical glomeruli (Horster and Thurau, 1968; Barger and Herd, 1973; Renkin and Gilmore, 1973; Valtin, 1977). In the Brattleboro' rat, a rat strain which exhibits hereditary diabetes insipidus (i.e. it cannot synthesise AVP), this heterogeneity of nephrons is reduced or absent but may be restored by exogenously administered AVP during their early development (Trinh-Trang-Tan *et al.*, 1981; Edwards *et al.*, 1982). It has recently been observed that chronic AVP administration to the adult Brattleboro' rat leads to the restoration of heterogeneity of glomerular structure and function, although acutely administered AVP has a lesser and more variable effect to increase SNGFR in deep nephrons and does not cause an acute increase in glomerular volume (Davis and Schnermann, 1971; Jamison *et al.*, 1973; Trinh-Trang-Tan *et al.*, 1984). Thus, AVP has complex actions on the glomerulus, producing an acute reduction in K_f (at least in superficial glomeruli) but also having a chronic trophic action to increase glomerular volume (and also presumably filtration surface area and thence K_f?) in deep nephrons.

Vasodilator Hormones

Intravenous infusion of a number of vasodilators including some prostaglandins (PGs), acetylcholine (ACh) and bradykinin (Bk) has been shown in both dog and rat to produce large increases in renal plasma flow rate and/or Q_A but little change in GFR and/or SNGFR; thus filtration fraction falls (Willis *et al.*, 1969; Baer *et al.*, 1970; Stein *et al.*, 1972; Strandhoy *et al.*, 1974). The most likely explanation for this observation would be that the vasodilator-induced reduction in blood pressure would be transmitted through to the glomerulus and the resulting fall in $\overline{\Delta P}$ would offset the effect of a rise in plasma flow rate (Q_A) to result in no net change in glomerular filtration rate. However, in micropuncture studies that directly tested this question, this was shown not to be the case. Rats studied in control hydropenic conditions and then during infusion of vasodepressor doses of ACh, Bk or prostaglandin E_1 (PGE_1) demonstrated constancy of $\overline{\Delta P}$ as well as SNGFR, despite a large increase in Q_A (Baylis *et al.*, 1976). Marked falls in the value of K_f with each of these vasodilators were the cause of the near constancy of SNGFR and the decline in single nephron filtration fraction (SNFF). Constancy of glomerular capillary hydraulic pressure, and thence $\overline{\Delta P}$, was the result of proportionally greater declines in the resistance of the afferent arterioles (R_A) than in the efferent resistance (R_E). In other studies on the rat, histamine and the non-specific vascular smooth-muscle paralysing agent, papaverine, have also been shown to evoke reductions in K_f (Deen *et al.*, 1972; Ichikawa and Brenner, 1979b).

The observation that both vasoconstrictors (i.e. AII and AVP) and vasodilators exert a directionally similar action on K_f is rather puzzling, but studies by Schor *et al.* (1981a) have provided an elegant explanation for this apparent disparity. It was found that the K_f-lowering action of prostacyclin, prostaglandin E_2 and cAMP could all be reversed by concomitant AII-receptor antagonism with saralasin, which strongly suggests that the primary agent evoking the reduction in K_f seen during renal vasodilatation is endogenously formed, locally acting AII. It is known that the PGs and cAMP exert a direct stimulating action on renin formation, both in the intact and isolated kidney and in the isolated glomerulus (McGiff *et al.*, 1970; Aiken and Vane, 1973; Needleman *et al.*, 1973; Beierwaltes *et al.*, 1980). Indeed, the renin-stimulating action of the PGs in the rat kidney is so intense that, at some doses and with some PGs, the underlying vasodilator action of the PGs may be obscured and appear as an apparent vasoconstriction manifested by falls in renal plasma flow rate due partly to concomitant renin release (Malik and McGiff, 1975; Gerber and Nies, 1979; Schor *et al.*, 1981a — see also Chapter 5).

Studies with PG synthesis inhibitors have indicated that under control mildly plasma-volume-expanded conditions and in hydropenia, PG inhibition in the rat has no net action on arterial blood pressure or glomerular renal haemodynamics, suggesting that endogenous PG production is not activated in these conditions (Finn and Arendshorst, 1976; Baylis and Brenner, 1978c). In many situations where the endogenous PG system *is* activated, there is also an elevation in renin-AII; not only does the PG system stimulate renin release but AII also provides a direct stimulus to increase PG production (McGiff *et al.*, 1970; Danon *et al.*, 1975; Gimbrone and Alexander, 1975). As indicated in the studies by Baylis and Brenner (1978c) and Finn and Arendshorst (1976), the PGs and AII exert mutually antagonistic actions on the renal vasculature due to their opposing vasodilator and vasoconstrictor actions. It has also been shown that in situations where both the AII and PG systems are endogenously elevated, such as in ureteral obstruction and chronic sodium depletion, the PGs exert a 'restraining' action on the vasoconstrictor actions of AII, and that in the presence of PG synthesis inhibitor a greatly magnified vasoconstrictor effect of AII becomes apparent (Ichikawa and Brenner, 1979a; Schor *et al.*, 1980).

By now it will be obvious that not only do a number of individual hormones exert direct actions on the glomerulus and the renal resistance vessels but also complex interactions occur between different vasoactive hormone systems.

Other Hormones

An effect of parathyroid hormone (PTH) on glomerular function was suggested by the observation that in plasma-loaded, acutely thyroparathyroidectomised rats, the value of K_f was significantly higher than in intact controls, although all the other determinants of glomerular ultrafiltration were similar. A dose-dependent reduction in K_f was observed in Thyroparathyroidectomised rats during infusion of PTH (Ichikawa *et al.*, 1978a). PTH has been shown to stimulate the synthesis of both cAMP and cGMP by glomeruli (Dousa *et al.*, 1977; Torres *et al.*, 1978), and since cAMP is capable of stimulating the intrarenal production of AII (Hofbauer *et al.*, 1978) it seemed reasonable to test whether the PTH-evoked fall in K_f might be mediated by AII. Accordingly, Schor *et al.* (1981a) investigated this possibility, and demonstrated that infusion of PTH with concomitant AII receptor antagonism with saralasin prevented the reduction in K_f seen with PTH alone. High levels of plasma calcium have also been shown to cause falls in K_f in intact but not in thyroparathyroidectomised rats (Humes *et al.*, 1978), suggesting that the reduced GFR seen in hypercalcaemic states (Bennett, 1970; Edwards *et al.*, 1974) might be the result of an excess of PTH.

It therefore seems that a number of different hormones can act on the glomerulus to produce alterations in the value of K_f and thus exert a potential influence on SNGFR (and GFR) by a direct action as well as indirectly by influencing afferent and/or efferent arteriolar resistances. A scheme by which these various hormones interact at the glomerulus has been proposed by Schor *et al.* (1981a) and is depicted in Figure 2.8. On the basis of the micropuncture and *in vitro* studies it is suggested that cAMP, PTH,

Figure 2.8: Pathways Showing Mechanisms by which the Glomerular Capillary Ultra-filtration Coefficient, K_f, May Be Lowered by Arginine Vasopressin (AVP), Angiotensin II (AII), Dibutyryl cAMP (DBcAMP), Parathyroid Hormone (PTH), Prostacyclin (PGI₂) and Prostaglandin E₂ (PGE₂)

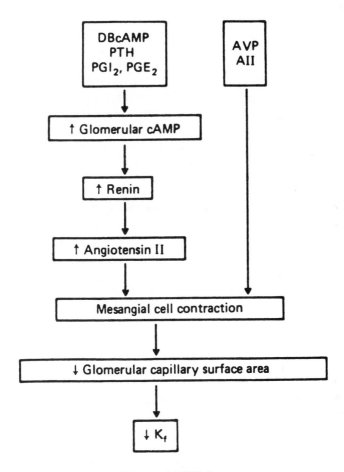

Reproduced with permission from Schor *et al.* (1981a)

prostacyclin (PGI₂) and PGE₂ (and possibly bradykinin, acetylcholine, etc., although these agents have not been explicitly tested) all produce a primary stimulus to glomerular cAMP production, which stimulates local, intraglomerular AII production, leading to mesangial contraction, reduction in filtering surface area and thus falls in K_f. Administered AII and either administered or endogenous AVP bypass the production of *locally* formed AII to exert a direct, contractile action on the glomerular mesangial cells. Thus, of all the multiplicity of hormones that have been shown to cause a fall in K_f, only two agents, i.e. AII and AVP, have been shown to exert a *direct* action to provoke mesangial contraction, and no agent has yet been described which alters glomerular water permeability.

Renal Nerves

As described earlier in this chapter, the kidney receives a rich adrenergic innervation. In the dog, acute renal denervation (under anaesthesia) has been reported to result in increased renal blood flow and GFR (Berne, 1952; Kamm and Levinsky, 1965; Sadowski *et al.*, 1979), but in the rat, little change in renal haemodynamics usually occurs after acute renal denervation when plasma volume is not contracted (Bello-Reuss *et al.*, 1975; DiBona and Rios, 1980; Pelayo *et al.*, 1983). In awake animals, only slight and usually statistically insignificant differences were seen in GFR and/or renal plasma flow rate in dogs and rats with chronic deverversation (Berne, 1952; Surtshin *et al.*, 1952; Sadowski *et al.*, 1979; Rogenes and Gottschalk, 1982). These observations have led to the general conclusion that in the intact, awake, unstressed animal, renal nerve activity has little tonic 'effect on renal haemodynamics (Smith, 1951; Gottschalk, 1979; O'Connor, 1982). It has been demonstrated in some studies that the stress of surgery and anaesthesia leads to an increase in sympathetically mediated vasoconstrictor tone (causing falls in GFR and renal plasma flow rate) in intact but not in denervated kidneys (Berne, 1952; Surtshin *et al.*, 1952), and that in awake dogs subjected to a frightening stimulus, activation of the renal sympathetics is presumed to lead to the observed reductions in renal blood flow that occur (see O'Connor, 1982). In recent micropuncture studies in the rat, the effect of α-adrenergic blockade (with phentolamine) on renal and systemic haemodynamics was investigated in rats anaesthetised either with a barbiturate anaesthetic (inactin) or with chloralose (Tucker *et al.*, 1982). Although α-adrenergic blockade lowered arterial blood pressure to a greater extent in barbiturate- vs. chloralose-anaesthetised rats (an effect predicted on the basis of the fact that chloralose is said not to increase adrenergic activity significantly), surprisingly, afferent and efferent arteriolar resistances were not affected by α-blockade in rats receiving either anaesthetic agent. However, studies in the chronically catheterised rat have provided persuasive evidence that the stress of acute surgery and anaesthesia leads to increases in renal vascular resistance (and consequent falls in GFR and renal plasma flow rate) in the anaesthetised compared with the awake state; the mechanism by which this occurs, i.e. whether neural or humoral, was not determined in this study (Walker *et al.*, 1983).

When the renal nerves are sectioned, in normal animals studied under anaesthesia, electrical stimulation of the cut nerve leads to renal vaso-constriction, the extent of which is determined by the frequency of stimulation (DiSalvo and Fell, 1971; Katz and Shear, 1975; Hermansson *et al.*, 1981;

Kon and Ichikawa, 1983). In micropuncture studies in the rat, an effort was made to determine the mechanism(s) by which both low-frequency (physiological) and high-frequency nerve stimulation influences SNGFR and its determinants (Kon and Ichikawa, 1983). It was found that at low stimulation frequencies, a small fall in SNGFR occurred which was not accompanied by significant reductions in Q_A or $\overline{\Delta P}$ but which was due to a neurally mediated decline in the glomerular capillary ultrafiltration coefficient, K_f. At high stimulation frequencies a greater decline in K_f was observed, together with large falls in SNGFR and Q_A in association with profound increases in both R_A and R_E. As the authors point out, a K_f-reducing effect of renal nerve stimulation may well be mediated by a reduction in surface area due to mesangial cell contraction, since the mesangium is contiguous with the juxtaglomerular apparatus, which receives a rich innervation.

Although acute renal denervation in the anaesthetised rat has generally been reported to produce no influence on SNGFR or its determinants as described above, Pelayo and Blantz have recently reported studies in which renal denervation was seen to produce measurable changes (Pelayo and Blantz, 1984). Rats were studied under the relatively volume-contracted condition of hydropenia (Maddox *et al.*, 1977; Ichikawa *et al.*, 1978b) in an attempt to stimulate renal sympathetic tone, since it is known that volume expansion (or repletion?) suppresses renal nerve activity (Schad and Seller, 1976). In acutely denervated kidneys, significant falls in K_f were observed compared with sham denervated controls; SNGFR was unaffected by denervation, however, since a marked rise in $\overline{\Delta P}$ also occurred which opposed the effect of the fall in K_f. Infusion of either AII receptor blockers or converting enzyme inhibitor normalised values of K_f and $\overline{\Delta P}$ (Pelayo and Blantz, 1984). These studies demonstrate that endogenous AII activity may be enhanced by renal denervation when the renal sympathetics were activated prior to the denervation. Indeed, it is known that the renal sympathetics provide a primary stimulus to renin release (DiBona, 1982). In more recent studies it has been found that circulating AII potentiates the action of renal nerve stimulation (Pelayo *et al.*, 1985).

Summary

This chapter has attempted to give some background on the recent advances in our understanding of the process of glomerular ultrafiltration, derived mainly from micropuncture and various types of *in vitro* studies. It will now be evident to the reader that the mechanisms by which SNGFR and therefore GFR are controlled are complex; the old notion that the glomerulus is a passive filter whose function is determined only by systemic haemodynamics and the renal vascular resistance is clearly no longer tenable in the face of overwhelming evidence to suggest that the glomerulus is also capable of synthesising and directly responding to a number of hormones. Some of the complex interactions between humoral and neural signals have also been described.

Much of the evidence reviewed here has dealt with the responses of the normal kidney to a variety of stimuli. It is striking that, despite profound and complex changes in the determinants of glomerular ultrafiltration, the SNGFR is maintained fairly constant during, for example, large changes in arterial blood pressure and the administration of potent vasoactive hormones. Marked alterations in SNGFR may be produced by acute changes in volume status, by manipulation of dietary protein intake and often as the result of some chronic, progressive disease process which somehow compromises the ability of the individual determinants of glomerular ultrafiltration to maintain SNGFR constant. The impaired glomerular responses to acute and chronic renal failure and to sustained periods of renal hyperfiltration have all been the subjects of recent reviews, and the reader is referred to the following articles: Hostetter *et al.* (1980), Brenner (1983) and Wilson and Blantz (1984).

Acknowledgements

The author is pleased to acknowledge the excellent secretarial assistance of Ms Janeen McCracken. This work was conducted while the author was the recipient of NIH grant HL 31933.

References

Aiken, J.W. and Vane, J.R. (1973) 'Intrarenal Prostaglandin Release Attenuates the Renal Vasoconstrictor Activity of Angiotensin', *J. Pharmacol. Exp. Ther.*, *184*, 678–87

Andreucci, V.E., Dal Canton, A., Corradi, A., Stanziale, R. and Migone, L. (1976). 'Role of the Efferent Arteriole in Glomerular Hemodynamics of Superficial Nephrons', *Kidney Int.*, *9*, 475–80

Arendshorst, W.J. and Beierwaltes, W.H. (1979) 'Renal and Nephron Hemodynamics in Spontaneously Hypertensive Rats', *Am. J. Physiol.*, *236*, F246–51

Arendshorst, W.J. and Finn, W.F. (1977) 'Renal Hemodynamics in the Rat before and during Inhibition of Angiotensin II', *Am. J. Physiol.*, *233*, F290–7

Arendshorst, W.J. and Gottschalk, C.W. (1974) 'Apparent Filtration Pressure Disequilibrium and Filtration Coefficient in the Rat Kidney', *Kidney Int.*, *6*, 18A

Arendshorst, W.J. and Gottschalk, C.W. (1980) 'Glomerular Ultrafiltration Dynamics: Euvolemic and Plasma Volume Expanded Rats', *Am. J. Physiol.*, *239*, F171–86

Arendshorst, W.J., Finn, W.F. and Gottschalk, C.W. (1975) 'Autoregulation of Blood Flow in the Rat Kidney', *Am. J. Physiol.*, *228*, 127–33

Asworth, C.T., Erdmann, R.R. and Arnold, B.S. (1960) 'Age Related Changes in the Renal Basement Membrane in Rats', *Am. J. Pathol.*, *36*, 165–80

Aukland, K. (1966) 'Heat Clearance in the Renal Medulla', *Acta Physiol. Scand.* (Suppl.), *277*, 18

Aukland, K., Tonder, K.H. and Naess, G. (1977) 'Capillary Pressure in Deep and Superficial Glomeruli of the Rat Kidney', *Acta Physiol. Scand.*, *101*, 418–27

Ausiello, D.A., Kreisberg, J.J., Roy, C. and Karnovsky, M.J. (1980) 'Contraction of Cultured Rat Glomerular Mesangial Cells after Stimulation with Angiotensin II and Arginine Vasopressin', *J. Clin. Invest.*, *65*, 754–60

Azar, S., Johnson, M.A. and Hertel, B. (1977) 'Single Nephron Pressures, Flows and Resistances in Hypertensive Kidneys with Nephrosclerosis', *Kidney Int. 12*, 28–40

Azar, S., Johnson, M.A., Scheinman, M.A., Bruno, J. and Tobian, L. (1979) 'Regulation of Glomerular Capillary Pressure and Filtration Rate in Young Kyoto Hypertensive Rats', *Clin. Sci.*, *56*, 203–9

Baer, P.G., Navar, L.G. and Guyton, A.C. (1970) 'Renal Autoregulation, Filtration Rate and Electrolyte Excretion during Vasodilation', *Am. J. Physiol.*, *219*, 619–25

Barger, A.C. and Herd, J.A. (1973) 'Renal Vascular Anatomy and Distribution of Blood Flow', in *Handbook of Physiology*, *section 8*, *Renal Physiology*, American Physiological Society, Washington, DC, pp.249–313

Baylis, C. (1979/80a) 'Effect of Imidazole on the Dynamics of Glomerular Ultrafiltration in the Rat', *Renal Physiol.*, *2*, 278–88

Baylis, C. (1979/80b) 'Effect of Early Pregnancy on Glomerular Filtration Rate and Plasma Volume in the Rat', *Renal Physiol.*, *2*, 333–9

Baylis, C. (1980) 'The Mechanism of the Increase in Glomerular Filtration Rate in the Twelve-day Pregnant Rat', *J. Physiol. (London)*, *305*, 405–14

Baylis, C. (1982) 'Glomerular Ultrafiltration in the Pseudopregnant Rat', *Am. J. Physiol.*, *243*, F300–5

Baylis, C. and Brenner, B.M. (1978a) 'Mechanism of the Glucocorticoid-induced Increase in Glomerular Filtration Rate', *Am. J. Physiol.*, *234*, F166–70

Baylis, C. and Brenner, B.M. (1978b) 'The Physiologic Determinants of Glomerular Ultrafiltration', *Rev. Physiol. Biochem. Pharmacol.*, *80*, 1–46

Baylis, C. and Brenner, B.M. (1978c) 'Modulation by Prostaglandin Synthesis Inhibitors of the Action of Exogenous Angiotensin II on Glomerular Ultrafiltration in the Rat', *Circ. Res.*, *43*, 889–98

Baylis, C. and Rennke, H.G. (1984) 'Repetitive Pregnancy: Physiologic Model of Hyper-filtration?', *Clin. Res.*, *32*, 441A

Baylis, C., Deen, W.M., Myers, B.D. and Brenner, B.M. (1976) 'Effects of Some Vasodilator Drugs on Transcapillary Fluid Exchange in Renal Cortex', *Am. J. Physiol.*, *230*, 1148–58

Baylis, C., Rennke, H.G. and Brenner, B.M. (1977b) 'Mechanisms of the Defect in Glomerular Ultrafiltration Associated with Gentamicin Administration', *Kidney Int.*, *12*, 344–53

Baylis, C., Ichikawa, I., Willis, W.T., Wilson, C.B. and Brenner, B.M. (1977a) 'Dynamics of Glomerular Ultrafiltration IX. Effects of Plasma Protein Concentration', *Am. J. Physiol.*, *232*, F58–71

Beaufils, M., Sraer, J., Lepreux, C. and Ardaillou, (1976) 'Angiotensin II Binding to Renal Glomeruli from Sodium-loaded and Sodium-depleted Rats', *Am. J. Physiol.*, *230*, 1187–93

Beeuwkes, R. (1971) 'Efferent Vascular Patterns and Early Vascular-Tubular Relations in the Dog Kidney', *Am. J. Physiol.*, *221*, 1361–74

Beierwaltes, W., Schryver, S., Olson, P. and Romero, J. (1980) 'Interaction of the Prostaglandin and Renin-Angiotensin Systems in Isolated Rat Glomeruli', *Am. J. Physiol.*, *239*, F602–08

Bello-Reuss, E., Colindres, R.E., Pastoriza-Munoz, E., Mueller, R.A. and Gottschalk, C.W. (1975) 'Effects of Acute Unilateral Renal Denervation in the Rat', *J. Clin. Invest.*, *56*, 208–17

Bennett, C.M. (1970) 'Urine Concentration and Dilution in Hypokalemic and Hypocalcemic Dogs'. *J. Clin. Invest.*, *49*, 1447–57

Berne, R.M. (1952) 'Hemodynamics and Sodium Excretion of Denervated Kidney in Anaesthetized and Unanaesthetized Dog', *Am. J. Physiol.*, *171*, 148–58

Blanc, E., Sraer, J., Sraer, J.D., Baud, L. and Ardaillou, R. (1978) 'Ca^{2+} and Mg^{2+} Dependence of Angiotensin II Binding to Isolated Rat Renal Glomeruli', *Biochem. Pharmacol.*, *27*, 517–24

Blantz, R.C. (1974) 'Effect of Mannitol on Glomerular Ultrafiltration in the Hydropenic Rat', *J. Clin. Invest.*, *54*, 1135–43

Blantz, R.C. (1975) 'The Mechanism of Acute Renal Failure after Uranyl Nitrate', *J. Clin. Invest.*, *55*, 621-35

Blantz, R.C. (1980) 'Segmental Renal Vascular Resistance: Single Nephron', *Ann. Rev. Physiol.*, *42*, 573–88

Blantz, R.C. and Tucker B.J. (1978) 'Measurements of Glomerular Dynamics', M. Martinez-Maldonado (ed.), *Methods in Pharmacology, Renal Pharmacology*, Plenum Press, New York, pp.141–63

Blantz, R.C., Israelit, A.H., Rector, F.C. Jr and Seldin, D.W. (1972) 'Relation of Distal Tubular NaCl Delivery and Glomerular Hydrostatic Pressure', *Kidney Int.*, *2*, 22–32

Blantz, R.C., Rector, F.C. Jr and Seldin, D.W. (1974) 'Effect of Hyperoncotic Albumin Expansion upon Glomerular Ultrafiltration in the Rat', *Kidney Int.*, *6*, 209–21

Blantz, R.C., Konnen, K.S. and Tucker, B.J. (1975) 'Glomerular Filtration Response to Elevated Ureteral Pressure in Both the Hydropenic and the Plasma-expanded Rat', *Circ. Res.*, *37*, 819–29

Blantz, R.C., Konnen, K.S. and Tucker, B.J. (1976) 'Angiotensin II Effects upon the Glomerular Microcirculation and Ultrafiltration Coefficient of the Rat', *J. Clin.*, *57*, 419–34

Blantz, R.C., Tucker, B.J., Gushwa, L.C. and Peterson, O.W. (1983) 'Mechanism of Diuresis Following Acute Modest Hyperglycemia in the Rat', *Am. J. Physiol.*, *244*, F185–94

Bohrer, M.P., Baylis, C., Robertson, C.R. and Brenner, B.M. (1977) 'Mechanisms of the Puromycin-induced Defect in the Transglomerular Passage of Water and Macromolecules', *J. Clin. Invest.*, *60*, 152–61

Bohrer, M.P., Baylis, C., Humes, H.D., Glassock, R.J., Robertson, C.R. and Brenner, B.M. (1978) 'Permselectivity of the Glomerular Capillary Wall. Facilitated Filtration of Circulating Polycations', *J. Clin. Invest.*, *61*, 72–8

Bonjour, J.P. and Malvin, R.L. (1974) 'Renal Extraction of PAH, GFR and $U_{Na}V$ in the Rat during Infusion of Angiotensin', *Am. J. Physiol.*, *216*, 554–8

Bonvalet, J.P., Bencsath, P. and De Rouffignac, C. (1972) 'Glomerular Filtration Rate of Superficial and Deep Nephrons during Aortic Constriction', *Am. J. Physiol.*, *222*, 599–606

Bowman, R.H. and Maack, T. (1974) 'Effect of Albumin Concentration and ADH on H_2O and Electrolyte Transport in Perfused Rat Kidney', *Am. J. Physiol.*, *226*, 426–30

Brenner, B.M. (1983) 'Hemodynamically Mediated Glomerular Injury and the Progressive Nature of Kidney Disease', *Kidney Int.*, *23*, 647–55

Brenner B.M., Troy, J.L. and Daugharty, T.M. (1971) 'The Dynamics of Glomerular Ultrafiltration in the Rat', *J. Clin. Invest.*, *50*, 1776–80

Brenner, B.M., Ueki, I.F. and Daugharty, T.M. (1972b) 'On Estimating Colloid Osmotic Pressure in Pre- and Post-glomerular Plasma in the Rat', *Kidney Int.*, *2*, 51–3

Brenner, B.M., Troy, J.L., Daugharty, T.M., Deen, W.M. and Robertson, C.R. (1972a) 'Dynamics of Glomerular Ultrafiltration in the Rat. II. Plasma-flow Dependence of GFR', *Am. J. Physiol.*, *223*, 1184–90

Briggs, J.P. and Wright, F.S. (1979) 'Feedback Control of Glomerular Filtration Rate: Site of the Effector Mechanism', *Am. J. Physiol.*, *236*, F40–7

Brown, G.P., Douglas, J. and Krontiris-Litowitz, J. (1980) 'Properties of Angiotensin II Receptors of Isolated Rat Glomeruli: Factors Influencing Binding Affinity and Comparative Binding of Angiotensin Analogs', *Endocrinology*, *106*, 1923–9

Burghardt, W., Schweisfurth, H. and Dahlheim, H. (1982) 'Juxtaglomerular Angiotensin II Formation', *Kidney Int.*, *22 (Suppl. 12)*, S–49

Caldicott, W.J.H., Taub, K.J., Margulies, S.S. and Hollenberg, N.K. (1981) 'Angiotensin Receptors in Glomeruli Differ from those in Renal Arteries', *Kidney Int.*, *19*, 687–93

Casellas, D. and Navar, L.G. (1984) '*In vitro* Perfusion of Juxtamedullary Nephrons in the Rat', *Am. J. Physiol.*, *246*, F349–58

Celio, M.R. (1982) 'Angiotensin II Immunoreactivity Coexisting with Renin in the Human Juxtaglomerular Epithelioid Cells', *Kidney Int.*, *22 (Suppl. 12)*, S30–2

Celio, M. and Inagami, T. (1981) 'Angiotensin II Immunoreactivity Coexists with Renin in the Juxtaglomerular Granular Cells of the Kidney', *Proc. Natl Acad. Sci. USA*, *78*, 3897

Chang, R.L.S., Deen, W.M., Robertson, C.R., Bennett, C.M., Glassock, R.J. and Brenner, B.M. (1976) 'Permselectivity of the Glomerular Capillary Wall. Studies of Experimental Glomerulonephritis in the Rat Using Neutral Dextran', *J. Clin. Invest.*, *57*, 1272–86

Chevalier, R.L. and Kaiser, R.L. (1983) 'Autoregulation of Renal Blood Flow in the Rat: Effects of Growth and Uninephrectomy', *Am. J. Physiol.*, *244*, F483–7

Collins, R.C. and Baylis, C. (1984) 'Effects of Angiotensin II (AII) Inhibition on Blood Pressure (AP) and Renal Hemodynamics in Late Pregnant (P) Rat', *Clin. Res.*, *32*, 444A

Conrad, K.P., Brinck-Johnson, T., Gellai, M. and Valtin, H. (1984) 'Renal Autoregulation in Chronically Catheterized Conscious Rats', *Am. J. Physiol.*, *247*, F229–33

Conger, J.D. and Burke, T.J. (1976) 'Effect of Anesthetic Agents on Autoregulation of Renal Hemodynamics in the Rat and Dog', *Am. J. Physiol.*, *230*, 652–7

Cox, J.W., Baehler, R.W., Sharma, H., O'Dorisio, T., Osgood, R.W., Stein, J.H. and Feriss, T.F. (1974) 'Studies on the Mechanism of Oliguria in a Model of Unilateral Acute Renal Failure', *J. Clin. Invest.*, *53*, 1546–58

Dal Canton, A., Conte, G., Esposito, C., Fuiano, G., Guasco, R., Russo, D., Sabbatini, M., Uccello, F. and Andreucci, V.E. (1982) 'Effects of Pregnancy on Glomerular Dynamics. Micropuncture Study in the Rat', *Kidney Int.*, *22*, 608–12

Danon, A., Chang, L.C.T., Sweetman, B.J., Nies, A.S. and Oates, J.A. (1975) 'Synthesis of Prostaglandins by the Rat Renal Papilla. Mechanism of Stimulation of Angiotensin II', *Biochem. Biophys. Acta.*, *388*, 71–83

Davis, J.M. and Schnermann, J. (1971) 'The Effect of Antidiuretic Hormone on the Distribution of Nephron Filtration Rate in Rats with Hereditary Diabetes Insipidus', *Pflügers Arch.*, *330*, 323–34

Davison, J.M. and Dunlop, W. (1980) 'Renal Hemodynamics and Tubular Function in Normal Human Pregnancy', *Kidney Int.*, *18*, 152–61

Deen, W.M., Robertson, C.R. and Brenner, B.M. (1972) 'A Model of Glomerular Ultrafiltration in the Rat', *Am. J. Physiol.*, *223*, 1178–83

Deen, W.M., Troy, J.L., Robertson, C.R. and Brenner, B.M. (1973) 'Dynamics of Glomerular Ultrafiltration in the Rat. IV. Determination of the Ultrafiltration coefficient', *J. Clin. Invest.*, *52*, 1500–8

Deen, W.M., Robertson, C.R. and Brenner, B.M. (1974b) 'Glomerular Ultrafiltration', *Fed. Proc.*, *33*, 14–20

Deen, W.M., Maddox, D.A., Robertson, C.R. and Brenner, B.M. (1974a) 'Dynamics of Glomerular Ultrafiltration in the Rat. VII. Response to Reduced Renal Mass', *Am. J. Physiol.*, *227*, 556–62

DiBona, G.F. (1982) 'The Functions of the Renal Nerves', *Rev. Physiol. Biochem. Pharmacol.*, *94*, 76–181

DiBona, G.F. and Rios, L.L. (1978) 'Mechanism of Exaggerated Diuresis in Spontaneously Hypertensive Rats', *Am. J. Physiol.*, *235*, F409–16

DiBona, G.F. and Rios, L.L. (1980) 'Renal Nerves in Compensatory Renal Response to Contralateral Renal Denervation', *Am. J. Physiol.*, *238*, F26–30

DiSalvo, J. and Fell, C. (1971) 'Changes in Blood Flow during Renal Nerve Stimulation', *Proc. Soc. Exp. Biol. Med.*, *136*, 150–3

Dousa, T.P. Barnes, L.D., Ong, S.H. and Steiner, A.L. (1977) 'Immunohistochemical Localization of 3',5'-Cyclic AMP and 3',5'-Cyclic GMP in Rat Renal Cortex: Effect of Parathyroid Hormone', *Proc. Natl Acad. Sci. USA*, *74*, 3569–73

Edwards, B.R., Sutton, R.A.L. and Dirks, J.H. (1974) 'Effect of Calcium Infusions on Renal Tubular Reabsorption in the Dog', *Am. J. Physiol.*, *227*, 13–18

Edwards, B.R., Mendel, D.B., Larochelle, F.T., Stern, P. and Valtin, H. (1982) 'Postnatal Development of Urinary Concentration Ability in Rats: Changes in Renal Anatomy and Neurohypophysial Hormones', in A. Spitzer (ed.), *The Kidney during Development. Morphology and Function*, McGraw-Hill, New York, pp. 233–40

Edwards, R.M. (1983) 'Segmental Effects of Norepinephrine and Angiotensin II on Isolated Renal Microvessels', *Am. J. Physiol*, *244*, F526–34

Eisenbach, G.M., Van Liew, J.B. and Boylan, J.W. (1975) 'Effect of Angiotensin on the Filtration of Protein in the Rat Kidney; a Micropuncture Study', *Kidney Int.*, *8*. 80–7

Ericson, A.C., Sjoquist, M. and Ulfendahl, H.R. (1982) 'Heterogeneity in Regulation of Glomerular Function', *Acta Physiol. Scand.*, *114*, 203–9

Evan, A.P. and Dail, W.G. (1977) 'Efferent Arterioles in the Cortex of the Rat Kidney', *Anat. Rec.*, *187*, 135

Farquhar, M.G., Lemkin, M.C., Rosenzweig, L.J. and Kanwar, Y.S. (1981) 'Nature, Composition, Function of Fixed Negatively Charged Sites in the Glomerulus', *Proc. 8th Int. Congr. Nephrol.*, *Athens*, Karger, Basel, pp. 116–29

Feld, L.G., Van Liew, J.B., Galaske, R.G. and Boylan, J.W. (1977) 'Selectivity of Renal Injury and Proteinuria in the Spontaneously Hypertensive Rat', *Kidney Int.*, *12*, 332–43

Finn, W.F. and Arendshorst, W.J. (1976) 'Effect of Prostaglandin Synthetase Inhibitors on Renal Blood Flow in the Rat', *Am. J. Physiol,* *231*, 1541–5

Foidart, J., Sraer, J.,DeLarue, F., Mahieu, P. and Ardaillou, R. (1980) 'Evidence for Mesangial Glomerular Receptors for Angiotensin II Linked to Mesangial Cell Contractility', *FEBS*

Lett., *121*, 333–9

Forster, R.P. and Maes, J.P. (1947) 'Effect of Experimental Neurogenic Hypertension on Renal Blood Flow and Glomerular Filtration Rates in Intact Denervated Kidneys of Unanesthetized Rabbits with Adrenal Glands Demedullated', *Am. J. Physiol.*, *150*, 534–40

Fourman, J. and Moffat, D.B. (1971). *The Blood Vessels of the Kidney*, Blackwell, Oxford

Freer, R.J. (1975) 'Calcium and Angiotensin Tachyphylaxis in Rat Uterine Smooth Muscle', *Am. J. Physiol.*, *228*, 1423–30

Gavras, H. and Gavras, I. (1981) 'The Renin-Angiotensin System in Hypertension', in B.M. Brenner, and J.H. Stein (eds), *Contemporary Issues in Nephrology*, Vol. 8., *Hypertension*, Churchill Livingstone, New York, pp. 65–99

Gellai, M. and Valtin, H. (1981) 'Autoregulation of Glomerular Filtration Rate and Renal Blood Flow in Conscious Rats', in K. Takacs (ed.), *Kidney and Body Fluids*, vol. 2, Acad. Kiado, Budapest, pp. 217–21

Gerber, J.G. and Nies, A.S. (1979) 'The Hemodynamic Effects of Prostaglandins in the Rat', *Circ. Res.*,*44*, 406–10

Gimbrone, M.A. Jr and Alexander, R.W. (1975) 'Angiotensin II Stimulation of Prostaglandin Production in Cultured Human Vascular Endothelium', *Science*, *189*, 219–20

Golenhofen, K. and Lammel, E. (1972) 'Selective Suppression of Some Components of Spontaneous Activity in Various Types of Smooth Muscle by Isoveratril (Verapamil)', *Pflügers Arch.*, *331*, 233–43

Gomez, D.M. (1951) 'Evaluation of Renal Resistances, with Special Reference to Changes in Essential Hypertension', *J. Clin. Invest.*, *30*, 1143–55

Gottschalk, C.W. (1979) 'Renal Nerves and Sodium Excretion', *Ann. Rev. Physiol.*, *41*, 229

Grangsjo, G. and Wolgast, M. (1972) 'The Pressure-Flow Relationship in Renal Cortical and Medullary Circulation', *Acta Physiol. Scand.*, *85*, 228–36

Haber, E. (1979) 'The Renin-Angiotensin System and Hypertension', *Kidney Int.*, *15*, 427–44

Hall, V. (1957) 'The Protoplasmic Basis of Glomerular Filtration' (Editorial), *Am. Heart J.*, *54*, 1–9

Heller, J. and Horacek, V. (1984) 'Kidney Function during Decreased Perfusion Pressure due to Aortic Clamping and Hemorrhagic Hypotension: a Single Nephron Study in Dog Kidney', *Renal Physiol.*, *7*, 90–101

Hermansson, K., Larson, M., Kallskog, O. and Wolgast, M. (1981) 'Influence of Renal Nerve Activity on Arteriolar Resistance, Ultrafiltration Dynamics and Fluid Reabsorption', *Pflügers Arch.*, *389*, 85–90

Hofbauer, K.G., Konrads, A., Schwartz, K. and Werner, U. (1978) 'Role of Cyclic AMP in the Regulation of Renin Release from the Isolated Perfused Rat Kidney', *Klin. Woch. enschr. Suppl. 1*, 56 51

Hollenberg, N.K., Epstein, M., Basch, R.I. and Merrill, J.P. (1969) ' "No Man's Land" of the Renal Vasculature. An Arteriographic and Hemodynamic Assessment of the Interlobar and Arcuate Arteries in Essential and Accelerated Hypertension', *Am. J. Med.*, *47*, 845–59

Hornych, H. and Richet, G. (1977) 'Dissociated Effect of Sodium Intake on Glomerular and Pressor Responses to Angiotensin', *Kidney Int.*, *11*, 28

Hornych, H., Beaufils, M. and Richet, G. (1972) 'The Effect of Exogenous Angiotensin on Superficial and Deep Glomeruli in the Rat Kidney', *Kidney Int.*, *2*, 336–43

Horster, M. and Thurau, K. (1968) 'Micropuncture Studies on the Filtration Rate of Single Superficial and Juxtamedullary Glomeruli in the Rat Kidney', *Pflügers Arch.*, *301*, 162–81

Hostetter, T.H., Wilkes, B.M. and Brenner, B.M. (1980) 'Mechanics of Impaired Glomerular Filtration in Acute Renal Failure', in B.M.Brenner and J.H. Stein (eds), *Contemporary Issues in Nephrology*, vol. 6, *Acute Renal Failure*, Churchill Livingstone, New York, pp. 52–78

Hostetter, T.H., Troy, J.L. and Brenner, B.M. (1981) 'Glomerular Hemodynamics in Experimental Diabetes Mellitus', *Kidney Int.*,*19*, 410–15

Humes, H.D., Ichikawa, I., Troy, J.L. and Brenner, B.M. (1978) 'Evidence for a Parathyroid Hormone-dependent Influence of Calcium on the Glomerular Ultrafiltration Coefficient', *J. Clin. Invest.*, *61*, 32–40

Ichikawa, I. (1982) 'Evidence for Altered Glomerular Hemodynamics during Acute Nephron Obstruction', *Am. J. Physiol.*, *242*, F580–5

Ichikawa, I. and Brenner, B.M. (1977) 'Evidence for Glomerular Actions of ADH and Dibutyryl Cyclic AMP in the Rat', *Am. J. Physiol.*, *233*, F102–17

Ichikawa, I. and Brenner, B.M. (1979a) 'Local Intrarenal Vasoconstrictor–Vasodilator Interactions in Mild Partial Ureteral Obstruction', *Am. J. Physiol.*, *236*, F131–40

Ichikawa, I. and Brenner, B.M. (1979b) 'Mechanisms of Action of Histamine and Histamine Antagonists on the Glomerular Microcirculation in the Rat', *Circ. Res.*, *45*, 737–45

Ichikawa, I., Humes, H.D., Dousa, T.P. and Brenner, B.M. (1978a) 'Influence of Parathyroid Hormone on Glomerular Ultrafiltration in the Rat', *Am. J. Physiol.*, *234*, F393–401

Ichikawa, I., Maddox, D.A., Cogan, M.A. and Brenner, B.M. (1978b) 'Dynamics of Glomerular Ultrafiltration in Euvolemic Munich-Wistar Rats', *Renal Physiol.*,*1*, 121–31

Ichikawa, I., Miele J.F. and Brenner, B.M. (1979) 'Reversal of Renal Cortical Actions of Angiotensin II by Verapamil and Manganese', *Kidney Int.*, *16*, 137–47

Ichikawa, I., Ferrone, R.A., Duchin, K.L., Manning, M., Dzau, V.J. and Brenner, B.M. (1983) 'Relative Contributions of Vasopressin and Angiotensin II in Two-kidney Goldblatt Hypertension', *Circ. Res.*, *53*, 592–602

Imbert, M., Chabardes, D. and Morel, F. (1974) 'Hormone-sensitive Adenylate-cyclase in Isolated Rabbit Glomeruli', *Mol. Cell. Endocrinol.*, *1*, 295–304

Intaglietta, M., Pawula, R.F. and Tompkins, W.R. (1970) 'Pressure Measurements in the Mammalian Microvasculature', *Microvasc. Res.*, *2*, 212–20

Jamison, R.L., Buerkert, J. and Lacy, F. (1973) 'A Micropuncture Study of Henle's Thin Loop in Brattleboro Rats', *Am. J. Physiol.*, *224*, 180–5

Kallskog, O., Lindbom, L.O., Ulfendahl, U.R. and Wolgast, M. (1975a) 'Kinetics of the Glomerular Ultrafiltration in the Rat Kidney. An Experimental Study',*Acta Physiol. Scand.*, *95*, 293

Kallskog, O., Lindbom, L.O., Ulfendahl, H.R. and Wolgast, M. (1975b) 'The Pressure-Flow Relationship of Different Nephron Populations in the Rat', *Acta Physiol. Scand.*, *94*, 289–300

Kamm, D.E. and Levinsky, N.G. (1965) 'The Mechanism of Denervation Diuresis', *J. Clin. Invest.*, *44*,93–102

Katz, M.A. and Shear, L. (1975) 'Effect of Renal Nerves on Renal Hemodynamics. I. Direct Stimulation and Carotid Occlusion', *Nephron*, *14*, 246–56

Kiil, F. (1974) 'Renal Autoregulation of Glomerular Filtration Rate: Evidence for the Transmural Pressure Hypothesis', *Proc. Int. Congr. Physiol. Sci., 26th, New Delhi*, *10*, 255–6

Kirkman, H. and Stowell, R.E. (1942) 'Renal Filtration Surface in the Albino Rat', *Anat. Rec.*, *82*, 373–89

Knox, F.G., Ott, C., Cuche, J.L., Gasser, J. and Haas, J. (1974) 'Autoregulation of Single Nephron Filtration Rate in the Presence and Absence of Flow to the Macula Densa', *Circ. Res.*, *34*, 836–42

Knutson, D.W., Chieu, F., Bennett, C.M. and Glassock, R.J. (1978) 'Estimation of Relative Glomerular Capillary Surface Area in Normal and Hypertrophic Rat Kidneys', *Kidney Int.*, *14*, 437–43

Kon, V. and Ichikawa, I (1983) 'Effector Loci for Renal Nerve Control of Cortical Microcirculation', *Am. J. Physiol.*, *245*, F545–53

Landis, E.M. and Pappenheimer, J.R. (1963) 'Exchange of Substances through the Capillary Walls', in *Handbook of Physiology, section II, vol. 2, Circulation*, American Physiological Society, Washington, DC, pp. 961–1034

Langer, G.A., Serena, S.D. and Nudd, L.M. (1975) 'Localization of Contractile-dependent Ca: Comparison of Mn and Verapamil in Cardiac and Skeletal Muscle', *Am. J. Physiol.*, *229*, 1003–7

Larson, M., Hermansson, K.and Wolgast, M. (1983) 'Hydraulic Permeability of the Peritubular and Glomerular Capillary Membranes in the Rat Kidney', *Acta Physiol. Scand.*, *117*, 251–61

Latta, H. (1973) 'Ultrastructure of the Glomerulus and Juxtaglomerular Apparatus', in J. Orloff and R.W. Berliner (eds), *Handbook of Physiology, section 8, Renal Physiology*, American Physiological Society, Washington DC, pp. 1–29

Leenen, F.H.H. and De Jong, W. (1981) 'Hypotensive Effect of Water Restriction in the Two-kidney One-clip Hypertensive Rat', *Am. J. Physiol.*, *241*, F525–31

Leenen, F.H.H., De Jong, W. and De Wied, D. (1973) 'Renal Venous and Peripheral Plasma Renin Activity in Renal Hypertension in the Rat', *Am. J. Physiol.*, *225*, 1513–18

Little, J.R. and Cohen, J.J. (1974) 'Effect of Albumin Concentration on Function of Isolated Perfused Rat Kidney', *Am. J. Physiol.*, *226*, 512–17

Lohmeier, T.E., Cowley, A.W.,Trippodo, N.C., Hall, J.E. and Guyton, A.C. (1977) 'Effects of Endogenous Angiotensin II on Renal Sodium Excretion and Renal Hemodynamics', *Am. J. Physiol.*, *233*, F388–95

Lowbridge, J., Manning, M., Haldar, J. and Sawyer, W.H. (1978) '[1-(β-Mercapto-β,β-Cyclopentamethylenepropionic acid), 4-Valine, 8-D-Arginine] Vasopressin, a Potent and Selective Inhibitor of the Vasopressor Response to Arginine Vasopressin', *J. Med. Chem.*, *21*, 313

Loyning, E.W. (1971) 'Effect of Reduced Perfusion Pressure on Intrarenal Distribution of Blood Flow in Dogs', *Acta Physiol. Scand.*, *83*, 191–202

McGiff, J.C., Crowshaw, K., Terragno, N.A. and Lonigro, A.J.(1970) 'Release of Prostaglandin-like Substance into Renal Venous Blood in Response to Angiotensin II', *Circ. Res.*, *26-7, Suppl. I*, I-121

Maddox, D.A., Deen, W.M. and Brenner, B.M. (1974a) 'Dynamics of Glomerular Ultra-filtration. *VI*. Studies in the Primate', *Kidney Int.*, *5*, 271–8

Maddox, D.A., Troy, J.L. and Brenner, B.M. (1974b) 'Autoregulation of Filtration Rate in the Absence of Macula Densa-Glomerulus Feedback', *Am. J. Physiol.*, *227*, 123–31

Maddox, D.A., Bennett, C.M. Deen, W.M., Glassock, R.J., Knudson, D., Daugharty, T.M. and Brenner, B.M. (1975) 'Determinants of Glomerular Filtration in Experimental Glomerulo-nephritis in the Rat', *J. Clin. Invest.*, *55*, 305

Maddox, D.A., Price, D.C. and Rector, F.C. Jr (1977) 'Effects of Surgery on Plasma Volume and Salt and Water Excretion in Rat', *Am. J. Physiol.*, *233*, F600–6

Mahieu, P.R., Foidart, J.B., DuBois, C.H., Dechenne, C.A. and Deheneffe, J. (1980) 'Tissue Culture of Normal Rat Glomeruli: Contractile Activity of the Cultured Mesangial Cells', *Invest. Cell. Pathol.*, *3*, 121

Malik, K.U. and McGiff, J.C. (1975) 'Modulation by Prostaglandins of Adrenergic Transmission on the Isolated Perfused Rabbit and Rat Kidney', *Circ. Res.*, *36* 599–609

Mason, J.C., Curry, F.E. and Michel, C.C. (1977) 'The Effects of Protein on the Filtration Coefficient of Individually Perfused Frog Mesenteric Capillaries', *Microvasc. Res.*, *13*, 185–202

Mendelsohn, F.O.A. (1980) 'Evidence for the Local Occurrence of Angiotensin II in Rat Kidney and its Modulation by Dietary Sodium Intake and Converting Enzyme Blockade', *Clin. Sci. Mol. Med.*,*57*, 173–9

Mendelsohn, F.A.O. (1982) 'Angiotensin II: Evidence for its Role as an Intrarenal Hormone', *Kidney Int.*, *22 (Suppl. 12)*, S78–81

Michels, L.D., Davidman, M. and Keane, W.F. (1981) 'Determinants of Glomerular Filtration and Plasma Flow in Experimental Diabetic Rats', *J. Lab. Clin. Med.*, *98*, 869–85

Moffat, D.B. (1981) 'New Ideas on the Anatomy of the Kidney', *J. Clin. Pathol.*, *34*, 1197–1206

Mohring, J., Mohring, B. and Maack, P.M. (1978) 'Plasma Vasopressin Concentrations and Effects of Vasopressin Antiserum on Blood Pressure in Rats with Malignant Two Kidney Goldblatt Hypertension', *Circ. Res.*, *42*, 17–22

Morgan, T., Davis, J. and Gillies, A. (1982) 'Release of Renin into the Circulation', *Kidney Int.*, *22 (Suppl. 12)*, S63–6

Moss, N.G. (1982) 'Renal Function and Renal Afferent and Efferent Nerve Activity', *Am. J. Physiol.*, *243*, F425–33

Müller-Suur, R., Persson, A.E.G. and Ulfendahl, H.R. (1982) 'Tubuloglomerular Feedback in Juxtamedullary Nephrons', *Kidney Int.*, *22 (Suppl. 12)*, S104–8

Myers, B.D., Deen, W.M. and Brenner, B.M. (1975a) 'Effects of Norepinephrine and Angiotensin II on the Determinants of Glomerular Ultrafiltration and Proximal Tubule Fluid Reabsorption in the Rat', *Circ. Res.*, *37*, 101

Myers, B.D., Deen, W.M., Robertson, C.R. and Brenner, B.M. (1975b) 'Dynamics of Glomerular Ultrafiltration in the Rat. VIII. Effects of Hematocrit', *Circ. Res.*, *36*, 425–35

Navar, L.G. (1970) 'Minimal Preglomerular Resistance and Calculation of Normal Glomerular Pressure', *Am. J. Physiol.*, *219*, 1658–64

Navar, L.G. (1978) 'Renal Autoregulation: Perspectives from Whole Kidney and Single Nephron Studies', *Am. J. Physiol.*, *234*, F357–70

Navar, L.G., Bell, P.D. and Burke, T.J. (1977a) 'Autoregulatory Responses of Superficial Nephrons and Their Association with Sodium Excretion during Arterial Pressure Alterations in the Dog', *Circ. Res.*, *41*, 487–96

Navar, L.G., Bell, P.D., White, B.W., Watts, R.L. and Williams, R.H. (1977b). 'Evaluation of the Single Nephron Glomerular Filtration Coefficient in the Dog', *Kidney Int.*, *12*, 137–49

Navar, L.G., La Grange, R.A., Bell, P.D., Thomas, C.E. and Ploth, D.W. (1979) 'Glomerular and Renal Hemodynamics during Converting Enzyme Inhibition (SQ 20881) in the Dog', *Hypertension*, *1*, 371–7

Needleman, P., Kaufman, A.H., Douglas, J.R., Johnson, E.M. and Marshall, G.R. (1973) 'Specific Stimulation and Inhibition of Renal Prostaglandin Release by Angiotensin Analogus', *Am. J. Physiol.*, *224*, 1415–19

Nizet, A. (1968) 'Influence of Serum Albumin and Dextran on Sodium and Water Excretion by the Isolated Dog Kidney', *Pflügers Arch. Ges. Physiol.*, *301*, 7–15

O'Connor, W.J. (1982) *Normal Renal Function*, Croom Helm, London

Oken, D.E. (1982) 'An Analysis of Glomerular Dynamics in Rat, Dog and Man', *Kidney Int.*, *22*, 136–45

Osborne, M., Droz, B., Meyer, P. and Morel, F. (1975) 'Angiotensin II Renal Localization in Glomerular Mesangial Cells by Autoradiography', *Kidney Int.*, *8*, 245–54

Osgood, R.W., Reineck, H.J. and Stein, J.H. (1981) 'Effect of Albumin Concentration (C_A) on Glomerular Ultrafiltration Coeffficient (K_f) in the Isolated Perfused Glomerulus', *Am. Soc. Nephrol.*, *14*, 119A

Osgood, R.W., Patton, M., Hanley, M.J., Venkatachalam, M., Reineck, H.J. and Stein, J.H. (1983) '*In vitro* Perfusion of the Isolated Dog Glomerulus', *Am. J. Physiol.*, *244*, F349–54

Osswald, H., Haas, J.A., Marchand, G.R. and Knox, F.G. (1979) 'Glomerular Dynamics in Dogs at Reduced Renal Artery Pressure', *Am. J. Physiol.*, *236*, F25–9

Ott, C. E., Marchand, G.R., Diaz-Buxo, J.A. and Knox, F.G. (1976) 'Determinants of Glomerular Filtration Rate in the Dog', *Am. J. Physiol.*, *231*, 235–9

Pelayo, J.C. and Blantz, R.C. (1984) 'Analysis of Renal Denervation in the Hydropenic Rat: Interactions with Angiotensin II', *Am. J. Physiol.*, *246*, F87–95

Pelayo, J.C., Ziegler, M.G., Jose, P.A. and Blantz, R.C. (1983) 'Renal Denervation in the Rat: Analysis of Glomerular and Proximal Tubular Function', *Am. J. Physiol.*, *244*, F70–7

Pelayo, J.C., Ziegler, M.G. and Blantz, R.C. (1985) 'Role of Angiotensin II in Adrenergic Induced Alterations in Glomerular Hemodynamics', *Am. J. Physiol.*, in press

Pullman, T.N., Alving, A.S., Dern, R.J. and Landowne, M. (1954) 'The Influence of Dietary Protein Intake on Specific Renal Functions in Normal Man', *J. Lab. Clin. Med.*, *44*, 320–32

Regoli, D. and Gauthier, R. (1971) 'Site of Action of Angiotensin and Other Vasoconstrictors on the Kidney', *Can. J. Physiol. Pharmacol.*, *49*, 608–12

Renkin, E.M. (1979) 'Relation of Capillary Morphology to Transport of Fluid and Large Molecules: a Review', *Acta Physiol. Scand., suppl. 463*, 81–91

Renkin, E.M. and Gilmore, J.P. (1973) 'Glomerular Filtration', in *Handbook of Physiology, section 8, Renal Physiology*, American Physiological Society, Washington, DC, pp. 185–248

Reubi, F.C., Weidmann, P., Hodler, J. and Cottier, P.T. (1978) 'Changes in Renal Function in Essential Hypertension', *Am. J. Med.*, *64*, 556–63

Robertson, C.R., Deen, W.M., Troy, J.L. and Brenner, B.M. (1972) 'Dynamics of Glomerular Ultrafiltration in the Rat. III. Hemodynamics and Autoregulation', *Am. J. Physiol.*, *223*, 1191–1200

Rogenes, P.R. and Gottschalk, C.W. (1982) 'Renal Function in Conscious Rats with Chronic Unilateral Renal Denervation', *Am. J. Physiol.*, *242*, F140–8

Ryan, G.B., Alcorn, D., Coghlan, J.P., Hill, P.A. and Jacobs, R. (1982) 'Ultrastructural Morphology of Granule Release from Juxtaglomerular Myoepithelial and Peripolar Cells', *Kidney Int.*, *22 (suppl. 12)*. S3–8

Sadowski, J., Kurkus, J. and Gellert, R. (1979) 'Denervated and Intact Kidney Responses to Saline Load in Awake and Anesthetized Dogs', *Am. J. Physiol.*, *237*, F262–7

Sakai, T., Harris, F.H., Marsh, D.J., Bennett, C.M. and Glassock, R.J. (1984) 'Extracellular Fluid Expansion and Autoregulation in Nephrotoxic Serum Nephritis in Rats', *Kidney Int.*, *25*, 619–28

Savin, V.J. (1983) 'Ultrafiltration in Single Isolated Human Glomeruli', *Kidney Int.*, *24*, 748–53

Savin, V.J. and Patak, R.V. (1982) 'Variation of Ultrafiltration Coefficient with Glomerular Size in Six Mammalian Species', *Kidney Int.*, *21*, 247

Savin, V.J. and Terreros, D.A. (1981) 'A Study of Filtration in Single Isolated Mammalian Glomeruli', *Kidney Int.*, *20*, 188–97

Schad,H. and Seller, H. (1976) 'Reduction of Renal Nerve Activity by Volume Expansion in Conscious Rats', *Pflügers Arch.*, *363*, 155–9

Schlondorff, D., Yoo, P. and Alpert, B.E. (1978) 'Stimulation of Adenylate Cyclase in Isolated Rat Glomeruli by Prostaglandins', *Am. J. Physiol.*, *235*, F458–64

Schor, N., Ichikawa, I. and Brenner, B.M. (1980) 'Glomerular Adaptations to Chronic Dietary Salt Restriction or Excess', *Am. J. Physiol.*, *238*, F428–36

Schor, N., Ichikawa, I. and Brenner, B.M. (1981a) 'Mechanisms of Action of Various Hormones and Vasoactive Substances on Glomerular Ultrafiltration in the Rat', *Kidney Int.*, *20*, 442–51

Schor, N., Ichikawa, I., Rennke, H.G., Troy, J.L. and Brenner, B.M. (1981b). 'Pathophysiology of Altered Glomerular Function in Aminoglycoside-treated Rats', *Kidney Int.*, *19*, 288–96

Schurek, H.J. and Alt, J.M. (1981) 'Effect of Albumin on the Function of the Perfused Rat Kidney', *Am. J. Physiol.*, *240*, F569–76

Schurek, H.J., Panzer, J., Wiemeyer, A., Kuhn, K., Aeikens, B. and Brod, J. (1982) 'Effect of Ageing on the Glomerular Capillaries, Blood Pressure and Renal Function', *Contr. Nephrol.*, *30*, 157

Schweitzer, G. and Gertz, K.H. (1979) 'Changes of Hemodynamics and Glomerular Utrafiltration in Renal Hypertension of Rats', *Kidney Int.*, *15*, 134–43

Selkurt, E.E., Hall, P.W. and Spencer, M.P. (1949) 'Influence of Graded Arterial Pressure Decrement on Renal Clearance of Creatinine, *p*-Aminohippurate and Sodium', *Am. J. Physiol.*, *159*, 369–78

Shea, S.M. Morrison, A.B. (1975) 'A Stereological Study of the Glomerular Filter in the Rat. Morphometry of the Slit Diaphragm and Basement Membrane', *J. Cell Biol.*, *67*, 436–43

Shipley, R.E. and Study, R.S. (1951) 'Changes in Renal Blood Flow, Extraction of Inulin, Glomerular Filtration Rate, Tissue Pressure and Urine Flow with Acute Alterations of Renal Artery Blood Pressure', *Am. J. Physiol.*, *167*, 676–88

Skorecki, K., Lawrence, W., Rennke, H., Alexander, R. and Brenner, B.M. (1981),'Regulation and Localization of Angiotensin II (AII) Binding to the Isolated Rat Renal Glomerulus', *Proc. 8th Int. Congr. Nephrol.*, *Athens*, Karger, Basel, p.169

Smith, H.W. (1951) *The Kidney: Structure and Function in Health and Disease*, Oxford University Press, Oxford

Snoei, H., Kucherer, H., Parekh, N., Wilhelm, K.R., Weis, S. and Steinhausen, M. (1984) 'Long and Short Pathways within the Glomerular Capillary Network in the Hydronephrotic Kidney of Rats', *Pflügers Arch.*, *40* (Suppl.), R42

Sraer, J., Baud, L., Cosyns, J., Verroust, P., Nivez, M. and Ardaillou, R. (1977) 'High Affinity Binding of ^{125}I-Angiotensin II to Rat Glomerular Basement Membranes', *J. Clin. Invest.*, *59*, 69–81

Stein, J.H., Congalbay, R.C., Marsh, D.L., Osgood, R.W. and Ferris, T.F. (1972) 'The Effect of Bradykinin on Proximal Tubular Sodium Reabsorption in the Dog: Evidence for Functional Nephron Heterogeneity', *J. Clin. Invest.*, *51*, 1709–21

Steiner, R.W. and Blantz, R.C. (1979)'Acute Reversal by Saralasin of Multiple Intrarenal Effects of Angiotensin II', *Am. J. Physiol.*, *237*, F386–91

Steiner, R.W., Tucker, B.J. and Blantz, R.C. (1979) 'Glomerular Hemodynamics in Rats with Chronic Sodium Depletion', *J. Clin. Invest.*, *64*, 503–12

Steiner, R.W., Tucker, B.J., Gushwa, L.C., Gifford, J., Wilson, C.B. and Blantz, R.C. (1982) 'Glomerular Hemodynamics in Moderate Goldblatt Hypertension in the Rat', *Hypertension*, *4*, 51–7

Strandhoy, J.W., Ott, C.E., Schneider, E.G., Willis, L.R., Beck, N.P., David, B.B. and Knox, F.G. (1974) 'Effect of Prostaglandin E_1 and E_2 on Renal Sodium Reabsorption and Starling Forces', *Am. J. Physiol.*, *226*, 1015–21

Surtshin, A., Barber Mueller, C. and White, H.L. (1952) 'Effect of Acute Changes in Glomerular Filtration Rate on Urine Flow Rate and Electrolyte Excretion. Mechanism of Denervation Diuresis', *Am. J. Physiol.*, *169*, 159–73

Taub, K.J., Caldicott, W.J.H. and Hollenberg, N.K. (1977) 'Angiotensin Antagonists with Increased Specificity for the Renal Vasculature', *Kidney Int.*, *59*, 528

Thomas, C.E., Bell, P.D. and Navar, L.G. (1979) 'Glomerular Filtration Dynamics in the Dog during Elevated Colloid Osmotic Pressure', *Kidney Int.*, *15*, 502–12

Thomson, B.I., Davison, J.M. and Kerr, D.N.S. (1983) 'Clinical Physiology of the Kidney: Tests of Renal Function and Structure', in D.S.Weatherall, J.D. Ledingham and D.A. Warrell (eds), *Oxford Textbook of Medicine*, Oxford University Press, Oxford

Tonder, K.H. and Aukland, K. (1979) 'Glomerular Capillary Pressure in the Rat. Validation of Pressure Measurement through Corticotomy', *Acta Physiol. Scand.*, *106*, 93–5

Thurau, K. (1964)'Renal Hemodynamics', *Am. J. Med.*, *36*, 698–719

Thurau, K., Gruner, A., Mason, J. and Dahlman, H. (1982) 'Tubular Signal for the Renin Activity in the Juxtaglomerular Apparatus', *Kidney Int.*, *22 (suppl. 12)*, S55–62

Torres, V.E., Northrup, T.E., Edwards, R.M., Shah, S.V. and Dousa, T.P. (1978) 'Modulation of Cyclic Nucleotides in Isolated Rat Glomeruli', *J. Clin. Invest.*, *62*, 1334–43

Trinh-Trang-Tan, M.M., Diaz, M., Grunfeld, J.P. and Bankir, l. (1981) 'ADH-dependent Nephron Heterogeneity in Rats with Hereditary Hypothalamic Diabetes Insipidus', *Am. J. Physiol.*, 240, F372–80

Trinh-Trang-Tan, M.M., Bouby, N., Doute, M. and Bankir, L. (1984) 'Effect of Long- and Short-term Antidiuretic Hormone Availability on Internephron Heterogeneity in the Adult Rat', *Am. J. Physiol.*, *246*, F879–88

Tucker, B.J. and Blantz, R.C. (1981) 'Effects of Glomerular Filtration Dynamics on the Glomerular Permeability Coefficient', *Am. J. Physiol.*, *240*, F245–54

Tucker, B.J. and Blantz, R.C. (1983) 'Mechanism of Altered Glomerular Hemodynamics during Chronic Sodium Depletion', *Am. J. Physiol.*, *244*, F11–18

Tucker, B.J. and Blantz, R.C. (1984) 'Effect of Furosemide Administration on Glomerular and Tubular Dynamics in the Rat', *Kidney Int.*, *26*, 112–21

Tucker, B.J., Steiner, R.W., Gushwa, L.C. and Blantz, R.C. (1978) 'Studies on the Tubuloglomerular Feedback System in the Rat. The Mechanism of Reduction in Filtration Rate with Benzolamide', *J. Clin. Invest.*, *62*, 993–1004

Tucker, B.J., Peterson, O.W., Ziegler, M.G. and Blantz, R.C. (1982) 'Analysis of Adrenergic Effects of the Anesthetics Inactin and α-Chloralose', *Am. J. Physiol.*, *243*, F253–9

Valtin, H. (1977) 'Structural and Functional Heterogeneity of Mammalian Nephrons', *Am. J. Physiol.*, *233*, F491–501

Vereerstaten, P. and Toussaint, C. (1969) 'Effects of Plasmaphoresis on Renal Hemodynamics and Sodium Excretion in Dogs', *Pflügers Arch. Ges. Physiol.*, *306*, 92–102

Walker, L.A., Buscemi-Bergin, M. and Gellai, M. (1983) 'Renal Hemodynamics in Conscious Rats: Effects of Anesthesia, Surgery and Recovery', *Am. J. Physiol.*, *245*, F67–74

Waugh, W.H. (1964) 'Circulatory Autoregulation in the Fully Isolated Kidney and in the Humorally Supported Isolated Kidney', *Circ. Res.*, *15*, *Suppl.I*, 1–156 to 1–69

Weinstein, S.W. and Szyjewicz, S. (1978) 'Superficial Nephron Tubular Vascular Relationships in the Rat Kidney', *Am. J. Physiol.*, *234*, F207–14

Willis, L.R., Ludens, J.H., Hook, J.B. and Williamson, H.E. (1969) 'Mechanism of Natriuretic Action of Bradykinin', *Am. J. Physiol.*, *217*, 1–5

Wilson, C.B. and Blantz, R.C. (1984) 'Nephroimmunopathology and Pathophysiology' (Editorial), *Am. J. Physiol.*, *248*, F319–31

Zimmerman, B.G., Abboud, F.M. and Eckstein, J.W. (1964) 'Effects of Norepinephrine and Angiotensin on Total and Venous Resistance in the Kidney', *Am. J. Physiol.*, *206*, 701–6

3 ION TRANSPORT IN THE LOOP OF HENLE

Eberhard Schlatter and Rainer Greger

Introduction

Function of the Loop of Henle

The main task of the loop of Henle is its function as a part of the countercurrent concentration system in the mammalian kidney. The loop of Henle generates the osmotic gradient in the kidney with increasing osmolarity from cortex to medulla. This osmotic gradient is the prerequisite to produce a highly concentrated urine. Furthermore, the loop of Henle also reabsorbs some of the remaining organic solutes and divalent cations from the luminal fluid, is capable of secreting potassium, and plays a role in lumen-fluid acidification.

Functional Differentiation of the Loop of Henle

The loop of Henle comprises functionally and morphologically different nephron segments: thick descending limb (pars recta), thin descending and ascending limb, and medullary and cortical thick ascending limb. The anatomical arrangement of the different segments and their ability to reabsorb ions via primary active pumps, secondary active transport systems, or passive permeation pathways, and the water permeability of the descending limb of the loop only, are responsible for the production of a diluted tubular fluid in the early distal tubule as compared with the plasma (Wirz et al., 1951). By these means a hyperosmotic interstitium is produced in the kidney.

In the last decade several studies using the technique of *in vitro* perfusion of isolated tubule segments have gathered much information on the identification and localisation of the different transport processes along the loop of Henle. The present brief review will concentrate on data obtained more recently on the *in vitro* perfused isolated tubule. Space limitation will make it necessary to focus on the main issues only. We therefore refer the reader to original reports and to recent excellent reviews on the various segments of the loop of Henle: pars recta (Berry and Warnock, 1982; Grantham, 1982; Schafer and Barfuss, 1982; Berry, 1983; Schafer and Work, 1984); thin descending and ascending limb (Kokko 1982; Imai et al., 1984b); and medullary and cortical thick ascending limb (Burg, 1982; Greger et al., 1984c, e; Hebert and Andreoli, 1984b; Imai, 1984a; Stokes, 1984; Greger, 1985b).

Thick Descending Limb of Henle (Pars Recta, PR)

Introduction

The pars recta segment can be subdivided morphologically and also with respect to its function into a superficial and a juxtamedullary portion. The pars recta has been studied most extensively with the technique of isolated *in vitro* perfused tubules, which was described first by Burg *et al.* (1966). Most data have been obtained for the rabbit. Recent studies of Barfuss and Schafer (1981a) and Volkl and Greger (1984) have, in addition, employed segments dissected from mouse and rat kidney. Functionally the pars recta is very similar to the convoluted proximal tubule. It reabsorbs Na$^+$ actively; however, its reabsorption rates for Na$^+$ and Cl$^-$ and also for water are only about 30 per cent of those observed in the proximal convoluted tubule (DeRouffignac and Morel, 1969; Grantham *et al.*, 1972). The pars recta segment is a typical low-resistance epithelium, characterised by a high permeability to water and to ions, allowing for high and essentially isotonic water flow across the epithelium. The transepithelial electrical resistance values reported for the pars recta are as low as those reported for the proximal convoluted tubule by Frömter (1981) and are, at about 10 ohm cm^2, the lowest reported for the entire nephron (Lutz *et al.*, 1973; H. Völkl and R. Greger, unpublished observations). Some of the properties of the superficial (SF) and juxta-medullary (JM) pars recta segment are listed in Table 3.1.

Permeability Properties of the Pars Recta

The pars recta has a high water permeability. Reported values range between 0.2 and 0.7 cm s^{-1} (Andreoli *et al.*, 1978; Schafer *et al.*, 1978b; Berry, 1983). Whereas most investigators agree on the range of the water permeability values, they disagree with respect to the route of water reabsorption. The paracellular route is supported by data of Gonzales *et al.* (1982) showing a transepithelial water permeability which is higher than the transcellular permeability. Furthermore, considerable amounts of chloride are reabsorbed by solvent drag (Schafer *et al.*, 1975, 1977; Andreoli *et al.*, 1979). If water flowed mainly cellularly, chloride reabsorption could not be explained by solvent drag. Other data of Berry (1983) and of Welling *et al.* (1983) on the basis of indirect evidence lead to the conclusion that the cellular water permeability is sufficiently high to account for the observed large water flow through the pars recta. The study by Berry (1983) assigns only some 5 to 10 per cent of the water flow to the paracellular route. All authors accept that the water permeability of the basolateral membrane is fairly high (Gonzales *et al.*, 1982; Persson and Spring, 1982; Berry, 1983; Welling *et al.*, 1983). Therefore, the question of where the water moves is dependent on reliable measurements of apical membrane permeability to water. If this is higher than that of the basolateral membrane, it is conceivable that a large fraction of water reabsorption moves transcellularly. If apical water permeability was of the

Table 3.1: Properties of the Pars Recta (PR) of the Proximal Tubule

Property	Superficial PR	Juxtamedullary PR
P_f (cm s^{-1})	0.2 to 0.7[16]; 0.4[1]	
P_{Na^+} (cm s^{-1} x 10^{-5})	2.3[13]; 2.6[9]	5.8[9]
P_{K^+} (cm s^{-1} x 10^{-5})	1.0[12]; 1.4[19,21]	5.2[19,21]
P_{Cl^-} (cm s^{-1} x 10^{-5})	5.6 to 8.7[2,9,13,19]	2.1[9,20]
$P_{HCO_3^-}$ (cm s^{-1} x 10^{-5})	0.4[13]; 2.0[17,20]	1.1[20]
P_{urea} (cm s^{-1} x 10^{-5})	1.4[8]	2.1[8]
P_{Na^+}/P_{Cl^-}	0.3[13]; 0.4[20]	2.0[20]
$P_{HCO_3^-}/P_{Cl^-}$	0.04[13]; 0.35[20]	0.53[20]
J_v (nl min^{-1} mm^{-1})	0.3 to 2.6[1,3,7,9,11,13-17,21]	0.6[9]
PD_{te} (mV)	−1.9 to +1.6[2,4,5,9,11,13-15,21]	−2.4[9]
PD_{bl} (mV)	−38 to −62[4,5,6,18]	
R_{te} (ohm cm^2)	8[11]; 13[19]	
I_{sc} (μA cm^{-2})	2.5[10]	

P_f, P_{Na^+}, P_{K^+}, P_{Cl^-}, $P_{HCO_3^-}$, P_{urea} = permeability coefficient for water, Na$^+$, K$^+$, Cl$^-$, HCO$_3^-$, and urea, respectively; J_v = reabsorptive volume flow; PD_{te}, PD_{bl} = potential difference across the epithelium and the basolateral membrane; R_{te} = transepithelial electrical resistance; I_{sc} = equivalent short-circuit current.

References

[1] Andreoli *et al.*, 1978. [2] Andreoli *et al.*, 1979. [3] Barfuss and Schafer, 1981b. [4] Bello-Reuss, 1982. [5] Biagi *et al.*, 1981a. [6] Biagi *et al.*,1981b. [7] Burg and Orloff, 1968. [8] Kawamura and Kokko, 1976. [9] Kawamura *et al.*, 1975. [10] Lutz *et al.*, 1973. [11] McKinney and Burg, 1977. [12] Schafer and Work, 1984. [13] Schafer *et al.*, 1974. [14] Schafer *et al.*, 1975. [15] Schafer *et al.*, 1978a. [16] Schafer *et al.*, 1978b. [17] Schafer *et al.*, 1981. [18] Völkl and Greger, 1984. [19] H. Völkl and R. Greger, unpublished observation. [20] Warnock and Burg, 1977. [21] Work *et al.*, 1982.

order of that for the basolateral membrane or smaller, only a fraction of the transepithelial water transport would take the transcellular route. In their recent estimates, Gonzales *et al.* (1984) claim that the apical water permeability is even lower than that of the basolateral membrane. In this case a large fraction of water transport will move paracellularly. Any indirect consideration, such as arguments based on solvent drag measurements or chloride pathways (Schafer *et al.*, 1975, 1977; Berry, 1983) appear secondary in this discussion, since many of the possible errors that overshadow the estimation of water permeability may also hamper the determination of the reflection coefficients.

Since the hydraulic conductance in this nephron segment is so high, a small osmotic gradient (a few milliosmoles) would be sufficient to drive the water flow observed in the pars recta. Even in the absence of an osmotic gradient, an effective driving force for passive water movement can be provided by the fact that the lumen fluid is concentrated with respect to chloride and depleted with respect to bicarbonate (McKinney and Burg, 1977; Schafer *et al.*, 1981). In addition it is depleted of organic compounds such as glucose and amino acids. Given the fact that the permeability ratio $P_{Cl^-}/P_{HCO_3^-}$ is considerably larger than unity (Schafer *et al.*, 1974; Warnock and Burg, 1977) and the reflection coefficient for bicarbonate is larger than that for chloride (Frömter *et al.*, 1973), this would drive water flow passively (Schafer *et al.*, 1975, 1978a; Andreoli *et al.*, 1979).

Using either 'natural' or artificial solutions in various perfusion experiments, volume reabsorption was shown (Schafer *et al.*, 1974, 1975, 1977, 1981; Barfuss and Schafer, 1981b) to be dependent on peritubular potassium, and inhibited by ouabain or cooling. Removal of bicarbonate or organic solutes from the perfusate, or addition of carbonic anhydrase inhibitors, reduced fluid reabsorption by 20 to 50 per cent (Schafer and Andreoli, 1976; McKinney and Burg, 1977). Thus, the reabsorption of fluid in the pars recta appears to be driven by an osmotic disequilibrium across the epithelium, which is generated by active reabsorption of solutes.

The passive permeability coefficients for sodium and potassium are about 2.5×10^{-5} and 1.2×10^{-5} cm sec^{-1}, respectively (Schafer *et al.*, 1974; Kawamura *et al.*, 1975; Work *et al.*, 1982; Schafer and Work, 1984) in the superficial pars recta, and have even higher values, 5.2×10^{-5} cm s^{-1}, in the juxtamedullary portion (Kawamura *et al.*, 1975; Work *et al.*, 1982; Schafer and Work, 1984). For the superficial as well as the juxtamedullary proximal straight tubule, a net potassium secretion has been reported by Wasserstein and Agus (1983) and Schafer and Work (1984). Considering the large K$^+$ permeability, especially in the juxtamedullary pars recta, this potassium secretion could be driven passively by a potassium concentration gradient from interstitium to lumen (Schafer and Work, 1984). Bicarbonate and urea permeabilities are similar in both portions (Schafer *et al.*, 1974, 1981; Kawamura and Kokko, 1976; Warnock and Burg, 1977), whereas the chloride permeability coefficient is larger in the superficial pars recta (Schafer *et al.*, 1974; Kawamura *et al.*, 1975; Warnock and Burg, 1977; Andreoli *et al.*, 1979). Permeability of magnesium in the pars recta is low compared with that of sodium. The small amount of magnesium transport observed in this nephron segment seems to occur by passive mechanisms (Quamme, 1982). The pars recta has been shown to be responsible for calcium reabsorption by Rocha *et al.* (1977), Rouse *et al.* (1980) and Ng *et al.* (1982), but little is known about the mechanism of this reabsorption.

The superficial pars recta has an anion-selective shunt pathway, with chloride more permeable than bicarbonate, whereas the juxtamedullary pars recta has a sodium-selective shunt pathway (Kawamura *et al.*, 1975; Jacobson and Kokko, 1976; Warnock and Burg, 1977, Berry *et al.*, 1978). Linear behaviour of the permselectivity ratio, over a wide range of transepithelial potential differences and independence of the polarity was shown by Schafer and Andreoli (1979). Also the permselectivity was independent of active transport. Thus, it appears likely that this permselectivity of the pars recta is due to properties of the paracellular shunt pathway rather than the transcellular route.

To evaluate the permeability properties of the individual cell membranes, intracellular measurements of the membrane potential together with concentration step experiments are needed. Only a few studies of this type have been reported thus far. Biagi *et al.* (1981a, b), Bello-Reuss (1982) and Völkl and Greger (1984) reported a potential difference across the basolateral membrane of −38 to −62 mV in the isolated rabbit and mouse pars recta. All studies agree that an increase in the bath potassium concentration leads to a depolarisation of the basolateral membrane potential, and therefore they all suggest a potassium conductance for this membrane. This potassium conductance can be blocked by barium (Bello-Reuss, 1982). Reduction of bicarbonate concentration in the bath depolarises the cell (Bello-Reuss, 1982; Biagi and Sohtell, 1983), which could be explained by a bicarbonate conductance of the basolateral membrane. Bello-Reuss (1982) excluded a sodium or chloride conductance of this membrane. Ouabain was reported to depolarise the basolateral membrane (Biagi *et al.*, 1981a, b; Völkl and Greger, 1984). This could be caused by the fall in intracellular potassium activity (Biagi *et al.*, 1981b) or, as was suggested recently by Völkl and Greger (1984), by a direct coupling between $(Na^+ + K^+)$ATPase activity and the magnitude of the basolateral potassium conductance in the pars recta of the mouse, in the sense that the potassium conductance was down-regulated with a reduction in the $(Na^+ + K^+)$ATPase activity. More direct proof of potassium conductance in the basolateral membrane of the rabbit pars recta was obtained in a study by Gögelein and Greger (1984) utilising the patchclamp technique in the perfused tubule. In addition another channel of as yet unidentified selectivity was found in the basolateral membrane (Gögelein and Greger, 1984).

Primary and Secondary Active Transport Systems

The transepithelial potential difference of the pars recta, although extensively studied, is still a matter of discussion. One reason for this is that in most studies different solutions were used on opposite sides of the epithelium. The values reported range between −2 mV and +2 mV (Schafer *et al.*, 1974, 1975, 1978a; Kawamura *et al.*, 1975; Andreoli *et al.*, 1979; Biagi *et al.*, 1981a; Bello-Reuss, 1982). If corrected for liquid junction potentials, all values should be slightly positive and then would correspond to the measurements of Frömter and Gessner (1974a, b) in the late proximal convoluted tubule under free-flow conditions *in vivo*. Using identical solutions on both epithelial sides, the transepithelial potential difference is lumen negative (Schafer *et al.*, 1974; Biagi *et al.*, 1981a). This indicates electrogenic transport of Na^+. This active transport potential difference can be abolished by removing peritubular potassium, by addition of ouabain to the bath perfusate (Schafer *et al.*, 1974; Biagi *et al.*, 1981a) or by removing substrates from the lumen perfusate

(Kokko, 1973).

The primary active pump for the isotonic reabsorption of water and NaCl in the pars recta is the basolateral $(Na^+ + K^+)$ATPase, which keeps the cellular potassium activity high and the sodium activity low. The sodium gradient from lumen to cell drives several sodium co-transport systems which transport sodium together with glucose, amino acids or phosphate (Tune and Burg, 1971; Hoffmann *et al.*, 1976; Barfuss and Schafer, 1979, 1981a, b; Biagi *et al.*, 1981a; Cheng and Sacktor, 1981). Compared with the reabsorption rates for these organic substances in the proximal convoluted tubule, the pars recta reabsorbs organic substances with a lower capacity but higher affinity (Berry, 1983). Therefore the pars recta is able to reduce the luminal glucose and amino acid concentration down to virtually zero (Barfuss and Schafer, 1979, 1981a; Barfuss *et al.*, 1980). The phosphate reabsorption in the pars recta is reduced by parathyrin (Lang *et al.*, 1977). Recently Turner and Moran (1982a, b) showed that this specific ability of the pars recta to generate extremely low lumen concentrations of organic substances may be intrinsic to the stoichiometry of the sodium-coupled systems. According to these studies one sodium per glucose is transported in the convoluted tubule but the ratio is two sodium per glucose in the pars recta. In addition, sodium-dependent uptake of amino acids from the basolateral side was demonstrated by Barfuss *et al.* (1980). The pars recta is also a major site of phosphate transport (Dennis *et al.*, 1976). Phosphate uptake from the lumen is a sodium-dependent process and seems to be electroneutral, i.e. two sodium per one phosphate (Hoffman *et al.*, 1976; Cheng and Sacktor, 1981). The exit mechanism for phosphate is still unclear.

There are so far no data from the pars recta about the existence of a sulphate-sodium co-transport system in the luminal membrane as has been shown by Dennis *et al.* (1976) and Ullrich *et al.* (1980) for the proximal convoluted tubule. The existence of Na^+/H^+ exchange in the luminal membrane was recognised by Murer *et al.* (1976) in vesicle preparations from brush border membranes of rat renal cortex, i.e. proximal convoluted and straight tubules. Other studies of Berry and Warnock (1982) and McKinney and Burg (1977) provide arguments that this Na^+/H^+ antiporter is present in the pars recta, too. This exchange system, with the help of membrane-bound carbonic anhydrase (Schafer and Andreoli, 1976) drives bicarbonate reabsorption. The nature of the exit step of bicarbonate across the basolateral membrane is still unclear.

Tune *et al.* (1969) measured the secretion rate of PAH. It was five times higher in the pars recta compared with the proximal convoluted tubule. PAH and several other organic anions are transported via one or even several common transport systems in the basolateral membrane and leave the cell across the luminal membrane possibly via another carrier system (Grantham, 1982). Figure 3.1 shows a possible cellular model for the pars recta segment.

Figure 3.1: Cellular Model for the Pars Recta. ⟶ = diffusion; ⟲ = carrier mediated transport; ⬤⟶ = active transport; X = amino acids, glucose, phosphate, sulphate; A⁻ = anion

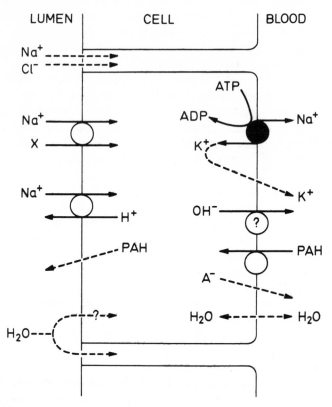

Pars Recta: Summary

(1) The pars recta is capable of reabsorbing Na^+ actively, driven by the basolateral $(Na^+ + K^+)$ATPase.

(2) Water is reabsorbed virtually iso-osmotically. A small ionic disequilibrium, caused by the preferential absorption of bicarbonate over chloride and the reabsorption of organic compounds, is sufficient to drive large amounts of fluid across the epithelium. This disequilibrium, however, has to be maintained by active transport of sodium. The route by which water is reabsorbed, i.e. paracellular or transcellular, is still controversial.

(3) The reabsorption of a multitude of solutes such as glucose, amino acids, phosphate and possibly also sulphate is coupled to the reabsorption of sodium, driven by the action of the basolateral $(Na^+ + K^+)$ATPase. The secondary active Na^+–dependent co-transport systems for these substances are located in the luminal membrane, and the exit mechanisms for these substances across the basolateral membrane seem to be coupled systems or possibly also conductive pathways.

(4) The mechanisms for the limited reabsorption of calcium and magnesium are still open. Calcium reabsorption, unlike that of magnesium, appears to be active.

(5) The pars recta also is a site of secretion of potassium driven by the potassium gradient across the epithelium.

(6) For the secretion of organic anions such as PAH, the pars recta is the major site along the entire nephron.

(7) The paracellular shunt permeability properties change along the pars recta or are different among the different nephron populations. Anion selectivity is predominant in the superficial portion, and sodium selectivity is typical for the juxtamedullary portion. So far, only potassium conductance has been demonstrated for the basolateral cell membrane.

Thin Descending Limb of Henle (tDLH)

Introduction

Wirz *et al.* (1951), Ullrich *et al.* (1955), Gottschalk and Mylle (1959) and Gottschalk *et al.* (1963) reported that the intraluminal fluid of the mammalian thin descending limb of Henle becomes more and more hypertonic as it reaches the bending point of the loop in the papilla. Several investigators have attempted to clarify the mechanism responsible for this increase along the thin descending limb. Mainly *in vivo* micropuncture and microperfusion techniques in the rat and hamster and more recently *in vitro* perfusion of isolated thin descending limbs of rabbit, rat and hamster kidney have been used. Two different hypotheses explaining the function of the thin descending limb have been put forward. The high concentration of the luminal fluid in the distal end of the thin descending limb compared with that in the proximal end may be due to absorption of water across this epithelium, which is relatively impermeable to solutes such as sodium and chloride or urea (Lassiter *et al.*, 1961; Marsh and Solomon, 1965; Jamison, 1968; Morgan and Berliner, 1968; Kokko, 1970, 1974; Marsh, 1970; Rocha and Kokko, 1973a; Abramov and Orci, 1980; Imai, 1984b; Imai *et al.*, 1984a, b). Alternatively, addition of such solutes to the lumen of the thin descending limb with an extremely low water permeability was postulated by Horster and Thurau (1968), DeRouffignac and Morel (1969), and Stoner and Roch-Ramel (1979). At any rate the thin descending limb seems to serve as an equilibration system, which equilibrates the lumen fluid with the increasing osmolality in the medullary interstitium and the vasa recta by solute or water fluxes.

Permeability Properties of the Thin Descending Limb of Henle's Loop

Several investigators have measured the permeabilities of the thin descending limb for sodium, potassium, calcium, phosphate, chloride, urea and water. Table 3.2 summarises these data. As can be seen from the data, the osmotic water permeability is rather high. This high water permeability may be an artefact, as Stoner and Roch-Ramel (1979) claim. They reported that the hydraulic permeability is low at low perfusion pressures, but that it increased with increasing perfusion pressure.

Table 3.2: Properties of the Thin Descending and Thin Ascending Limb of Henle's Loop (tDLH, tALH)

		tDLH	tALH
P_f	(cm s⁻¹ x 10⁻³)	3.1[8]; 14.8 to 26.6[2]	0[2,4,9]
P_{Na^+}	(cm s⁻¹ x 10⁻⁵)	0.17 to [a]4.2[1,6,7,10]; [b]45[6]	24.9 to 87.6[2,4,9]
P_{K^+}	(cm s⁻¹ x 10⁻⁵)	2.5[10]	80[2]
$P_{Ca^{2+}}$	(cm s⁻¹ x 10⁻⁵)	0.8[11]	1.09[11]
P_{Cl^-}	(cm s⁻¹ x 10⁻⁵)	[a]1.3[6]; [b]4.2[6]	44 to 196[2,3,4,9,11]
$P_{PO_4^{3-}}$	(cm s⁻¹ x 10⁻⁵)	0.5[11]	0.67[11]
P_{urea}	(cm s⁻¹ x 10⁻⁵)	1.4 to [b]1.5[6-8]; [a]7.4[6]	6.7 to 22.8[2,4,9]
P_{Na^+}/P_{Cl^-}	(cm s⁻¹ x 10⁻⁵)	[b]0.7[6]; [a]1.0 to 4.0[6]	0.2[4,9]; 0.4[2]
J_v	(nl min⁻¹ mm⁻¹)	−0.29 to −22.6[6,7,12]	0[2,4,9]
PD_{te}	(mV)	0[6,7,10]	0[2,4,9]
R_{te}	(ohm cm²)	700[1]	very low[5]

$P_f, P_{Na^+}, P_{K^+}, P_{Ca^{2+}}, P_{Cl^-}, P_{PO_4^{3-}}, P_{urea}$ = permeability coefficients for water, Na⁺, K⁺, Ca⁺⁺, Cl⁻, PO₄³⁻, urea respectively; J_v = reabsorptive volume flow with osmotic gradient across the epithelium; PD_{te}, R_{te} = transepithelial potential difference and electrical resistance respectively; a = short-looped tDLH; b = long-looped tDLH.

References

[1] Abramov and Orci, 1980. [2] Imai, 1977a. [3] Imai, 1984b. [4] Imai and Kokko, 1974. [5] Imai and Kokko, 1976. [6] Imai et al.,, 1984a. [7] Kokko, 1970. [8] Kokko, 1970. [9] Kokko, 1972. [10] Rocha and Kokko, 1973a. [11] Rocha et al., 1977. [12] Stoner and Roch-Ramel, 1979

With respect to the permeability coefficients for sodium, potassium and urea, there is close agreement among the different studies. All these permeabilities as well as that to chloride, calcium and phosphate are low (Kokko, 1970, 1972; Rocha and Kokko, 1973a; Rocha et al., 1977; Stoner and Roch-Ramel, 1979; Abramov and Orci, 1980; Shareghi and Agus, 1982; Imai et al., 1984a). As this is also true for urea (Kokko, 1972; Stoner and Roch-Ramel, 1979; Imai et al., 1984a), which is accumulated in the medullary interstitium, an osmotic driving force for water movement from lumen to interstitium will be generated. However, although urea permeability is low in the thin descending limb, it will still allow for a limited passive inward transport of urea into the lumen. This was shown by Stoner and Roch-Ramel (1979) in the rabbit in *in vitro* perfusion studies, and by Marsh (1970) in the intact kidney of the hamster. Despite an outward-directed NaCl gradient in the thin descending limb, little if any passive movement of NaCl occurs out of the lumen because the permeabilities to sodium and chloride are very limited (Kokko, 1970; Marsh, 1970; Rocha and Kokko, 1973; Abramov and Orci, 1980; Imai *et al.*, 1984a). In sharp contrast to these findings, DeRouffignac and Morel (1969) reported *in vivo* microperfusion studies in *Psammomys* kidney, in which the increase in osmolarity of the luminal fluid was a consequence of NaCl addition (85 per cent) rather than of water withdrawal (15 per cent).

Recently Imai (1984b) and Imai *et al.* (1984a,b) also reported qualitative functional differences between long- and short-looped thin descending limbs. Although these authors find the same high water permeability for both segments, the sodium and chloride permeabilities are lower in the descending limb of short-looped nephrons than in the long-looped nephrons. The urea permeability on the other hand is lower in the thin descending limb of long-looped nephrons. These differences between the thin descending limbs of short- and long-looped nephrons are found in hamster and rat, but to a much lesser extent in rabbit.

In addition to the above discussed permeability properties there is further evidence that the thin descending limb of Henle's loop is an epithelium with a high transepithelial resistance. In fact, the value of some 700 ohm cm² reported by Abramov and Orci (1980) is the highest measured for any nephron segment including the collecting duct. This finding is in good agreement with electron micrographs of this nephron segment, which show numerous strands of the tight junctions (Welling and Welling, 1976).

Transepithelial Potential Difference

Electrical measurements of Kokko (1970), Rocha and Kokko (1973a) and Imai *et al.* (1984a, b) in the isolated perfused thin descending limb seem to indicate that this segment does not generate a transepithelial potential difference when perfused with identical solutions on both epithelial sides. This is in good agreement with the earlier findings of Windhager (1964) in *in vivo* experiments in the hamster, and also with *in vivo* data from the rat (Hogg and Kokko, 1978). The latter study demonstrated a small lumen-positive transepithelial potential difference of +1.9 mV in the last part of the thin descending limb before it reaches the hairpin bend. This small potential difference is probably a diffusion potential caused by a chloride concentration gradient directed from lumen to blood, as it reversed its polarity when the chloride gradient was inwardly directed. The absence of a transepithelial potential difference renders unlikely the existence of active transport of solutes in this nephron segment. Furthermore, Kokko (1970) did not find any change in sodium concentration of the lumen perfusate between the perfusion and collection end of the *in vitro* perfused rabbit thin descending limb of Henle's loop with identical solutions in bath and lumen. Further support comes from measurements by Katz *et al.* (1979) and Garg *et al.* (1981) of the $(Na^+ + K^+)$ATPase activity, indicating that $(Na^+ + K^+)$ATPase activity is very low (100 to 240 pmol P_i mm^{-1} h^{-1}) in the cells of the thin descending limb.

tDLH: Summary

Presently available experimental data would lead to the following conclusions as to the properties of the mammalian thin descending limb of Henle:

(1) It is a high-resistance epithelium, probably because the tight junctions are complex and inhibit solute permeation.
(2) There is little or no active NaCl transport, and consequently no measurable active transport potential.
(3) Permeabilities for sodium, potassium, chloride and urea, but also for calcium and phosphate, are low.
(4) The water permeability on the other hand is high.
(5) Quantitative differences in the permeability ratios are reported between the thin descending limbs of long- and short-looped nephrons and also among different species.

Thus, the thin descending limb of Henle's loop serves as a simple passive equilibration system within the countercurrent concentration system of the kidney. It does not by itself contribute to the generation of interstitial hypertonicity. The lumen fluid of the thin descending limb is osmotically equilibrated with the vasa recta and the interstitium, mainly by osmotically induced water removal and to a lesser degree by passive urea influx following the concentration gradient for urea. Differences in the passive permeabilities between sodium and urea lead to a tubular fluid which has a higher NaCl concentration but a lower urea concentration when compared with the interstitium and the vasa recta in the papilla.

Thin Ascending Limb of Henle (tALH)

Introduction

A long-standing debate exists about whether the thin ascending limb of Henle is capable of active transport, and thus could be a source for the development of the corticomedullary concentration gradient to drive the countercurrent system. There is some conflicting data, which on the one hand suggest that at least part of the NaCl movement is an active process (Windhager, 1964; Jamison *et al.*, 1967; Marsh and Azen, 1975). On the other hand several studies of Marsh and Solomon (1965), Stephenson (1966, 1972), Morgan and Berliner (1968), Sakai *et al.* (1971), Kokko and Rector (1972), Imai and Kokko (1974, 1976), Kokko (1974, 1982), Imai (1977a) and Hogg and Kokko (1978) exclude the existence of active processes in this nephron segment. In accordance with these data, Garg *et al.* (1981) and Katz *et al.* (1979) demonstrated that the thin ascending limb of Henle has virtually no (Na$^+$+K$^+$)ATPase activity.

Permeability Properties of the Thin Ascending Limb of Henle

Marsh and Solomon (1965), Morgan and Berliner (1968), Marsh (1970) and Sakai *et al.* (1971), using the *in vivo* microperfusion technique, and studies in the isolated perfused thin ascending limb of Henle (Imai and Kokko, 1974; Imai, 1977a) have concluded that the thin ascending limb has an immeasurably small water permeability. The TF/P ratio for inulin does not change along this nephron segment (Marsh, 1970). In an earlier study, Marsh and Solomon (1965) were unable to demonstrate any reabsorption of fluid in split droplet microperfusion experiments. The osmolality of the tubule fluid falls along the thin ascending limb of Henle (Marsh, 1970). The difference in the lumen osmolality between the thin descending and the thin ascending limb of Henle is mainly a difference in the concentration of NaCl, which accounts for 91 per cent of this osmolality difference (Sakai *et al.*, 1965). Imai and Kokko (1976) showed that the reabsorption of sodium from the thin ascending limb was independent of sodium concentration. The sodium efflux thus occurs most likely via diffusion out of the lumen (Marsh and Solomon, 1965; Marsh, 1970; Imai and Kokko, 1974, 1976; Kokko, 1974). Marsh and Solomon (1965), Imai and Kokko (1974, 1976), Kokko (1974, 1982). Hogg and Kokko (1978), Imai and Kokko (1974, 1976), Kokko (1974, 1982) and Marsh and Solomon (1965) showed that chloride transport also was passive following the concentration gradient for this ion.

Several groups (Sakai *et al.*, 1971; Imai and Kokko, 1974; Kokko, 1974, 1982; Rocha *et al.*, 1977), using mainly *in vitro* perfused isolated thin ascending limb segments, measured passive permeability coefficients for sodium, potassium, chloride, urea and also calcium and phosphate. Table 3.2 summarises these data. The striking differences between the thin descending and thin ascending limb of Henle are:

(1) The high osmotic water permeability in the thin descending limb and the low value in the thin ascending limb epithelium, which for all practical purposes is impermeable to water.
(2) The permeability coefficients for sodium and chloride are extremely high, ranging from 25×10^{-5} to 88×10^{-5} cm sec^{-1} for sodium, and from 44×10^{-5} to 196×10^{-5} cm sec^{-1} for chloride in the thin ascending limb, but they are low in the thin descending limb.
(3) Urea permeability is moderate but still 10 to 15 times higher in the ascending limb than in the thin descending limb. Permeabilities for calcium and phosphate are low and virtually identical in the thin descending and ascending limbs of Henle.

The absence of any active transport process in the thin ascending limb of Henle is further strengthened by measurements of the transepithelial potential difference. First measurements in *in vivo* microperfusion experiments showed a lumen negative potential difference across the epithelium of about -10 mV. Windhager (1964) explained this voltage as an active transport potential,

Marsh and Solomon (1965) as a diffusion potential. Marsh and Martin (1977) and Hogg and Kokko (1978) reported a lumen positive potential difference of 1–2 mV, which was dependent on the polarity of the chloride gradient. All these data are biased by the fact that only the lumen compartment was defined with respect to the ionic composition. In fact all measurements in the isolated *in vitro* perfused thin ascending limb of Henle with identical solutions in bath and lumen have failed to show any potential differences across the epithelium (Imai and Kokko, 1974; Kokko, 1974; Imai, 1977a).

tALH Response to Hormones

In several studies an attempt was made to evaluate whether the thin ascending limb of Henle responds to antidiuretic hormone, as do the medullary thick ascending limb and the collecting duct. Although ADH-dependent adenylate cyclase activity was found in the thin ascending limb of Henle, only a very limited increase of water permeability was reported by Imbert *et al.* (1975), Morel *et al.* (1976), Chabardes *et al.* (1978), Imbert-Teboul (1978) and Imai and Kusano (1982). There was clearly no effect on chloride transport (Imai and Kusano, 1982). Thus, the role of this adenylate cyclase in the thin ascending limb of Henle still awaits further elucidation.

tALH: Summary

In conclusion, the majority of reports favour the view that the thin ascending limb of Henle, like the thin descending limb, is a passive equilibration system. However, the permeability characteristics of the thin ascending limb epithelium are just the opposite of those of the thin descending limb epithelium: an extremely low hydraulic permeability contrasts with very high sodium and chloride permeabilities. The urea permeability is moderate.

The lumen fluid delivered out of the thin descending limb is highly concentrated with respect to sodium and chloride and rather less concentrated with respect to urea. NaCl leaves the lumen following the concentration gradients across the epithelium. Little urea enters the lumen. As the thin ascending limb of Henle is impermeable to water, the equilibration with the interstitium occurs via solute efflux from the lumen.

The thin descending and the thin ascending limb of Henle serve as countercurrent diffusion systems. Neither segment performs active transport work utilising metabolic energy. These nephron segments, therefore, do not by themselves create the corticomedullary concentration gradient.

Thick Ascending Limb of Henle (TAL)

Introduction

In general the mechanisms by which ions are transported across the epithelium of the thick ascending limb of Henle are identical for the medullary portion (mTAL) and the cortical portion (cTAL) of this nephron segment. Thus, these two portions of the loop of Henle will be discussed together.

The permeability of the thick ascending limb to water is minimal. Early studies by Burg and Green (1973) and Rocha and Kokko (1973a) with the isolated perfused thick ascending limb demonstrated this low water permeability, which was confirmed by Hall and Varney (1980) and Sasaki and Imai (1980). It holds for all three species studied so far, i.e. rabbit, rat and mouse. Morel *et al.* (1976, 1981), Ng *et al.* (1982) and Shareghi and Agus (1982) demonstrated an ADH-dependent adenylate cyclase in the mouse and rat medullary thick ascending limb. In contrast to the mammalian collecting duct (Grantham and Burg, 1972; Schafer and Andreoli, 1972), the thick ascending limb does not increase its water permeability but it increases active transport of NaCl in response to antidiuretic hormone (Hall and Varney, 1980; Sasaki and Imai, 1980; Hebert *et al.*, 1981a, DeRouffignac *et al.*, 1983; Schlatter and Greger, 1985).

As the water-impermeable thick ascending limb reabsorbs high amounts of NaCl, it serves as a diluting segment. This had been deduced by Wirz *et al.* (1951) from *in vivo* micropuncture data, which showed that luminal fluid in the early distal convoluted tubule was hypotonic with respect to the interstitium.

Permeability Properties of the Thick Ascending Limb of Henle

Some of the properties of the thick ascending limb are shown in Tables 3.3 and 3.4. The passive permeability to water of the thick ascending limb of Henle is close to zero in both portions (Burg and Green, 1973; Rocha and Kokko, 1973b, 1974; Horster, 1978; Hall and Varney, 1980; Sasaki and Imai, 1980; Hebert *et al.*, 1981a), and it is very low for urea in both portions (Rocha and Kokko, 1974; Knepper and Vurek, 1982). The urea permeability is some $1–2 \times 10^{-5}$ cm s^{-1}. For chloride the permeability is 1×10^{-5} cm s^{-1} (Burg and Green, 1973; Rocha and Kokko, 1973b; Hall and Varney, 1980; Hebert *et al.*, 1981a). The sodium and potassium permeabilities are considerably larger (2–6 and $5–61 \times 10^{-5}$ cm s^{-1}, respectively) (Burg and Green, 1973; Rocha and Kokko, 1973b; Hebert *et al.*, 1981a, 1984; Shareghi and Agus, 1982; Stokes, 1982). From diffusion-potential measurements across the epithelium of this nephron segment it was deduced that the paracellular shunt pathway, composed of the tight junctions and lateral spaces, is cation selective (Burg and Green, 1973; Greger, 1981a; Hebert *et al.*, 1981a). The permeability ratio of P_{Na^+} over P_{Cl^-} is between 2 and 6 (Burg and Green, 1973; Rocha and Kokko, 1973b; Greger, 1981a; DiStefano *et al.*, 1984). Greger (1981a) also determined the sequence of the shunt permselectivity: $P_{K^+} > P_{Na^+} > P_{Rb^+} = P_{Li^+} > P_{Cs^+} > P_{Cl^-}$. DiStefano *et al.* (1984) demonstrated that the cation selectivity of the tight junctions was reduced by increases above 2.5 mmol litre^{-1} in luminal or peritubular calcium or magnesium concentrations. With 5 mmol litre^{-1} calcium or magnesium, the P_{Na^+}/P_{Cl^-} ratio decreased from 4 to about 2.

Table 3.3: Properties of the Medullary Thick Ascending Limb of Henle's Loop (mTAL)

		Without ADH			With ADH		
		Rabbit	Mouse	Rat	Rabbit	Mouse	Rat
P_f	(cm s^{-1} x 10^{-3})	0[8]; low[9]	0.6 to 2.3[2,4,10]	low[10]	low[9]	0.1[4]; low[2,10]	low[10]
P_{Na^+}	(cm s^{-1} x 10^{-5})	6.3[8]	2.3[4]			2.5[4]; 5[6]	
P_{K^+}	(cm s^{-1} x 10^{-5})	61.3[14]					
$P_{Ca^{++}}$	(cm s^{-1} x 10^{-5})	2.1[15]					
P_{Cl^-}	(cm s^{-1} x 10^{-5})	1.0[8]	1.0[4]; 1.1[2]			1.2[4]; 1.4[2]	
P_{urea}	(cm s^{-1} x 10^{-5})	0.86[9]	2.2[4]		0.63[9]		
P_{Na^+}/P_{Cl^-}		6.3[8]	2.2[4]			1.6[4]	
PD_{te}	(mV)	3 to 7[8,9,14]	4 to 6[2,4,5,6,10,11,14]	4 to 6[7,10,12]	5[9]	7 to 12[2,4,6,10,11]	5[10]
PD_{bl}	(mV)		-50[3]; -83[11]			-40[4]; -68[11]	
R_{te}	(ohm cm^2)	25[1]	11 to 24[4,6,11]			11 to 20[4,6,11]	
I_{sc}	(μA cm^{-2})		280 to 450[4,6,11]			660 to 970[4,6,11]	

P_f, P_{Na^+}, P_{K^+}, $P_{Ca^{++}}$, P_{Cl^-}, P_{urea} = permeability coefficients for water, Na$^+$, K$^+$, Ca^{2+}, Cl$^-$ and urea, respectively; PD_{te}, PD_{bl} = potential difference across the epithelium and the basolateral membrane, respectively; R_{te} = electrical transepithelial resistance; I_{sc} = equivalent short-circuit current.

References

[1] Greger, 1985b. [2] Hall and Varney, 1980. [3] Hebert and Andreoli, 1984. [4] Hebert *et al.*, 1984. [5] Hebert *et al.*, 1981a. [6] Hebert *et al.*, 1981b. [7] Imai, 1977b. [8] Rocha and Kokko, 1973b. [9] Rocha and Kokko, 1974. [10] Sasaki and Imai, 1980. [11] Schlatter and Greger, 1985. [12] Stoner and Trimble, 1982. [13] Stokes, 1979. [14] Stokes, 1982. [15] Suki *et al.*, 1980.

Table 3.4: Properties of the Cortical Thick Ascending Limb of Henle's Loop (cTAL)

		Rabbit	Rat	Mouse
P_f	(cm s^{-1} x 10^{-3})	1.1[2]; 2.8[10]		
P_{Na^+}	(cm s^{-1} x 10^{-5})	2.8[2]		6.3[5]
P_{K^+}	(cm s^{-1} x 10^{-5})	4.7[14]		
$P_{Ca^{2+}}$	(cm s^{-1} x 10^{-5})	0.8 to 1.3[1,12,14,16]		
$P_{Mg^{2+}}$	(cm s^{-1} x 10^{-5})	0.5[14]		
P_{Cl^-}	(cm s^{-1} x 10^{-5})	1.4[2]		5.1[5]
P_{urea}	(cm s^{-1} x 10^{-5})	2.0[13]		
P_{Na^+}/P_{Cl^-}		2.0 to 3.6[2,4,7]		1.4[5]
PD_{te}	(mV)	3 to 8[1,2,7,11,14-16]	6 to 9[6]	7.4[9]; 8[5]
PD_{bl}	(mV)	−69[8]		
R_{te}	(ohm cm^2)	25[2]; 34[8]		
I_{sc}	(μA cm^{-2})	206[8]; 280[2];		

P_f, P_{Na^+}, P_{K^+}, $P_{Ca^{2+}}$, $P_{Mg^{2+}}$, P_{Cl^-}, P_{urea} = permeability coefficients for water, Na$^+$, K$^+$, Ca^{2+}, Mg^{2+}, Cl$^-$ and urea, respectively; PD_{te}, PD_{bl} = potential difference across the epithelium and the basolateral membrane, respectively; R_{te} = electrical transepithelial resistance; I_{sc} = equivalent short-circuit current.

References

[1] Bourdeau and Burg, 1979. [2] Burg and Green, 1973. [3] Burg *et al.*, 1973. [4] DiStefano *et al.*, 1984. [5] Friedman and Andreoli, 1982. [6] Good *et al.*, 1984. [7] Greger, 1981a. [8] Greger and Schlatter, 1983a, 1985. [9] Hebert *et al.*, 1981a. [10] Horster, 1978. [11] Imai, 1977b. [12] Imai, 1978. [13] Knepper and Vurek, 1982. [14] Shareghi and Agus, 1982. [15] Stokes, 1979. [16] Suki *et al.*, 1980.

Experiments analysing diffusion potentials across the lumen or basolateral membrane (Greger, 1981c, Greger and Schlatter, 1983a, b; Hebert and Andreoli, 1984a, Hebert *et al.*, 1984) show that the luminal membrane of both the medullary and the cortical portion of the thick ascending limb is almost exclusively potassium conductive (transference number for K$^+$ between 0.9 and 1). This potassium conductance of the apical membrane of the thick ascending limb can be blocked by barium, which then leads to a marked increase in the resistance across this membrane and across the entire epithelium (Greger and Schlatter, 1983a, 1985).

The basolateral membrane potential responds with a depolarisation if the peritubular potassium concentration is increased or if the peritubular chloride concentration is reduced (Greger, 1981c; Greger and Schlatter, 1983b). These data were explained by a chloride conductance in parallel with a non-conductive KCl exit system. The exit system for potassium cannot be a conductance as the inhibition of this system by barium has no effect on the conductivity of the basolateral membrane. Considerations based on circular current analysis also render unlikely the existence of a quantitatively important basolateral potassium conductance. The existence of a basolateral chloride conductance was also shown by Hebert and Andreoli (1984a) and Hebert *et al.* (1984) for the mouse medullary thick ascending limb. Recently Wittner *et al.* (1984a), DiStefano (1985) and Greger (1985b) showed that this basolateral chloride conductance in the thick ascending limb of mouse and rabbit can be blocked by anthracene-9-COOH and more completely by diphenylamine-2-COOH.

There is no evidence for phosphate transport in the thick ascending limb of Henle (Rocha *et al.*, 1977; Shareghi and Agus, 1982). Calcium and magnesium are reabsorbed in this nephron segment. However, the mechanism of reabsorption is still a matter of discussion. Bourdeau and Burg (1979) and Shareghi and Agus (1982) reported that the calcium as well as magnesium fluxes across the rabbit cortical thick ascending limb are voltage dependent, and thus could be explained merely by diffusion. On the other hand, Rocha *et al.* (1977), Imai (1978), Suki *et al.* (1980), and Suki and Rouse (1981) found even higher calcium fluxes both in the presence and absence of a positive transepithelial voltage.

Transepithelial Potential Difference and Resistance in the Thick Ascending Limb of Henle

As a result of the different conductances of the luminal (potassium permeable) and the basolateral (chloride permeable) membrane in the *in vitro* isolated thick ascending limb of Henle a lumen-positive transepithelial potential difference is found. With identical solutions on both epithelial sides the transepithelial potential difference ranges from $+3$ to $+8$ mV (lumen positive) in the cortical (Burg *et al.*, 1973; Imai, 1977b; Bourdeau and Burg, 1979; Stokes, 1979; Suki *et al.*, 1980; Greger, 1981a; Friedman and Andreoli, 1982; Shareghi and Agus, 1982; Good *et al.*, 1984) and $+3$ to $+12$ m V in the medullary portion (Rocha and Kokko, 1973b, 1974; Imai, 1977b; Hall and Varney, 1980; Sasaki and Imai, 1980; Hebert *et al.*, 1981a, 1984; Schlatter and Greger, 1985) of rabbit, rat and mouse.

The transepithelial resistance of the thick ascending limb measured electrically is surprisingly low for an epithelium which is virtually impermeable to water. The values reported by Hebert *et al.* (1981a, 1984), and by Schlatter and Greger (1985) range between 11 and 24 ohm cm^2 in the mouse medullary and 25 ohm cm^2 in the rabbit medullary portion (Greger, 1985b). In the rabbit cortical thick ascending limb the transepithelial resistance is 25–34 ohm cm^2 (Burg and Green, 1973; Greger, 1981a) and 18 ohm cm^2 in that of the mouse (Friedman and Andreoli, 1982).

Primary and Secondary Active Transport Systems in the Thick Ascending Limb of Henle

The primary active (i.e. energy-consuming) process in the reabsorption of NaCl in the cortical and medullary portion of the thick ascending limb of Henle is the ATP-dependent (Na$^+$+K$^+$) pump (Greger, 1981b; Hebert *et al.*,

1981a). ATP generation is strictly dependent on metabolic substrates in this nephron segment (Wittner *et al.*, 1984b). The metabolism is aerobic. Within three minutes after the removal of substrates, a decrease in the equivalent short-circuit current and a concomitant depolarisation of the cell potential have been reported. This indicates that the thick ascending limb cells have high NaCl transport rates but small energy pools. Substrate removal, however, is without effect if active NaCl transport is inhibited in these cells by loop diuretics such as furosemide (Greger *et al.*, 1984b, c).

In the luminal membrane of the thick ascending limb a one-sodium, two-chloride, one-potassium co-transport system was demonstrated by Greger and Schlatter (1981) and Greger *et al.* (1983a). This co-transport system was first described for the Ehrlich ascites tumour cell by Geck *et al.*, 1980. The dependence of the short-circuit current, i.e. the active NaCl reabsorption, in the cortical thick ascending limb of the rabbit on sodium, potassium and chloride concentration is shown in Figure 3.2. The apparent affinities to sodium, potassium and chloride are 3–4, 1 and 50 mmol litre^{-1}, respectively.

Figure 3.2: Sodium, Chloride and Potassium Dependence of Equivalent Short-circuit Current in Isolated Perfused cTAL Segments

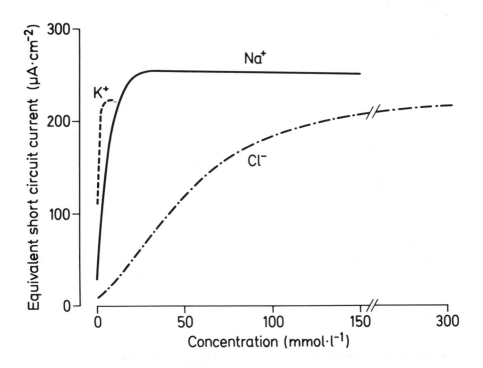

Source: Greger and Schlatter (1983b)

Similar affinity values for sodium and chloride are also reported from studies in vesicles prepared from luminal membranes of medullary thick ascending limb cells (Koenig *et al.*, 1983). Evidence for a 1 : 2 : 1 stoichiometry for the Na : Cl : K co-transport system in the luminal membrane of the thick ascending limb can be summarised as follows:

(1) The Hill coefficients dereived from the kinetic studies in the entire epithelium (Greger *et al.*, 1983a) and in membrane vesicles (Koenig *et al.*, 1983) are 1 for sodium and 2 for chloride.
(2) This co-transporter is electrically neutral (Greger *et al.*, 1983a), which makes necessary the participation of one potassium.

The sensitivity of this $Na^+2Cl^-K^+$ co-transport system towards loop diuretics, such as furosemide, bumetanide or piretanide, was shown by Burg *et al.* (1973), Eveloff *et al.* (1980, 1981), Sasaki and Imai (1980), Greger and Frömter (1981), Schlatter *et al.* (1983), and Hebert and Andreoli (1984a). Currently evidence is accumulating that this carrier is present in several epithelia or cells transporting NaCl. So far it has been postulated for the diluting segment of amphibia and freshwater teleosts (Oberleithner *et al.*, 1982a, b; Hoshi *et al.*, 1983; Nishimura *et al.*, 1983a, b), the shark rectal gland (Hannafin *et al.*, 1983; Greger and Schlatter, 1984a), the fish intestine (Mush *et al.*, 1982), the rabbit colon (Heintze *et al.*, 1983), the trachea (Shorofsky *et al.*, 1982; Welsh *et al.*, 1982; Welsh 1983), the cornea (Reuss *et al.*, 1983), avian and human erythrocytes (Dunn, 1970; Wiley and Cooper, 1974; Dunham *et al.*, 1980; Palfrey *et al.*, 1980; Bakker–Grunwald, 1981; Chipperfield, 1981; Haas *et al.*, 1982), Ehrlich ascites tumour cells (Geck *et al.*, 1980), cultured MDCK kidney cells (Aiton and Simmons, 1983), ganglion cells (Ballanyi *et al.*, 1984), glial cells (Johnson *et al.*, 1982), the squid axon (Russell, 1983), the frog skin (Mills, 1985; Ussing, 1985) the gall bladder (Davis and Finn, 1983), the operculum of fish (Degnan *et al.*, 1977), and the pancreas (Peterson and Maruyama, 1984).

Direct proof for the stoichiometry of one Na : two Cl : one K for this co-transport system was obtained recently by Greger and Schlatter (1984b) for the chloride-secreting epithelium of the shark rectal gland. It was shown that the initial rate of decline in intracellular chloride activity was twice as rapid as that of sodium after inhibition of the co-transport system by furosemide.

The mouse and rat cortical thick ascending limb, unlike the rabbit cortical thick ascending limb or the medullary portion of mouse and rabbit, seems to possess additional carrier systems in the luminal membrane: Na^+/H^+ and Cl^-/OH^- antiporters (Friedman and Andreoli, 1982; Good *et al.*, 1984). In this segment the presence of bicarbonate increases NaCl reabsorption, although no measurable net reabsorption of bicarbonate was noted. This portion of the NaCl reabsorption (bicarbonate dependent) is SITS (4-acetamido-4′-isothiocyanostilbene-2,2′-disulphonic acid) or ethoxzola mide inhibitable (Friedman and Andreoli, 1982). The absence of bicarbonate transport in the rabbit cortical and the mouse medullary thick ascending limb was demonstrated by Hebert *et al.* (1981a), Iino and Burg (1981) and Greger *et al.* (1982). On the other hand, Good *et al.* (1984) demonstrated bicarbonate and ammonia reabsorption in the rat cortical and medullary thick ascending limb. Another co-transport system in the thick ascending limb is the above mentioned (p. 101) electroneutral KCI exit in the basolateral membrane (Greger and Schlatter, 1983b). Other carrier systems typical for the proximal tubule, such as sodium-glucose or sodium-amino acid co-transport systems, do not apparently exist in the thick ascending limb (Schlatter and Greger, 1982). On the other hand, there is recent evidence for carrier systems for the uptake of various substrates in the basolateral membrane (Wittner *et al.*, 1984b).

TAL Response to Hormones

Morel *et al.* (1976, 1981) demonstrated an adenylate cyclase activity dependent on ADH, calcitonin, glucagon and isoprenaline in the mouse and rat thick ascending limb, but not in that of rabbit or man. This adenylate cyclase is confined to the medullary portion and does not occur in the cortical portion. The adenylate cyclase is ADH dependent and increases cellular cAMP, which in turn regulates NaCl reabsorption (Hall and Varney, 1980; Sasaki and Imai, 1980; Hebert *et al.* 1981a, 1984; Schlatter and Greger, 1985). This was postulated many years ago from measurements of ADH-dependent adenylatecyclase, but it took almost ten years until measurements of NaCl-reabsorption and equivalent short-circuit current verified this hypothesis. ADH increases the transepithelial potential difference and decreases the transepithelial resistance, and increases NaCl transport about twofold (Hall and Varney, 1980; Hebert *et al.*, 1981a, Schlatter and Greger, 1985). The mechanism responsible for this action of cAMP has been a matter of controversy. In reports by Hebert and Andreoli (1984a) and Hebert *et al.* (1984) based on transepithelial and unpaired transmembrane voltage measurements, it was argued that cAMP primarily increases the number of active apical potassium channels and $Na^+2Cl^-K^+$ co-transporter molecules. These authors also found an increase in basolateral chloride conductance. On the other hand, there is clear evidence from other chloride-transporting epithelia that the stimulation of this transport via cAMP leads to an increase in the chloride conductance (Frizzell *et al.*, 1979; Shorofsky *et al.*, 1982; Welsh *et al.*, 1982; Petersen and Reuss, 1983). Recently, Greger *et al.* (1984d, 1985) showed, for the shark rectal gland, that cAMP stimulates NaCl secretion primarily via an increase in the chloride conductance. Furthermore, in paired experiments Schlatter and Greger (1985) demonstrated that ADH and cAMP increase the basolateral chloride conductance of the mouse medullary thick ascending limb. This led to a depolarisation of the potential difference across this membrane. These authors were also able to demonstrate that, as in the shark rectal gland, this effect of cAMP on the chloride conductance is the primary event, i.e. primary to an activation of both the co-transport system and the $(Na^++K^+)ATPase$ and the increase in luminal potassium conductance (Schlatter and Greger 1985, Greger, 1985a). The fractional resistance of the basolateral membrane decreases upon stimulation even when the luminal co-transport system and therefore also the (Na^++K^+) ATPase are inhibited by furosemide.

TAL: Summary

Using the cellular model for the thick ascending limb shown in Figure 3.3 one can explain NaCl reabsorption in this nephron segment as follows:

(1) The $(Na^++K^+)ATPase$ is the only energy-consuming process. It keeps the cellular sodium activity low and cellular potassium activity high (Greger *et al.*, 1984a).

(2) Sodium, chloride and potassium enter the luminal membrane following their chemical gradients mediated by a specific carrier system. This co-transport system is sensitive to loop diuretics.

(3) Potassium that is above the equilibrium concentration in the cell leaves the cell passively via the luminal conductance for this ion.

(4) Chloride leaves the cell passively via the basolateral chloride conductance by the electrochemical driving force, as chloride is above equilibrium in the cell (Greger *et al.*, 1983b), and via the electroneutral KCl exit. The basolateral chloride conductance is regulated by ADH in the medullary portion of the thick ascending limb of mouse and rat.

(5) The difference in membrane potentials between the potassium-permeable luminal membrane and the chloride-permeable basolateral membrane results in a lumen positive potential difference across the epithelium. This potential drives part of the sodium through the cation-selective paracellular shunt.

(6) Thus, all the chloride but only half of the sodium is reabsorbed in the thick ascending limb of Henle transcellularly; the other half is reabsorbed paracellularly. Therefore, only half a sodium per one NaCl reabsorbed is transported actively, i.e. with consumption of ATP. This renders the thick ascending limb of Henle a very efficiently reabsorbing epithelium.

(7) In the isolated preparation there is almost no potassium reabsorption; however, *in vivo* the thick ascending limb reabsorbs potassium driven by the lumen positive potential difference.

(8) The thick ascending limb is a major site of magnesium and calcium reabsorption, which is regulated by parathyroid hormone and calcitonin.

(9) The cortical portion of the mouse and rat thick ascending limb has the capability to acidify the lumen fluid by a net bicarbonate reabsorption rate exceeding that for ammonium.

Figure 3.3: Cellular Model for the Thick Ascending Limb of Henle. ------→ = diffusion, ⟶ = carrier-mediated transport, ⟶ = active transport. The cell has a negative potential of −72 mV relative to the bath (= interstitial fluid), and the lumen has a potential of + 6 mV relative to the bath

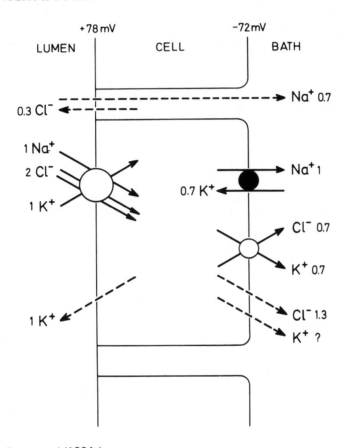

Source: Greger *et al.* (1984e)

Acknowledgement

Work from the authors' laboratory quoted in this article was supported by Deutsche Forschungsgemeinschaft GR 480/6-8.

References

Abramov, M. and Orci, L. (1980) 'On the "Tightness" of the Rabbit Descending Limb of the Loop of Henle — Physiological and Morphological Evidence', *Int. J. Biochem.*, *12*, 23–7

Aiton, J.F. and Simmons, N.L. (1983) 'Effect of Ouabain upon Diuretic-sensitive K^+ Transport in Cultured Cells. Evidence for Separate Modes of Operation of the Transporter', *Biochem. Biophys. Acta, 734*, 279–89

Andreoli, T.E., Schafer, J.A. and Troutman, S.L (1978) Perfusion Rate Dependence of Transepithelial Osmosis in Isolated Proximal Convoluted Tubules: Estimation of the Hydraulic Conductance', *Kidney Int., 14*, 263–9

Andreoli, T.E., Schafer, J.A., Troutman, S.L. and Watkins, M.L. (1979) 'Solvent Drag Component of Cl^- Flux in Superficial Proximal Straight Tubules: Evidence for a Paracellular Component of Isotonic Fluid Absorption', *Am. J. Physiol., 237*, F455–62

Bakker-Grunwald, T. (1981) 'Hormone Induced Diuretic-sensitive Potassium Transport in Turkey Erythrocytes is Anion Dependent', *Biochim. Biophys. Acta, 641*, 427–31

Ballanyi, K., Grafe, P. and ten Bruggencate, G. (1984) 'GABA-action and Chloride Transport in Rat Sympathetic Ganglia', *Pflügers Arch., 400*, R37

Barfuss, D.W. and Schafer, J.A. (1979) 'Active Amino Acid Absorption by Proximal Convoluted and Straight Tubules', *Am. J. Physiol., 236*, F149–62

Barfuss, D.W. and Schafer,J.A. (1981a) 'Differences in Active and Passive Glucose Transport along the Proximal Nephron', *Am. J. Physiol., 240*, F322–32

Barfuss, D.W. and Schafer, J.A. (1981b) 'Collection and Analysis of Absorbate from Proximal Straight Tubules', *Am. J. Physiol., 241*, F597–604

Barfuss, D.W., Mays, J.M. and Schafer, J.A. (1980) 'Peritubular Uptake and Transepithelial Transport of Glycine in Isolated Proximal Tubules', *Am. J. Physiol., 238*, F324–33

Bello-Reuss, E. (1982) 'Electrical Properties of the Basolateral Membrane of the Straight Portion of the Rabbit Proximal Renal Tubule', *J. Physiol., 326*, 49–63

Berry, C.A. (1983) 'Water Permeability and Pathways in the Proximal Tubule', *Am. J. Physiol., 245*, F279–94

Berry, C.A. and Warnock, D.G. (1982) 'Acidification in the *in vitro* Perfused Tubule', *Kidney Int., 22*, 507–18

Berry, C.A., Warnock, D.G. and Rector, F.C. Jr (1978) 'Ion Selectivity and Proximal Salt Reabsorption', *Am. J. Physiol., 235*, F234–45

Biagi, B. and Sohtell, M. (1983) 'pH and Bicarbonate Effects on Membrane Potentials in the Proximal Tubule of the Rabbit', *Fed. Proc., 42*, 303

Biagi, B., Kubota, T., Sohtell, M. and Giebisch, G. (1981a) 'Intracellular Potentials in Rabbit Proximal Tubules Perfused *in vitro*', *Am. J. Physiol., 240*, F200–10

Biagi, B., Sohtell, M. and Giebisch, G. (1981b) 'Intracellular Potassium Activity in the Rabbit Proximal Straight Tubule', *Am. J. Physiol., 241*, F677–86

Bourdeau, J.E. and Burg, M.B. (1979) 'Voltage Dependence of Calcium Transport in the Thick Ascending Limb of Henle's Loop', *Am. J. Physiol., 236*, F357–64

Burg, M.B. (1982) 'Thick Ascending Limb of Henle's Loop', *Kidney Int., 22*, 454–64

Burg, M.B., and Green, N. (1973) 'Function of the Thick Ascending Limb of Henle's Loop', *Am. J. Physiol., 224*, 659–68

Burg, M.B. and Orloff, J. (1968) 'Control of Fluid Absorption in the Renal Proximal Tubule', *J. Clin. Invest., 47*, 2016–24

Burg, M., Grantham, J., Abramow, M. and Orloff, J. (1966) 'Preparation and Study of Fragments of Single Rabbit Nephrons', *Am. J. Physiol., 210*, 1293–8

Burg, M., Stoner, L., Cardinal, J. and Green, N. (1973) 'Furosemide Effect on Isolated Perfused Tubules', *Am. J. Physiol., 225*, 119–24

Chabardes, D., Imbert-Teboul, M., Gagnan-Brunette, M. and Morel, F. (1978) 'Different Hormonal Target Sites along the Mouse and Rabbit Nephrons', in W.G. Guder and U. Schmidt (eds), *Biochemical Nephrology*, Huber, Bern, pp.447–54

Cheng, L. and Sacktor, B. (1981) 'Sodium Gradient-dependent Phosphate Transport in Renal Brush Border Membrane Vesicles', *J. Biol. Chem., 256*, 1556–64

Chipperfield, A.R. (1981) 'Chloride Dependence of Frusemide- and Phloretin-sensitive Passive Sodium and Potassium Fluxes in Human Red Cells', *J. Physiol., 312*, 435–44

Davis, C.W. and Finn, A.L. (1983) 'Na, K, Cl Cotransport in *Necturus* Gallbladder', *Fed. Proc., 42*, 988

Degnan, K.J., Karnaky, K.J., and Zadunaisky, J.A. (1977) 'Active Chloride Transport in the *in vitro* Opercular Skin of a Teleost (*Fundulus heteroclitus*), a Gill-like Epithelium Rich in Chloride Cells', *J. Physiol., 251*, 155–91

Dennis, V.W., Woodhall, P.B. and Robinson, R.R. (1976) 'Characteristics of Phosphate Transport in Isolated Proximal Tubule', *Am. J. Physiol.*, *231*, 979–85

DeRouffignac, C. and Morel, F. (1969) 'Micropuncture Study of Water, Electrolytes, and Urea Movements along the Loop of Henle in *Psammomys*', *J. Clin. Invest.*, *48*, 474–86

DeRouffignac, C., Corman, B. and Roinel, N. (1983) 'Stimulation by Antidiuretic Hormone of Electrolyte Tubular Reabsorption in Rat Kidney', *Am. J. Physiol.*, *244*, F156–64

DiStefano, A., Wittner, M., Gebler, B. and Greger, R. (1984) 'Increased Ca^{++} or Mg^{++} Reduces the Na^+-Conductance of the Paracellular Pathway in Isolated Perfused Cortical Thick Ascending Limbs of Henles Loop (cTAL) of Rabbit Kidney', *Pflügers Arch.*, *400*, 84

DiStefano, A., Wittner, M., Schlatter, E., Lang, H.J., Englert, H. and Greger, R. (1985) 'Diphenylamine-2-carboxylate, a Blocker of the Cl^--conductive Pathway in Cl^- Transporting Epithelia', *Pflügers Arch.*, in press

Dunham, P.B., Stewart, G.W. and Ellory, J.C. (1980) 'Chloride-activated Passive Potassium Transport in Human Erythrocytes', *Proc. Natl Acad. Sci. USA*, *77*, 1711–15

Dunn, M.J. (1970) 'The Effect of Transport Inhibitors on Sodium Outflux and Influx in Red Blood Cells: Evidence for Exchange Diffusion', *J. Clin. Invest.*, *49*, 1804–14

Eveloff, J., Bayerdörffer, E., Haase, W. and Kinne, R. (1980) 'Biochemical and Physiological Studies on Cells Isolated from the Medullary Thick Ascending Limb of Henle's Loop', *Int. J. Biochem.*, *12*, 55–9

Eveloff, J., Bayerdörffer, E., Silva, P. and Kinne, R.(1981) 'Sodium Chloride Transport in the Thick Ascending Limb of Henle's Loop. Oxygen Consumption Studies in Isolated Cells', *Pflügers Arch.*, *389*, 263–70

Friedman, P.A. and Andreoli, T.E. (1982) 'CO_2-stimulated NaCl Absorption in the Mouse Renal Cortical Thick Ascending Limb of Henle. Evidence for Synchronous Na^+/H^+ and Cl^-/HCO_3^- Exchange in Apical Plasma Membranes', *J. Gen. Physiol.*, *80*, 683–711

Frizzell, R.A., Field, M. and Schultz, S.G. (1979) 'Sodium-coupled Chloride Transport by Epithelial Tissues', *Am. J. Physiol.*, *236*, F1–8

Frömter, E. (1981) 'Electrical Aspects of Tubular Transport of Organic Substances', in R. Greger, F. Lang and S. Silbernagl (eds), *Renal Transport of Organic Substances*, Springer-Verlag, Berlin, pp. 30–44

Frömter, E. and Gessner, K. (1974a) 'Free-flow Potential Profile along Rat Kidney Proximal Tubule', *Pflügers Arch.*, *351*, 69–83

Frömter, E. and Gessner, K. (1974b) 'Active Transport Potentials, Membrane Diffusion Potentials and Streaming Potentials Across Rat Kidney Proximal Tubule', *Pflügers Arch.*, *351*, 85–98

Frömter, E., Rumrich, G. and Ullrich, K.J. (1973) 'Phenomenologic Description of Na^+, Cl^- and HCO_3^- Absorption from Proximal Tubules of the Rat Kidney', *Pflügers Arch.*, *343*, 189–220

Garg, L., Knepper, M. and Burg, M. (1981) 'Mineralocorticoid Stimulation of Na-K-ATPase in Nephron Segments', *Kidney Int.*, *19*, 241

Geck, P., Pietrzyk, C., Burckhardt, B.C., Pfeiffer, B. and Heinz, E. (1980) 'Electrically Silent Cotransport of Na^+, K^+ and Cl^- in Ehrlich Cells', *Biochim. Biophys. Acta*, *600*, 432–47

Gögelein, H. and Greger, R. (1984) 'Single Channel Recordings from Basolateral and Apical Membranes of Renal Proximal Tubules', *Pflügers Arch.*, *401*, 424–6

Gögelein, H. and Greger, R. (1985) 'Putative Anion Channels in the Basolateral and Luminal Membrane of the Rabbit Proximal Tubule', *Pflügers Arch.*, *403*, R10

Gonzales, E., Carpi-Medina, P. and Whittembury, G. (1982) 'Cell Osmotic Water Permeability of Isolated Rabbit Proximal Straight Tubules', *Am. J. Physiol.*, *242*, F321–30

Gonzales, E., Carpi-Medina, P., Linares, H. and Whittembury, G. (1984) 'Osmotic Water Permeability of the Apical Membrane of Proximal Straight Tubular (PST) Cells', *Pflügers Arch.*, *402*, 337–9

Good, D.W., Knepper, M.A. and Burg, M.B. (1984) 'Ammonia and Bicarbonate Transport by Thick Ascending Limb of Rat Kidney', *Am. J. Physiol.*, *247*, F35–44

Gottschalk, C.W. and Mylle, M. (1959) 'Micropuncture Study of the Mammalian Urinary Concentrating Mechanism: Evidence for the Countercurrent Hypothesis', *Am. J. Physiol.*, *196*, 927–36

Gottschalk, C.W., Lassiter, W.E., Mylle, M., Ullrich, K.J., Schmidt-Nielsen, B., O'Dell, R. and

108   *Ion Transport in the Loop of Henle*

Pehling, G. (1963) 'Micropuncture Study of Composition of Loop of Henle Fluid in Desert Rodents', *Am. J. Physiol.*, *204*, 532–5

Grantham, J.J. (1982) 'Studies of Organic Anion and Cation Transport in Isolated Segments of Proximal Tubules', *Kidney Int.*, *22*, 519–525

Grantham, J.J. and Burg, M.B. (1972) Effect of Vasopressin and Cyclic AMP on the Permeability of Isolated Collecting Ducts', *Am. J. Physiol.*, *211*, 255–9

Grantham, J.J., Qualizza, P.B. and Welling, L.W. (1972) 'Influence of Serum Proteins on Net Fluid Reabsorption of Isolated Proximal Tubules', *Kidney Int.*, *2*, 66–75

Greger, R. (1981a) 'Cation Selectivity of the Isolated Perfused Cortical Thick Ascending Limb of Henle's Loop of Rabbit Kidney', *Pflügers Arch.*, *390*, 30–7

Greger, R. (1981b) 'Chloride Reabsorption in the Rabbit Cortical Thick Ascending Limb of the Loop of Henle. A Sodium-dependent Process', *Pflügers Arch.*, *390*, 38–43

Greger, R. (1981c) 'Coupled Transport of Na^+ and Cl^- in the Thick Ascending Limb of Henle's Loop of Rabbit Nephron', *Scand. Audiol. Suppl.*, *14*, 1–15

Greger, R. (1985a) 'Chloride Transporting Epithelia — Cellular Mechanisms — Regulation', *Pflügers Arch.*, *403*, R5

Greger, R. (1985b) 'Ion Transport in the Thick Ascending Limb of Henle's Loop of the Mammalian Nephron', *Physiological Rev.*, *65*, pp. 760–97

Greger, R. and Frömter, E. (1981) 'Time Course of Ouabain and Furosemide Effects on Transepithelial Potential Difference in Cortical Thick Ascending Limbs of Rabbit Nephrons', in L. Takacs (ed.), *Kidney and Body Fluids*, *11*, Pergamon Press, Oxford, pp. 375–9

Greger, R. and Schlatter, E. (1981) 'Presence of Luminal K^+, a Prerequisite for Active NaCl Transport in the Cortical Thick Ascending Limb of Henle's Loop of Rabbit Kidney', *Pflügers Arch.*, *392*, 92–4

Greger, R. and Schlatter, E. (1983a) 'Properties of the Lumen Membrane of the Cortical Thick Ascending Limb of Henle's Loop of Rabbit Kidney', *Pflügers Arch.*, *396*, 315–24

Greger, R. and Schlatter, E. (1983b) 'Properties of the Basolateral Membrane of the Cortical Thick Ascending Limb of Henle's Loop of Rabbit Kidney. A Model for Secondary Active Chloride Transport', *Pflügers Arch.*, *396*, 325–34

Greger, R. and Schlatter, E. (1984a) 'Mechanism of NaCl Secretion in the Rectal Gland of Spiny Dogfish (*Squalus acanthias*). I. Experiments in Isolated *in vitro* Perfused Rectal Gland Tubules', *Pflügers Arch.*, *402*, 63–75

Greger, R. and Schlatter, E. (1984b) 'Mechanism of NaCl Secretion in Rectal Gland Tubules of Spiny Dogfish (*Squalus acanthias*). II: Effects of Inhibitors', *Pflügers Arch.*, *402*, 364–75

Greger, R., Schlatter, E., Weidtke, C. and Wittner, M. (1982) 'Active NaCl Transport in the Cortical Thick Ascending Limb of Henle's Loop (cTAL) of Rabbit Nephron Does not Require the Presence of Bicarbonate', *Pflügers Arch.*, *394*, 65

Greger, R., Schlatter, E. and Lang, F. (1983a) 'Evidence for Electroneutral Sodium Chloride Co-transport in the Cortical Thick Ascending Limb of Henle's Loop of Rabbit Kidney', *Pflügers Arch.*, *396*, 308–14

Greger, R., Oberleithner, H., Schlatter, E., Cassola, A.C. and Weidtke, C. (1983b) 'Chloride Activity in Cells of Isolated Perused Cortical Thick Ascending Limbs of Rabbit Kidney', *Pflügers Arch.*, *399*, 29–34

Greger, R., Schlatter, E. and Wittner, M. (1984b) 'Cellular Mechanism of Action of Furosemide-like Diuretics in the Thick Ascending Limb of the Loop of Henle', in J.B. Puschett and A. Greenberg (eds), *Diuretics, Chemistry, Pharmacology, and Clinical Applications*, Elsevier, Amsterdam, pp. 215–21

Greger, R., Weidtke, C., Schlatter, E., Wittner, M. and Gebler, B. (1984a) 'Potassium Activity in Cells of Isolated Perfused Cortical Thick Ascending Limbs of Rabbit Kidney', *Pflügers Arch.*, *401*, 52–7

Greger, R., Wittner, M., Schlatter, E. and DiStefano, A. (1984c) '$Na^+2Cl^-K^+$-Cotransport in the Thick Ascending Limb of Henle's Loop and Mechanism of Action of Loop Diuretics', in T. Hoshi (ed.), *Coupled Transport in Nephron*, Miura Foundation, Tokyo, pp. 96–118

Greger, R., Schlatter, E., Wang, F. and Forrest, J.N. Jr (1984d) 'Mechanism of NaCl Secretion in Rectal Gland Tubules of Spiny Dogfish (*Squalus acanthias*). III: Effects of Stimulation of Secretion by Cyclic AMP', *Pflügers Arch.*, *402*, 376–84

Greger, R., Wittner, M., Schlatter, E., Gebler, B., Weidtke, C. and DiStefano, A. (1984e)

'Sodium Chloride Reabsorption in the Thick Ascending Limb of the Loop of Henle', in R.R. Robinson (ed), *Nephrology*, vol.1, Springer-Verlag, Berlin, pp. 224–42

Greger, R., Schlatter, E. and Gögelein, H. (1985) 'Cl⁻-channels in the Apical Cell Membrane of the Rectal Gland "Induced" by cAMP', *Pflügers Arch.*, *403*, 446–8

Haas, M. Schmidt, W.F. III and McManus, T.J. (1982) 'Catecholamine-stimulated Ion Transport in Duck Red Cells. Gradient Effects in Electrically Neutral (Na + K + 2Cl) Co-transport', *J. Gen. Physiol.*, *80*, 125–47

Hall, D.A. and Varney, D.M. (1980) 'Effect of Vasopressin on Electrical Potential Difference and Chloride Transport in Mouse Medullary Thick Ascending Limb of Henle's Loop', *J. Clin. Invest.*, *66*, 792–802

Hannafin, J., Kinne-Saffran, E., Friedman, D. and Kinne, R. (1983) 'Presence of a Sodium Potassium Chloride Cotransport System in the Rectal Gland of *Squalus acanthias*', *J. Membrane Biol.*, *75*, 73–83

Hebert, S.C. and Andreoli, T.E. (1984a) 'The Effects of Antidiuretic Hormone on Cellular Conductive Pathways in Mouse Medullary Thick Ascending Limbs of Henle. II. Determinants of the ADH-mediated Increases in Transepithelial Voltage and in Net Cl⁻ Absorption', *J. Membrane Biol.*, *80*, 221–33

Hebert, S.C. and Andreoli, T.E. (1984b) 'Control of NaCl Transport in the Thick Ascending Limb', *Am. J. Physiol.*, *15*, F745–56

Hebert, S.C., Culpepper, R.M. and Andreoli, T.E. (1981a) 'NaCl Transport in Mouse Medullary Thick Ascending Limbs. I. Functional Nephron Heterogeneity and ADH-stimulated NaCl Cotransport', *Am. J. Physiol.*, *241*, F112–431

Hebert, S.C., Culpepper, R.M. and Andreoli, T.E. (1981b) 'NaCl Transport in Mouse Medullary Thick Ascending Limbs. II. ADH Enhancement of Transcellular NaCl Cotransport; Origin of Transepithelial Voltage', *Am. J. Physiol.*, *241*, F432–42

Hebert, S.C., Friedman, P.A. and Andreoli, T.E. (1984) 'The Effects of Antidiuretic Hormone on Cellular Conductive Pathways in Mouse Medullary Thick Ascending Limbs of Henle. I. ADH Increases Transcellular Conductance Pathways', *J. Membrane Biol.*, *80*, 201–19

Heintze, K., Stewart, C.P. and Frizzell, R.A. (1983) 'Sodium-dependent Chloride Secretion across Rabbit Descending Colon', *Am. J. Physiol.*, *244*, G357–65

Hoffmann, N., Thees, M. and Kinne, R. (1976) 'Phosphate Transport by Isolated Renal Brush Border Vesicles', *Pflügers Arch.*, *362*, 147–56

Hogg, R.J. and Kokko, J.P. (1978) 'Comparison between the Electrical Potential Profile and the Chloride Gradients in the Thin Limbs of Henle's Loop in Rats', *Kidney Int.*, *14*, 428–36

Horster, M. (1978) 'Loop of Henle Functional Differentiation *in vitro* Perfusion of the Isolated Thick Ascending Segment', *Pflügers Arch.*, *378*, 15–24

Horster, M. and Thurau, K. (1968) 'Micropuncture Studies on the Filtration Rate of Single Superficial and Juxtamedullary Glomeruli in the Rat Kidney', *Pflügers Arch.*, *301*, 162–81

Hoshi, T., Kuramochi, G. and Yoshitomi, K. (1983) 'Lumen-positive Chloride Transport Potential in the Early Distal Tubule of *Triturus* Kidney: its Absolute Dependence on the Presence of Na⁺ and K⁺ in the Luminal Fluid', *Jap. J. Physiol.*, *33*, 855–61

Iino, Y. and Burg, M.B. (1981) 'Effect of Acid-Base Status *in vivo* on Bicarbonate Transport by Rabbit Renal Tubules *in vitro*', *Jap. J. Physiol.*, *31*, 99–107

Imai, M. (1977a) 'Function of the Thin Ascending Limb of Henle of Rats and Hamsters Perfused *in vitro*', *Am. J. Physiol.*, *232*, F201–9

Imai, M. (1977b) 'Effect of Bumetanide and Furosemide on the Thick Ascending Limb of Henle's Loop of Rabbits and Rats Perfused *in vitro*', *Eur. J. Pharmacol.*, *41*, 409–16

Imai, M. (1978) 'Calcium Transport across the Rabbit Thick Ascending Limb of Henle's Loop Perfused *in vitro*', *Pflügers Arch.*, *374*, 255–63

Imai, M. (1984a) 'Regulation of Ion Transport in the Thick Ascending Limb of Henle's Loop', in T. Hoshi (ed), *Coupled Transport in Nephron*, Miura Foundation, Tokyo, pp. 119–30

Imai, M. (1984b) 'Functional Heterogeneity of the Descending Limb of Henle's Loop: II. Interspecies Differences among Rabbits, Rats, and Hamsters', *Pflügers Arch.*, *402*, 393–401

Imai, M. and Kokko, J.P. (1974) 'Sodium Chloride, Urea, and Water Transport in the Thin Ascending Limb of Henle. Generation of Osmotic Gradients by Passive Diffusion of Solutes', *J. Clin. Invest.*, *53*, 393–402

Imai, M. and Kokko, J.P. (1976) 'Mechanism of Sodium and Chloride Transport in the Thin Ascending Limb of Henle', *J. Clin. Invest.*, *58*, 1054–60

Imai, M. and Kusano, E. (1982) 'Effects of Arginine Vasopressin on the Thin Ascending Limb of Henle's Loop of Hamsters', *Am. J. Physiol.*, *243*, F167–72

Imai, M., Hayashi, M. and Araki, M. (1984a) 'Functional Heterogeneity of the Descending Limbs of Henle's Loop: I. Internephron Heterogeneity in the Hamster Kidney', *Pflügers Arch.*,*402*, 385–92

Imai, M., Hayashi, M., Araki, M. and Tabei, K. (1984b) 'Function of the Thin Limbs of Henle's Loop', in R.R. Robinson (ed.), *Nephrology*, vol. 1, Springer-Verlag, Berlin, pp. 196–207

Imbert, M., Chabardes, D., Montegut, M., Clique, A. and Morel, F. (1975) 'Vasopressin-dependent Adenylate Cyclase in Single Segments of Rabbit Kidney Tubule', *Pflügers Arch.*, *357*, 173–86

Imbert-Teboul, M., Chabardes, D., Montegut, M., Clique, A. and Morel, F. (1978) 'Vasopressin-dependent Adenylate Cyclase Activities in the Rat Kidney Medulla: Evidence for Two Separate Sites of Action', *Endocrinology*, *102*, 1254–61

Jacobson, H.R. and Kokko, J.P. (1976) 'Intrinsic Differences in Various Segments of the Proximal Convoluted Tubule', *J. Clin. Invest.*, *57*, 818–25

Jamison, R.L. (1968) 'Micropuncture Study of Segments of Thin Loop of Henle in the Rat', *Am. J. Physiol.*, *215*, 236–42

Jamison, R.L., Bennett, C.M. and Berliner, R.W. (1967) 'Countercurrent Multiplication by the Thin Loops of Henle', *Am. J. Physiol.*, *212*, 357–66

Johnson, J.H., Dunn, D.P. and Rosenberg, R.N. (1982) 'Furosemide-sensitive K^+ Channel in Glioma Cells but not Neuroblastoma Cells in Culture', *Biochim. Biophys. Res. Comm.*, *109*, 100–5

Katz, A.I., Doucet, A. and Morel, F. (1979) 'Na-K-ATPase Activity along the Rabbit, Rat, and Mouse Nephron', *Am. J. Physiol.*, *237*, F114–20

Kawamura, S. and Kokko, J.P.(1976) 'Urea Secretion by the Straight Segment of the Proximal Tubule', *J. Clin. Invest.*, *58*, 604–12

Kawamura, S., Imai, M., Seldin, D.W. and Kokko, J.P. (1975) 'Characteristics of Salt and Water Transport in Superficial and Juxtamedullary Straight Segments of Proximal Tubules', *J. Clin. Invest.*, *55*, 1269–77

Knepper, M.A. and Vurek, G.G. (1982) 'Urea Transport in Isolated, Perfused Cortical Thick Ascending Limbs and Proximal Straight Tubules from Rabbits', *Kidney Int.*, *21*, 280

Koenig, B., Ricapito, S. and Kinne, R. (1983) 'Chloride Transport in the Thick Ascending Limb of Henle's Loop: Potassium Dependence and Stoichiometry of the NaCl Cotransport System in Plasma Membrane Vesicles', *Pflügers Arch.*, *399*, 173–9

Kokko, J.P. (1970) 'Sodium Chloride and Water Transport in the Descending Limb of Henle', *J. Clin. Invest.*, *49*, 1838–46

Kokko, J.P. (1972) 'Urea Transport in the Proximal Tubule and the Descending Limb of Henle', *J. Clin. Invest.*, *51*, 1999–2008

Kokko, J.P. (1973) 'Proximal Tubule Potential Difference. Dependence on Glucose, HCO_3 and Amino Acids', *J. Clin. Invest.*, *52*, 1362–7

Kokko, J.P. (1974) 'Membrane Characteristics Governing Salt and Water Transport in the Loop of Henle', *Fed. Proc.*, *33*, 25–30

Kokko, J.P. (1982) 'Transport Characteristics of the Thin Limbs of Henle', *Kidney Int.*, *22*, 449–54

Kokko, J.P. and Rector, F.C. Jr (1972) 'Countercurrent Multiplication System without Active Transport in Inner Medulla', *Kidney Int.*, *2*, 214–23

Lang, F., Greger, R., Marchand, G. and Knox, F. (1977) 'Saturation Kinetics of Phosphate Reabsorption in Rats', in S.G. Massry and E. Ritz (eds), *Phosphate Metabolism*, Plenum Press, New York, pp.153–5

Lassiter, W.E., Gottschalk, C.W. and Mylle, M. (1961) 'Micropuncture Study of Net Transtubular Movement of Water and Urea in Nondiuretic Mammalian Kidney', *Am. J. Physiol.*,*200*, 1139–46

Lutz, M.D., Cardinal, J. and Burg, M.B.(1973) 'Electrical Resistance of Renal Proximal Tubule Perfused *in vitro*', *Am. J. Physiol.*, *225*, 729–34

McKinney, T.D. and Burg, M.B. (1977) 'Bicarbonate and Fluid Absorption by Renal Proximal Straight Tubules', *Kidney Int.*, *12*, 1–8

Marsh, D.J. (1970) 'Solute and Water Flows in Thin Limbs of Henle's Loop in the Hamster Kidney', *Am. J. Physiol., 218*, 824–31

Marsh, D.J. and Azen, S.P. (1975) 'Mechanism of NaCl Reabsorption by Hamster Thin Ascending Limbs of Henle's Loop', *Am. J. Physiol., 228*, 71–9

Marsh, D.J. and Martin, C.M. (1977) 'Origin of Electrical PDs in Hamster Thin Ascending Limbs of Henle's Loop', *Am. J. Physiol., 232*, F348–57

Marsh, D.J. and Solomon, S. (1965) 'Analysis of Electrolyte Movement in Thin Henle's Loops of Hamster Papilla', *Am. J. Physiol., 208*, 1119–28

Mills, J. (1985) 'Ion Transport Pathways in the Exocrine Glands of the Frog Skin', *Pflügers Arch.*, in press

Morel, F., Chabardes, D. and Imbert, M. (1976) 'Functional Segmentation of the Rabbit Distal Tubule by Microdetermination of Hormone-dependent Adenylate Cyclase Activity', *Kidney Int., 9*, 264–77

Morel, F., Imbert-Teboul, M. and Chabardes, D. (1981) 'Distribution of Hormone Dependent Adenylate Cyclase in the Nephron and its Physiological Significance', *Ann. Rev. Physiol., 43*, 569–81

Morgan, T. and Berliner, R.W. (1968) 'Permeability of the Loop of Henle, Vasa Recta, and Collecting Duct to Water, Urea, and Sodium', *Am. J. Physiol., 215*, 108–15

Murer, H., Hopfer, U. and Kinne, R. (1976) 'Sodium/Proton Antiport in Brush-border Membrane Vesicles Isolated from Rat Small Intestine and Kidney', *Biochem. J., 154*, 597–604

Mush, M.W. Orellana, S.A., Kimberg, L.S., Field, M., Hahn, D.R., Krasny, E.J. and Frizzell, R.A. (1982) 'Na$^+$-K$^+$-Cl$^-$ Co-transport in the Intestine of a Marine Teleost', *Nature (Lond.). 300*, 351–3

Ng, R.C.K., Peraino, R.A. and Suki, W.N. (1982) 'Divalent Cation Transport in Isolated Tubules', *Kidney Int., 22*, 492–7

Nishimura, H., Imai, M. and Ogawa, M. (1983a) 'Sodium Chloride and Water Transport in the Renal Distal Tubule of the Rainbow Trout', *Am. J. Physiol., 244*, F247–54

Nishimura, H., Imai, M. and Ogawa, M. (1983b) 'Transepithelial Voltage in the Reptilian- and Mammalian-types Nephrons from Japanese Quail', *Fed. Proc., 42*, 304

Oberleithner, H., Guggino, W. and Giebisch, G. (1982a) 'Mechanism of Distal Tubular Chloride Transport in *Amphiuma* Kidney', *Am. J. Physiol., 242*, F331–9

Oberleithner, H., Guggino, W. and Giebisch, G. (1982a) 'Mechanism of Distal Tubular Chloride Furosemide Sensitive Transport System in the Kidney', *Klin. Wochenschr.,60*, 1173–9

Palfrey, H.C., Feit, P.W. and Greengard, P. (1980) 'cAMP-stimulated Transport in Avian Erythrocytes: Inhibition by Loop Diuretics', *Am. J. Physiol., 238*, C139–48

Persson, B. and Spring, K.R. (1982) 'Gallbladder Epithelial Cell Hydraulic Water Permeability and Volume Regulation', *J. Gen. Physiol., 79*, 481–505

Peterson, K.U. and Reuss, L. (1983) 'Cyclic AMP-induced Chloride Permeability in the Apical Membrane of *Necturus* Gallbladder Epithelium', *J. Gen. Physiol., 81*, 705–29

Peterson, O.H. and Maruyama, Y. (1984) 'Calcium-activated Potassium Channels and their Role in Secretion', *Nature (Lond.), 307*, 693–6

Quamme, G.A. (1982) 'Magnesium Transport in Isolated Proximal Straight Tubules of the Rabbit', *Kidney Int., 21*, 139

Reuss, L., Reinach, P., Weinmam, S.A. and Grady, T.P. (1983) 'Intracellular Ion Activities and Cl$^-$ Transport Mechanism in Bullfrog Corneal Epithelium', *Am. J. Physiol., 244*, C336–47

Rocha, A.S. and Kokko, J.P. (1973a) 'Membrane Characteristics Regulating Potassium Transport out of the Isolated Perfused Descending Limb of Henle', *Kidney Int., 4*, 326–30

Rocha, A.S. and Kokko, J.P. (1973b) 'Sodium Chloride and Water Transport in the Medullary Thick Ascending Limb of Henle; Evidence for Active Chloride Transport', *J. Clin. Invest., 52*, 612–23

Rocha, A.S. and Kokko, J.P. (1974) 'Permeability of Medullary Nephron Segments to Urea and Water: Effect of Vasopressin', *Kidney Int., 6*, 379–87

Rocha, A.S., Magaldi, J.B. and Kokko, J.P. (1977) 'Calcium and Phosphate Transport in Isolated Segments of Rabbit Henle's Loop', *J. Clin. Invest., 59*, 975–83

Rouse, D., Ng, R.C.K. and Suki, W.N. (1980) 'Calcium Transport in the Pars Recta and Thin Descending Limb of Henle of the Rabbit, Perfused *in vitro*', *J. Clin. Invest., 65*, 37–42

Russell, J.M. (1983) 'Cation-coupled Chloride Influx in Squid Axon. Role of Potassium and

Stoichiometry of the Transport Process', *J. Gen. Physiol.*, *81*, 909–25

Sakai, F., Jamison, R.L. and Berliner, R.W. (1965) 'A Method for Exposing the Rat Renal Medulla *in vivo*: Micropuncture of the Collecting Duct', *Am. J. Physiol.*, *209*, 663–8

Sakai, F., Tadokoro, M. and Teraoka, M. (1971) 'Experimentelle Untersuchungen Über die Funktion des Nierenmarks mit der Micropunktionsmethode', *Tokyo J. Med. Sci.*, *79*, 1–30

Sasaki, S. and Imai, M.(1980) 'Effects of Vasopressin on Water and NaCl Transport across the *in vitro* Perfused Medullary Thick Ascending Limb of Henle's Loop of Mouse, Rat, and Rabbit Kidneys', *Pflügers Arch.*, *383*, 215–21

Schafer, J.A. and Andreoli, T.E. (1972) 'Cellular Constraints to Diffusion. The Effect of Antidiuretic Hormone on Water Flows in Isolated Mammalian Collecting Tubules', *J. Clin. Invest.*, *51*, 1264–78

Schafer, J.A. and Andreoli, T.E. (1976) 'Anion Transport Processes in the Mammalian Superficial Proximal Straight Tubule', *J. Clin. Invest.*, *58*, 500–13

Schafer, J.A. and Andreoli, T.E. (1979) 'Rheogenic and Passive Na^+ Absorption by the Proximal Nephron', *Ann. Rev. Physiol.*, *41*, 211–27

Schafer, J.A. and Barfuss, D.W. (1982) 'The Study of Pars Recta Function by the Perfusion of Isolated Tubule Segments', *Kidney Int.*, *22*, 434–48

Schafer, J.A. and Work, J. (1984) 'Transport Properties of the Pars Recta', in R.R. Robinson (ed), *Nephrology*, vol. 1, Springer-Verlag, Berlin, pp. 186–95

Schafer, J.A., Troutman, S.L. and Andreoli, T.E. (1974) 'Volume Reabsorption, Transepithelial Potential Differences, and Ionic Permeability Properties in Mammalian Superficial Proximal Straight Tubules', *J. Gen. Physiol.*, *64*, 582–607

Schafer, J.A., Patlak, C.S. and Andreoli, T.E. (1975) 'A Component of Fluid Absorption Linked to Passive Ion Fluxes in the Superficial Pars Recta', *J. Gen Physiol.*, *66*, 445–71

Schafer, J.A., Patlak, C.S. and Andreoli, T.E. (1977) 'Fluid Absorption and Active and Passive Ion Flows in the Rabbit Superficial Pars Recta', *Am. J. Physiol.*, *233*, F154–67

Schafer, J.S., Troutman, S.L., Watkins, M.L. and Andreoli, T.E. (1978a) 'Volume Absorption in the Pars Recta. I. "Simple" Active Na^+ Transport', *Am. J. Physiol.*, *234*, F332–9

Schafer, J.A., Patlak, C.S., Troutman, S.L. and Andreoli, T.E. (1978b) 'Volume Absorption in the Pars Recta. II. Hydraulic Conductivity Coefficient', *Am. J. Physiol.*, *234*, F340–8

Schafer, J.A., Troutman, S.L., Watkins, M.L. and Andreoli, T.E. (1981) 'Flow Dependence of Fluid Transport in the Isolated Superficial Pars Recta: Evidence that Osmotic Disequilibrium between External Solutions Drives Isotonic Fluid Absorption', *Kidney Int.*, *20*, 588–97

Schlatter, E. and Greger, R. (1982) 'Metabolic Substrates for Maintaining Active Transport in the Isolated Cortical Thick Ascending Limb (cTAL) of Rabbit Kidney', *Pflügers Arch.*, *394*, 64

Schlatter, E. and Greger, R. (1985) 'cAMP Increases the Basolateral Cl^- Conductance in the Isolated Perfused Medullary Thick Ascending Limb of Henle's Loop (mTAL) of the Mouse', *Pflügers Arch.*, in press.

Schlatter, E., Greger, R. and Weidtke, C. (1983) 'Effect of "high ceiling" Diuretics on Active Salt Transport in the Cortical Thick Ascending Limb of Henle's Loop of Rabbit Kidney. Correlation of Chemical Structure and Inhibitory Potency', *Pflügers Arch.*, *396*, 210–17

Shareghi, G.R. and Agus, Z.S. (1982) 'Magnesium Transport in the Cortical Thick Ascending Limb of Henle's Loop of the Rabbit', *J. Clin. Invest.*, *69*, 759–69

Shorofsky, S.R., Field, M. and Fozzard, H.A. (1982), 'The Cellular Mechanism of Active Chloride Secretion in Vertebrate Epithelia: Studies in Intestine and Trachea', *Phil. Trans. R. Soc. London*, *B299*, 597–607

Stephenson, J.L. (1966) 'Concentration in Renal Counterflow Systems', *Biophys. J.*, *6*, 539–51

Stephenson, J.L. (1972) 'Concentration of Urine in Central Core Model of the Renal Counterflow System', *Kidney Int.*, 85–94

Stokes, J.B. (1979) 'Effect of Prostaglandin E_2 on Chloride Transport across the Rabbit Thick Ascending Limb', *J. Clin. Invest.*, *64*, 495–502

Stokes, J.B. (1982) 'Consequences of Potassium Recycling in the Renal Medulla. Effects on Ion Transport by the Medullary Thick Ascending Limb of Henle's Loop', *J. Clin. Invest.*, *70*, 219–29

Stokes, J.B. (1984) 'Regulation of NaCl Transport by the Loop of Henle', in R.R. Robinson (ed.) *Nephrology*, vol. 1, Springer-Verlag, Berlin, pp. 208–23

Stoner, L.C. and Roch-Ramel, F. (1979) 'The Effects of Pressure on the Water Permeability of the Descending Limb of Henle's Loops of Rabbits', *Pflügers Arch.*, *382*, 7–15

Stoner, L.C. and Trimble, M.E. (1982) 'Effects of MK-196 and Furosemide on Rat Medullary Thick Ascending Limbs of Henle *in vitro*', *J. Pharmacol. Exp. Ther.*, *221*, 715–20

Suki, W.N. and Rouse, D. (1981) 'Hormonal Regulation of Calcium Transport in Thick Ascending Limb Renal Tubules', *Am. J. Physiol.*, *241*, F171–4

Suki, W.N., Rouse, D., Ng, R.C.K. and Kokko, J.P. (1980) 'Calcium Transport in the Thick Ascending Limb of Henle. Heterogeneity of Function in the Medullary and Cortical Segments', *J. Clin Invest.*, *66*, 1004–9

Tune, B.M. and Burg, M.B. (1971) 'Glucose Transport by Proximal Renal Tubules', *Am. J. Physiol.*, *221*, 580–5

Tune, B.M., Burg, M.B. and Patlak, C.S. (1969) 'Characteristics of *p*-Amino Hippurate Transport in Proximal Renal Tubules', *Am. J. Physiol.*, *217*, 1057–65

Turner, R.J. and Moran, A. (1982a) 'Heterogeneity of Sodium-dependent D-Glucose Transport Sites along the Proximal Tubule: Evidence from Vesicle Studies', *Am. J. Physiol.*, *242*, F406–14

Turner, R.J. and Moran, A. (1982b) 'The Sodium: Glucose Stoichiometry of Renal Brushborder Membrane D-Glucose Reabsorption', *Fed. Proc.*, *41*, 1010

Ullrich, K.J., Drenckhahn, F.O. and Jarausch, K.H.(1955) 'Untersuchungen zum Problem der Harnkonzentrierung und -verdünnung. Über das osmotische Verhalten von Nierenzellen und die begleitende Elektrolytanhäufung im Nierengewebe bei verschiedenen Diuresezuständen', *Pflügers Arch.*, *261*, 62–77

Ullrich, K.J., Rumrich, G. and Klöss, S. (1980) 'Active Sulfate Reabsorption in the Proximal Convolution of the Rat Kidney: Specificity, Na^+ and HCO_3^- Dependence', *Pflügers Arch.*, *383*, 159–63

Ussing, H.H. (1985) 'Volume Regulation of the Frog Skin Epithelium', *Pflügers Arch.*, in press

Völkl, H. and Greger, R. (1984) '$(Na^+ + K^+)$-ATPase Activity Controls the Basolateral K^+ Conductance in the Mouse Proximal Tubule', *Pflügers Arch.*, *402*, 6

Warnock, D.G. and Burg M.B. (1977) 'Urinary Acidification: CO_2 Transport by the Rabbit Proximal Straight Tubule', *Am. J. Physiol.*, *232*, F20–5

Wasserstein, A.G. and Agus, Z.S. (1983) 'Potassium Secretion in the Rabbit Proximal Straight Tubule', *Am. J. Physiol.*, *245*, F167–74

Welling, L.W. and Welling, D.J. (1976) 'Shape of Epithelial Cells and Intercellular Channels in the Rabbit Proximal Nephron', *Kidney Int.*, *9*, 385–94

Welling, L.W., Welling, D.J. and Ochs, T.J. (1983) 'Video Measurement of Basolateral Membrane Hydraulic Conductivity in the Proximal Tubule', *Am. J. Physiol.*, *245*, F123–9

Welsh, M.J. (1983) 'Intracellular Chloride Activities in Canine Tracheal Epithelium', *J. Clin. Invest.*, *71*, 1392–1401

Welsh, M., Smith, P.L. and Frizzell, R.A. (1982) 'Chloride Secretion by Canine Tracheal Epithelium: II. The Cellular Electrical Potential Profile', *J. Membrane Biol.*, *70*, 227–38

Wiley J.S. and Cooper, R.A.(1974) 'A Furosemide-sensitive Cotransport of Sodium plus Potassium in the Human Red Cell', *J. Clin. Invest.*, *53*, 745–55

Windhager, E.E. (1964) 'Electrophysiological Study of Renal Papilla of Golden Hamsters', *Am. J. Physiol.*, *206*, 694–700

Wirz, H., Hargitay, B. and Kuhn, W. (1951) 'Lokalisation des Konzentrierungsprozesses in der Niere durch direkte Kryoskopie', *Helv. Physiol. Pharmacol. Acta*, *9*, 196–362

Wittner, M., Greger, R., DiStefano, A., Gebler, B. and Meyer, C. (1984a) 'Inhibitors of the Basolateral Cl^--conductance in Isolated Perfused Cortical Thick Ascending Limbs of Henle Loops (cTAL) of Rabbit Nephrons', *Pflügers Arch.*, *400*, 86

Wittner, M., Weidtke, C., Schlatter, E., DiStefano, A., and Greger, R. (1984b) 'Substrate Utilization in the Isolated Perfused Cortical Thick Ascending Limb of Rabbit Nephron', *Pflügers Arch.*, *402*, 52–62

Work, J., Troutman, S.L. and Schafer, J.A. (1982) 'Transport of Potassium in the Rabbit Pars Recta', *Am. J. Physiol.*, *242*, F226–37

4 TUBULOGLOMERULAR FEEDBACK MECHANISMS: INTERRELATIONSHIPS BETWEEN TUBULAR FLOW AND GLOMERULAR FILTRATION RATE

D. A. Häberle and J. M. Davis

Introduction

Renal solute and water balance is a dynamic steady state, the achievement of which results from a very precise control of tubular flow rate — the theme of this article, tubular epithelial transport activity, and, additionally, from the interaction between these two parameters.

The flow of the glomerular filtrate through the nephron is a hydrodynamic phenomenon which, in theory, could be controlled by regulation of either the driving force for fluid flow, or the series of flow resistances along the nephron, or both. The ultimate driving force for tubular flow is the hydrostatic pressure in the glomerular capillaries, and the major flow resistances are the filtration barrier itself, the loop of Henle and the collecting duct system. Whereas the latter two resistances appear not to be regulated by any specific mechanisms (Steven, 1977), both the apparent resistance of the filtration barrier (as expressed in the filtration coefficient K_f) and the hydrostatic pressure in the glomerular capillaries are under the control of an intricate regulator system.

Although this system has defied many an investigative effort to unravel it, the numerous studies have nevertheless revealed complex interrelationships between tubular flow and glomerular filtration dynamics. These include, first, what might be termed a 'hydrodynamic negative feedback'; secondly, an autoregulatory mechanism, which may well reside within the vascular elements of the glomerular pole itself; and, thirdly, a humorally mediated negative-feedback loop operating via the macula densa (the mechanism referred to in the literature as 'the' tubuloglomerular feedback mechanism).

To date, the vast majority of investigations in this area have analysed the individual components of this involved system of interacting mechanisms, and indeed the experimental protocols have mostly neglected the possibility of mutual interaction between the component studied and the other components. It is more the intention of this chapter to focus on the phenomenology and interactions of the various mechanisms and the dependency of their activities on extracellular fluid volume and composition than to analyse in detail the individual components. For the latter, the reader is referred to recent excellent reviews (Baylis and Brenner, 1978, Navar, 1978; Wright and Briggs, 1979; Navar et al., 1980; Schnermann et al., 1980; Blantz and Pelayo, 1984).

Hydrodynamic Effects of Tubular Flow on Glomerular Filtration

From Bowman's space, the onward flow of filtrate is essentially driven by the hydrostatic pressure gradient between this site and the renal pelvis. The pressure in Bowman's space is determined by proximal tubular compliance and intratubular volume, which in turn is defined by the rate of volume inflow (i.e. the glomerular filtration rate), proximal tubular fluid reabsorption and the flow resistances in the subsequent segments of the nephron. As already noted, these resistances appear not to be regulated by any specific mechanisms, and thus variations in the rate of fluid reabsorption by any of the nephron segments should be reflected in changes in proximal tubular pressure, particularly if it is assumed that glomerular filtration rate remains constant. Thus it may be expected that when fractional fluid reabsorption is low, for example during water diuresis (Ichikawa and Brenner, 1977), mannitol diuresis (Gottschalk and Mylle, 1957; Blantz, 1974) drug-induced diuresis (Krause *et al.*, 1967) or saline diuresis (Andreucci *et al.*, 1971a), proximal tubular pressure would be high, and vice versa.

The interaction between intratubular pressure and the rate of filtrate formation is defined by the filtration equation:

$$\text{GFR} = K_f[\,(P_{gc} - P_{bs}) - \pi_{\overline{gc}}\,]$$

where GFR represents glomerular filtration rate; P_{gc} and $\pi_{\overline{gc}}$ the glomerular capillary hydrostatic and oncotic pressures respectively, the latter averaged along the capillary length; and P_{bs} the hydrostatic pressure in Bowman's space. The pressure term is simplified to $P_{\overline{uf}}$, the mean effective filtration pressure. Since the mean effective filtration pressure is, in fact, only of the order of a few mmHg (see Chapter 2; and review by Baylis and Brenner, 1978), variations in intratubular pressure might well be expected to have considerable influence on glomerular filtration (see also Steven, 1974; Hartupee *et al.*, 1981). Thus simply because of the structural and functional relationships of the various tubular segments, variations in fractional fluid reabsorption should lead to inverse variations of glomerular filtration rate by virtue of the concomitant changes in intratubular pressure, even in the absence of any specific regulatory mechanism.

This inverse interaction between intratubular hydrodynamics and glomerular filtration dynamics results in steady states which can be estimated by model calculations based on the filtration model of Deen *et al.* (1972). The results of these calculations are shown in Figure 4.1. In this figure, three unbroken lines, labelled A, B and C, represent the relationship between intratubular pressure and glomerular filtration rate calculated from three sets of experimentally measured filtration determinants taken from the literature (the data are taken from the control groups of all relevant studies quoted by Baylis and Brenner, 1978). The closed triangles thus represent the values of

Figure 4.1: The Relationship between Single Nephron Filtration Rate (SNGFR) and Proximal Intratubular Pressure (P_{tub}) calculated from the Filtration Model of Deen *et al.* (1972) for Three Sets of Filtration Determinants (A,B,C). K_f and arterial protein concentration $C_{prot_{art}}$ were held constant at the values shown for all curves; P_{gc} and Q_{gpf} were fixed at the values shown for each curve; SNGFR and P_{tub} are indicated by the closed triangles (▲). The inset shows the database from which the three sets of determinants were arbitrarily selected. The data points are the mean values for control animals from all the relevant studies quoted by Baylis and Brenner (1978). The dotted lines indicate the hypothetical increase in intratubular pressure which would result from decreasing proximal fractional reabsorption from 60 per cent to 25 per cent; the open triangles (△) indicate the new steady states reached after this change. For explanation see text.

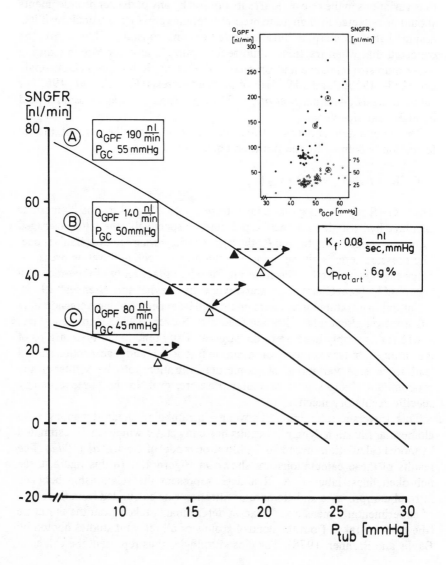

intratubular pressure and GFR from these data sets, and the remaining filtration determinants (glomerular plasma flow Q_{gpf}, arterial protein concentration, P_{gc} and K_f) were held constant at the values indicated in the figure. It should be noted that variations of glomerular filtration rate at constant glomerular plasma inflow necessarily imply variations in filtration fraction and hence plasma outflow through the efferent arteriole. For simplification, it was initially assumed that efferent arteriolar resistance is not actively regulated and, hence, that changes in efferent arteriolar resistance do not affect glomerular capillary pressure or K_f (for details, see appendix). These calculations reveal what was derived intuitively above, namely, that even without any specific regulatory mechanisms, glomerular filtration rate is quite sensitive to changes in intratubular pressure. This effect is more pronounced, i.e. the curve is steeper, at high values of glomerular capillary pressure and plasma flow (curve A), than at low values (curve C) where the mean effective filtration pressure declines to zero by the end of the glomerular capillary (filtration pressure equilibrium). Also shown in this figure is the influence of variations in proximal tubular fluid reabsorption on intratubular pressure and glomerular filtration rate. Fractional fluid reabsorption is assumed to fall from 60 per cent to 25 per cent; the increase in intratubular hydrostatic pressure due to the increased flow through the resistance offered by the loop of Henle is calculated by the Navier-Stokes equations (see appendix). Starting from the real data points (the closed triangles), the horizontal arrows represent the hypothetical increase in intratubular pressure which would occur if the filtration rate were assumed to remain constant. However, as just noted, this rise in pressure will depress glomerular filtration rate and, *ipso facto,* lead to a fall in loop of Henle flow rate and thus intratubular pressure. Accordingly, both glomerular filtration rate and intratubular pressure decline in parallel to new steady-states on the tubular pressure–glomerular filtration rate curve indicated by the open triangles.

In summary, variations in tubular fluid reabsorption will be partially compensated by a negative 'hydrodynamic' feedback without any additional regulatory mechanisms.

Intrinsic Regulatory Properties of the Glomerulus

A clue to the existence of a further mechanism is delivered by a comparison of the curves shown in Figure 4.1 with those determined experimentally by Seiller and Gertz (1977). This comparison reveals that, in the absence of fluid flow through the loop of Henle and, consequently, any humorally mediated tubuloglomerular feedback influences (see subsequent section on the tubuloglomerular feedback mechanism), an experimentally induced increase in intratubular pressure causes a much smaller decrease in glomerular filtration rate than would be predicted by the model calculations just described. In Seiller and Gertz's study, glomerular filtration rate (GFR) decreased linearly in response to increasing intratubular pressure (ITP) according to the equation $GFR = (38.8 \pm 7.5) - (0.92 \pm 0.28)$ ITP. Thus, at an intratubular hydrostatic pressure of zero, glomerular filtration rate would be 38.8 nl min^{-1}, whereas, at a pressure of 41.7 ± 3.8 mmHg, glomerular filtration would cease. The discrepancy between these experimental results (compare also Andreucci *et al.*, 1971b; Brenner *et al.*, 1971) and the model predictions might be explained by the presence of a glomerular mechanism that adjusts the glomerular capillary pressure and/or K_f in proportion to changes in intratubular hydrostatic pressure. Evidence for this proposal can be drawn from the observations of Ichikawa (1982a). In this study, glomerular capillary pressure was measured in nephrons in which flow through the loop of Henle had been experimentally prevented and in which the glomerular filtrate was allowed to escape through a hole in the proximal tubule. When the escape of the filtrate was subsequently prevented, leading to a rise in intratubular pressure to stop-flow levels, glomerular capillary pressure also increased. An explanation suggested by these authors is that when the formation of the glomerular filtrate is opposed by an increase of intratubular hydrostatic pressure, filtration fraction declines and efferent arteriolar plasma outflow rises. If efferent arteriolar resistance either remains unaltered or even increases, due to some intrinsic autoregulatory properties (in contrast to the simplifying assumption made above in the model calculations), glomerular capillary pressure must increase and total glomerular blood flow decrease. Such an intrinsic autoregulatory capability of the vascular elements of the glomerular pole was indeed observed in experiments in rats in which stop-flow pressure was measured during experimentally induced alterations of systemic blood pressure. In the absence of the humorally mediated tubuloglomerular feedback mechanism (loop of Henle flow was prevented by the proximal tubular block), stop-flow pressure, and thus presumably glomerular capillary pressure, was either independent (Gertz *et al.*, 1966) or only partially dependent (Moore, 1984) on systemic blood pressure over the autoregulatory range.

In summary, this intrinsic glomerular autoregulatory mechanism interacts with glomerular and tubular hydrodynamics in such a manner as to at least partially counteract the hydrodynamic effect of changes of intratubular pressure on glomerular filtration rate.

The Humorally Mediated Tubuloglomerular Feedback Mechanism

Although the concept of a humorally mediated mechanism located at the macula densa and controlling glomerular filtration rate was first formulated 40 years ago (Goormaghtigh, 1945), the key experimental observations which kindled research interest in such a mechanism were those of Thurau, Schnermann and co-workers some 20 years later (Thurau and Schnermann, 1965; Schnermann *et al.*, 1970). These workers showed that the filtration rate in an individual nephron decreases when the flow rate through the macula densa segment of the early distal tubule is increased, and vice versa. The tubular signal is thought to be the load-dependent sodium chloride transport rate at the macula densa (Schnermann and Briggs, 1982) and the effector mechanism a humorally mediated alteration in glomerular haemodynamics, probably including a change in glomerular capillary pressure itself (Bell *et al.*, 1984; Briggs, 1984)

Although many of the characteristics and subordinate mechanisms of this regulatory loop have been elucidated by subsequent extensive investigation, almost all such studies have been carried out with the control loop interrupted ('open loop') and the mechanism thus isolated from the possibility of mutual interaction with the other mechanisms previously described. This condition is unavoidable in protocols in which glomerular filtration rate is measured by quantitative proximal fluid collection during simultaneous experimental variation of flow rate and/or fluid composition in the loop of Henle. Despite the fact that this mechanism can be shown to participate in the regulation of glomerular filtration rate in the free-flowing nephron, in which the control loop is intact ('closed loop'), little is known of its behaviour or characteristics under these closed loop conditions.

A recent attempt to gain insight into the normal operation of this mechanism and its interaction with other mechanisms was made by studying the relationship between tubular flow and hydrostatic pressure in free-flowing nephrons, i.e. under closed-loop conditions, when fluid delivery into the loop of Henle of the nephron is experimentally changed. The essence of the protocol is the estimation of an unknown flow rate in free-flowing nephrons from the measurement of the intratubular pressure (Häberle and Davis, 1982a). Since the protocol is complex, the method will first be described in some detail, and the results and their theoretical implications will then be summarised. The operation of the three-phase protocol is shown in Figure 4.2. In phase I, Figure 4.2A, late proximal tubular flow in a free-flowing nephron was varied by either addition or partial withdrawal of tubular fluid by means of a microperfusion-suction pump incorporating a micropressure transducer (Lohfert *et al.*, 1971). Transducer output and pump flow rate were recorded on an X–Y recorder yielding a curve showing the pressure at the perfusion site as a function of the instantaneous pump flow rate (Figure 4.2B, curve 1). The actual loop of Henle inflow during this phase is unknown, since it consists of an unknown native component plus or minus the pumped component. The actual flows are estimated by subsequently 'calibrating' the loop of Henle flow resistance in phase II (Figure 4.2A) by repeating the perfusion after blockade of the proximal tubule with a long, viscous, oil block and recording again the pressure-flow relationship (Figure 4.2B, curve II). Under these circumstances, the pump flow rate is now the actual loop inflow. During this phase, several timed quantitative collections of early proximal tubule fluid were also made allowing the tubuloglomerular feedback curve with the control loop 'open' or

120   *Tubuloglomerular Feedback Mechanisms*

Figure 4.2: (A) Protocol Employed to Investigate the Tubuloglomerular Feedback Mechanism in its Operating ('Closed Loop') State by Varying Loop of Henle Inflow by Means of a Microperfusion-Suction Pump with Simultaneous Registration of Proximal Tubular Pressure (Häberle and Davis, 1982a). In Phase I this is carried out in the free-flowing nephron; in Phase II, with the proximal tubule blocked, and with simultaneous measurement of early proximal flow rate; in Phase III (not shown) the microperfusion-pressure system is calibrated. (B) Pressure-Flow Curves Obtained with this Protocol. $\dot{V}$ is pump flow rate (negative values indicate fluid withdrawal). I, II and III indicate the curves obtained in the respective protocol phases. (C) Relationship between Early Proximal Flow Rate (EPFR) and Loop of Henle Perfusion Rate Gained from Phase II of Protocol. For explanation see text.

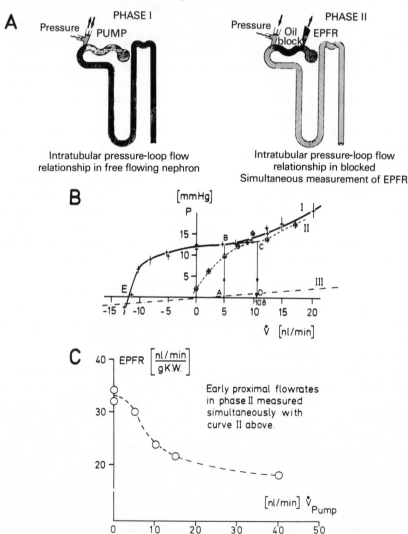

From Häberle and Davis (1982a), with permission

interrupted to be constructed (Figure 4.2C). Finally, in phase III (not shown in Figure 4.2A), the microperfusion system itself is calibrated yielding a pressure-flow relationship (Figure 4.2B, curve III) which must be taken into account in the analysis of the other curves. The method of data analysis is best illustrated by an example in Figure 4.2B. The aim is to construct the closed-loop feedback curve, which requires that the loop of Henle inflow and the early proximal flow in the free-flowing nephron be known. Starting at point A on the abscissa in Figure 4.2B, where the pump was infusing 5 nl min^{-1}, the first unknown is the actual loop of Henle inflow at this point. A perpendicular is raised to B, the intratubular free-flow pressure at this unknown flow rate. Next, a line, parallel to the microperfusion system calibration curve III, is extended across to curve II (the 'calibration curve' for the isolated loop of Henle and distal nephron) at point C, which is the corresponding intratubular pressure achieved when the loop was being perfused at a known rate by the pump alone. The corresponding flow rate is then given by dropping the perpendicular to D on the abscissa, 10.8 nl min^{-1}. Thus the actual loop inflow at point A was 10.8 nl min^{-1} of which the pump was contributing 5 nl min^{-1} and the native late proximal flow $10.8 - 5.0 = 5.8$ nl min^{-1}. It now remains to calculate the corresponding early proximal flow rate, which can only be done indirectly by estimating the hypothetical late proximal 'TF/P$_{inulin}$'. This is possible since there is one condition under which both late and early proximal flow rates are known: namely zero loop of Henle flow. The corresponding early proximal flow rate is the zero loop flow value taken from the curve in Figure 4.2C — the open loop feedback curve (33 nl min^{-1}); the late proximal flow is assumed to be the pump collection rate in phase 1 at which all the fluid is being collected and intratubular pressure is zero (Figure 4.2B, curve 1, point E on the abscissa, 13 nl min^{-1}). The TF/P$_{inulin}$ in this instance is thus $33/13 = 2.54$. Now assuming that this ratio remains constant during feedback-induced changes of GFR (the condition of glomerulotubular balance), early proximal flow rate in the original example is simply the product of the native late proximal flow and this 'TF/P$_{inulin}$' ratio, i.e. $5.8 \times 2.54 = 14.7$ nl min^{-1}. Extending this analysis through the phase I curve thus allows the closed-loop feedback curve to be constructed.

The results from these experiments are summarised in Figure 4.3 and allow two major conclusions to be drawn. First, a striking feature of the late proximal pressure-flow curves in the free-flowing nephron (Figure 4.3A) is the plateau phase extending approximately ± 5 nl min^{-1} either side of the spontaneous free-flow late proximal flow rate (zero pump flow rate). That is, simulation of a change in proximal tubular reabsorption (compare also Figure 4.1) by infusing or withdrawing up to 5 nl min^{-1} reveals almost complete compensation by the nephron, such that intratubular pressure and, hence, distal delivery, remain practically unaltered. The second conclusion is drawn from a comparison (Figure 4.3C) of the open and closed feedback curves from phases II and I,

Figure 4.3: Summary of Results Gained with the Protocol Illustrated in Figure 4.2 (Häberle and Davis, 1982a). A. Relationship between late proximal pressure and pump flow rate in free-flowing nephrons (Phase I). B. Relationship between early proximal flow rate and loop of Henle perfusion rate in blocked proximal tubules in Phase II ('open loop' feedback curve). EPFR is expressed as a percentage of the value at zero loop perfusion. The dotted line is the regression line C. The relationship between early proximal flow rate and loop of Henle inflow in free-flowing nephrons ('closed loop' feedback curve), derived from the plateau phase of the pressure flow curves from Phase I (Figures 4.2B and 4.3A). The closed circles indicate the naturally occurring EPFR and loop of Henle inflow. The dotted line is the open-loop feedback curve from Figure 4.3B

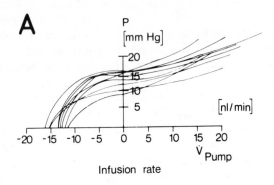

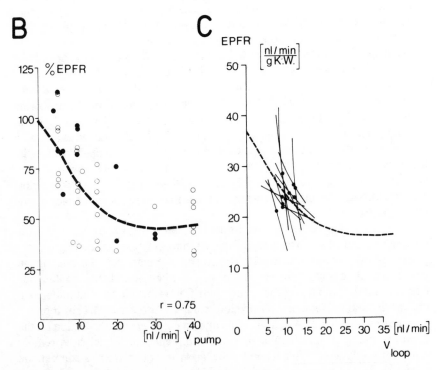

From Häberle and Davis (1982a), with permission

respectively. The open-loop data are shown in Figure 4.3B, together with the calculated regression line representing the open-loop feedback curve. This line is reproduced in Figure 4.3C for comparison with the closed-loop curves. The latter, drawn from the plateau phase of the pressure-flow relationship in the free-flowing nephron as described above, represents the 'integrated' feedback response of early proximal flow to variations of loop of Henle inflow, since all mechanisms may interact freely. The spontaneously occurring early and late proximal flow rates in an individual nephron define the so-called 'operating point' of the feedback system. These points are indicated for the closed-loop curves in Figure 4.3C by the closed circles. Interestingly, when the loop of Henle is experimentally perfused at a rate corresponding to the spontaneous late proximal flow in the free-flowing nephron, an early proximal flow rate is found which is also similar to that occurring spontaneously. In other words, the closed-loop operating points lie on or close to the open-loop feedback curve. Although by no means conclusive, this finding is consistent with the view that the tubuloglomerular feedback mechanism is the main regulatory mechanism for control of filtration rate in the free-flowing nephron. Further support for this concept is the disappearance of the plateau phase from the pressure-flow curves under conditions in which the feedback is inhibited (see below).

Further inspection of Figure 4.3C reveals, however, that the slope of the majority of closed-loop feedback curves is considerably steeper than that of the tubuloglomerular feedback curve obtained under open-loop conditions. This may imply that glomerular filtration rate in the free-flowing nephron is more perfectly controlled by the various feedback mechanisms acting together than by the tubuloglomerular feedback mechanism operating alone under open-loop conditions. The explanation for this finding is not immediately apparent. One possible explanation may be found in the methods. Early proximal hydrostatic pressure during the open-loop measurements in which the tubular fluid is quantitatively collected may well be lower than that during the free-flow measurements. In view of the earlier discussion, one might speculate that a decreased intratubular pressure in some way reduces the sensitivity of the glomerular filtration process to the tubuloglomerular feedback signal.

Resetting of the Tubuloglomerular Feedback Mechanism During Chronic Volume Expansion

In rats chronically volume expanded by a high-salt diet, these systems appear to be much less effective (see Figures 4.4 and 4.6). This is concluded first from experiments employing a modified form of the conventional 'open-loop' protocol for investigation of the tubuloglomerular feedback mechanism, which show a humoral inhibition of the macula densa mechanism (Häberle and

Davis, 1984). Secondly, studies using the 'closed loop' or pressure-flow protocol as described previously not only confirm the above but also reveal an additional alteration in the characteristics of the filtration mechanism. These two groups of experiments and their interpretation are the substance of this section.

Tubuloglomerular Resetting: Open Loop Studies

That the resetting of the macula densa mechanism apparently results from the appearance of an inhibitory principle in tubular fluid is shown by experiments (Häberle and Davis, 1984) summarised in Figure 4.4. In rats fed a high-salt diet (10 g NaCl per 100 g food) for two weeks, plasma volume increased from 4.7 ± 0.8 to 6.2 ± 0.6 ml per 100 g body weight (Häberle and Davis, 1982b). Tubuloglomerular feedback response was assessed in control and in salt-loaded rats by measuring early proximal flow rate during experimental loop of Henle perfusion at rates of 0, 10 or 40 nl min^{-1}. Loop perfusion fluids were either Ringer's solution or late proximal tubular fluid, harvested immediately before and by means of a microperfusion-suction pump, from both volume-expanded and control rats. In the chronically salt-loaded rats (Figure 4.4, left-hand panel), loop perfusion with homologous tubular fluid elicited no significant tubuloglomerular feedback response. Perfusion with tubular fluid from control rats or with Ringer's solution, however, elicited a response similar to that seen in the control animals (Figure 4.4, right-hand panel). Conversely, loop perfusion with tubular fluid from high-salt rats in control animals resulted in a resetting of the tubuloglomerular feedback response in a similar manner to that seen in the volume-expanded rats. Thus, first, the feedback response to the two different tubular fluids is different, and the same difference is seen in both groups of rats. This implies that the high salt intake has changed the composition of the tubular fluid, but not those characteristics of the juxtaglomerular apparatus which determine the tubuloglomerular feedback response under open-loop conditions (compare also Schnermann *et al.*, 1975, 1979; Mason *et al.*, 1979). Secondly, since the feedback response to the high-salt tubular fluid differs from those to both control tubular fluid and Ringer's solution, whereas the latter two are similar to each other, it may be inferred that the chronic high-salt diet has induced the appearance of a principle in the tubular fluid which reversibly inhibits the mediation of the feedback response by the juxtaglomerular apparatus from the macula densa site.

Interestingly enough, this principle was not detectable during comparable, but acute, expansion of plasma and extracellular volume by iso-oncotic plasma and Ringer's infusion (Davis *et al.*, 1984). The results of these experiments, employing a protocol similar to that just described, are shown in Figure 4.5. It is obvious that tubular fluid from both normal and volume-expanded rats elicits similar feedback responses in each group of rats, implying that the fluids do not differ in their composition (as far as the presence

Figure 4.4: The Response of Early Proximal Flow Rate (EPF) to Loop of Henle Perfusion in Rats Fed either a High-salt Diet (Left-hand Panel) or a Control, Low-salt Diet (Right-hand Panel). Loops of Henle were perfused with either tubular fluid, previously harvested from high-salt rats (●) or low-salt rats (○), or with Ringer's solution (Δ). EPF is expressed as a percentage of the value at zero loop perfusion

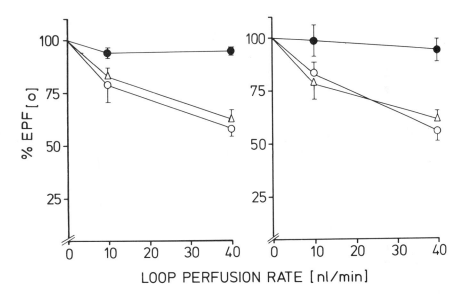

HIGH SALT RATS   LOW SALT RATS

● HIGH SALT TUBULAR FLUID
○ LOW SALT TUBULAR FLUID
Δ RINGER'S SOLUTION

From Häberle and Davis (1984)

of an inhibitor is concerned). On the other hand, the response to both fluids appears to be modestly attenuated in the volume-expanded rats, compared with the control rats. This apparent difference between the two groups of rats implies that acute volume expansion, in contrast to chronic volume expansion, may indeed alter some of those properties of the juxtaglomerular apparatus determining the feedback response. A possible explanation for the attenuated response is a fall in plasma protein concentration in some of the volume-expanded rats, despite the expansion with iso-oncotic plasma. Colloid osmotic pressure variations have been reported to exert a strong modifying influence on the tubuloglomerular feedback mechanism (Persson *et al.*, 1979).

Figure 4.5: The Response of Early Proximal Flow Rate (EPF) to Loop of Henle Perfusion in Rats Acutely Volume Expanded with Iso-oncotic Ringer's Solution (Right-hand Panel) and in Control Rats (Left-hand Panel). Loops of Henle were perfused wtih tubular fluid previously harvested from the control or acutely volume-expanded rats. EPF is expressed as a percentage of the value at zero loop perfusion. The closed circles (●) indicate loop perfusion with the homologous tubular fluid, open circles (○) with the heterologous tubular fluid

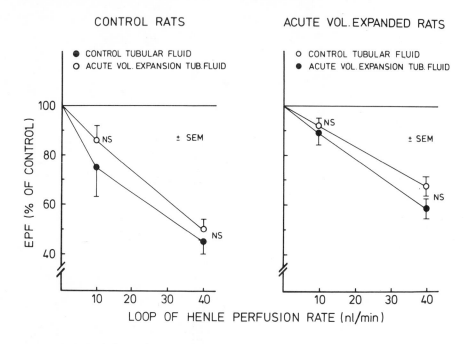

Resetting of Tubuloglomerular Feedback and Glomerular Vascular Characteristics. Closed Loop Studies

Inactivation of the tubuloglomerular feedback mechanism in chronic volume expansion should also be reflected in the pressure-flow relationships of free-flowing nephrons in which the loop of Henle inflow is experimentally varied as described in Figure 4.2 (the 'closed-loop' protocol). Figure 4.6 (lower panel) shows that in rats fed a high-salt diet (4 g NaCl per 100 g food) for two weeks, addition or withdrawal of late proximal tubular fluid is accompanied by continuous changes of intratubular pressure, i.e. the constant pressure or plateau phase seen in this relationship in normal animals (upper panel) is missing. In other words, variations in loop of Henle inflow are no longer compensated by appropriate variations in GFR (such that intratubular pressure remains constant), meaning that the feedback mechanism is inhibited.

These curves reveal two further characteristics of tubuloglomerular interaction during chronic volume expansion. First, analysis of the curves by

Figure 4.6: Late Proximal Pressure Flow Curves Obtained with the Protocol Described in Figure 4.2. Upper panel: control animals (from Figure 4.3B). Lower panel: curves from animals fed a high-salt diet for two weeks

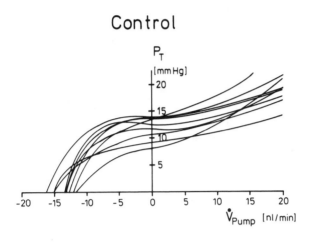

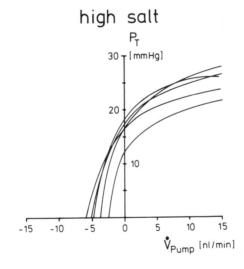

Upper panel from Häberle and Davis (1982a)

the method described for Figure 4.2 shows that late proximal delivery rates remain constant, or even tend to fall, when loop of Henle inflow and hence intratubular pressure are reduced by tubular fluid withdrawal. Secondly, the late proximal delivery rates at zero intratubular pressure (and, consequently, zero loop of Henle flow, in turn meaning interruption of the feedback loop, i.e. 'open' loop) are considerably lower in the volume-expanded rats than in the normal rats. In contrast, with the loop closed, late proximal flow rates are comparable in both groups of animals. Since the proximal tubular fractional reabsorption of the glomerular filtrate in chronically salt-loaded rats is either the same or reduced compared with normal rats (Wright *et al.*, 1969; Willis *et al.*, 1972; Sonnenberg, 1973; Kaufmann *et al.*, 1976), the relative constancy of late proximal delivery in closed-loop conditions and the lower late proximal flow in open-loop conditions probably reflect similar differences in GFR between the volume-expanded and normal animals. A possible explanation for these findings is that the high salt intake, besides the induction of a principle inhibiting the feedback mechanism, also induces a mechanism which preserves the ability of the glomerulus to maintain glomerular filtration rate constant in the face of alterations in intratubular pressure, as described by Seiller and Gertz (1977) for normal rats. In other words, glomerular dynamics have apparently been changed in such a manner as to replace the throttling effect of the tubuloglomerular feedback mechanism by some glomerular mechanism keeping GFR at a 'normal' level. Such an interpretation is consistent with other observations in chronically salt-loaded rats. In normal rats, the nephron filtration rate determined by quantitative collection from the proximal tubule is higher than that determined by quantitative collection from the distal tubule of the same nephron (for literature see Ploth *et al.*, 1978; Wright and Briggs, 1979; Schnermann *et al.*, 1984), as might be expected from the elimination of the tubuloglomerular feedback signal during the proximal collection (i.e. loop of Henle flow is prevented). This filtration rate difference between proximal and distal collections is not seen in chronically salt-loaded animals, indicating that the tubuloglomerular feedback mechanism is no longer operating (Dev *et al.*, 1974; Kaufmann *et al.*, 1976; Moore *et al.*, 1979). Furthermore, at comparable blood pressure, nephron filtration rates in chronically salt-loaded rats are closer to those measured distally in normal rats (Dev *et al.*, 1974), and indeed whole kidney GFR is only marginally increased during chronic salt loading (Reinhardt and Behrenbeck, 1967; Wright *et al.*, 1969; Willis *et al.*, 1972; Sonnenberg, 1973; Davis *et al.*, 1974; Dev *et al.*, 1974; Marchand *et al.*, 1977; Schor *et al.*, 1980; Häberle and Davis, 1982b). It must be emphasised that this is not true for acute volume expansion in which plasma protein concentration falls (for literature see Earley and Schrier, 1973). That the filtration rate fails to rise substantially in chronic volume expansion, as might be expected if the feedback mechanism were totally inhibited, could be explained if some other mechanism were simultaneously induced, presumably glomerular in nature, keeping GFR 'normal'.

That this additional mechanism is probably glomerular is suggested by two further observations. First, a high salt intake is accompanied by a greater rise in renal blood flow than in glomerular filtration rate so that filtration fraction falls (Marchand *et al.*, 1977). If it is assumed that the filtration coefficient K_f remains constant, the above findings would imply that the mean effective filtration pressure and renal vascular resistance had fallen, presumably as the result of decreased efferent arteriolar vascular resistance. Secondly, in a study (Schor *et al.*,1980) in which glomerular filtration dynamics of single nephrons in mildly salt-loaded and salt-deprived rats were compared, glomerular capillary pressure and K_f in the salt-loaded group were substantially decreased in comparison to the values in the salt-deprived group. Additionally, efferent arteriolar resistance was proportionately more reduced than that of the afferent arteriole. Consequently, filtration pressure equilibrium was probably achieved in the salt-loaded group, which may well explain the fact that glomerular filtration rate remained stable when intratubular hydrostatic pressure was altered in the absence of an operating tubuloglomerular feedback mechanism.

The mechanisms underlying the alterations of the glomerular vascular characteristics are not known. Since, however, in the study of Schor *et al.*, (1980), the effects of the increased salt intake on glomerular filtration dynamics are paralleled by decreases of the prostaglandin and renin activities in the region of the glomerular vascular pole (Sraer *et al.*, 1982; DeRouffignac *et al.*, 1974; Davila *et al.*, 1978; Gillies and Morgan, 1978); and, further, since the activation of the tubuloglomerular feedback mechanism is believed to reduce the rate of glomerular filtration by a stimulation of the *local* angiotensin II formation (Ploth and Roy, 1982), one could speculate that the inability of salt-loaded rats to increase glomerular filtration, after humoral inhibition of the tubuloglomerular feedback mechanism, to levels comparable with those in normal rats under open-loop conditions may result from the decrease of prostaglandin activity. When the tubuloglomerular feedback mechanism under these circumstances is nevertheless activated by experimental loop of Henle perfusion with Ringer's solution, less angiotensin II would be needed to induce a vasoconstriction adequate to reduce glomerular filtration to a similar extent to that in salt-deprived animals, and hence, despite the reduced renin activity during high salt intake, similar feedback responses can be achieved.

Summary and Future Directions

The experiments described in the foregoing provide evidence that the kidney is able to maintain a stable glomerular filtration rate in the face of intratubular hydrostatic pressure changes (for example due to altered fluid reabsorption) in both normal and chronically salt-loaded animals. The mechanisms underlying this regulation are not known, but some of the observations point to autoregulatory characteristics within the vascular elements of the glomerulus.

In addition to this mechanism, the kidney possesses a mechanism for control of the distal tubular salt and fluid delivery which is apparently switched off during chronic high salt intake by an inhibitor present in the tubular fluid. The mechanism itself appears to operate normally when stimulated with artificial solutions or tubular fluid from normal animals. This mechanism appears to be able to compensate for proximal tubular fluid reabsorption changes by appropriate changes of glomerular filtration rate at practically constant intratubular hydrostatic pressure, and is certainly involved in the maintenance of autoregulation of glomerular filtration and renal blood flow.

Two problems would seem especially worthy of future investigations. First, during normal salt intake, glomerular filtration and renal blood flow are almost perfectly autoregulated when the tubuloglomerular feedback mechanism is operating. When analysed under open-loop conditions, however, the slope of the tubuloglomerular feedback curve is too flat to explain such a perfect regulation. Two possibilities might be taken into consideration: namely, whether or not the tubuloglomerular feedback mechanism affects the autoregulatory responsiveness of the glomerular vascular elements, and whether or not the sensititivy of the tubuloglomerular feedback mechanism is considerably greater in the 'operating mode' than is suggested by analysis under 'open loop' conditions. The second problem is that the mechanisms responsible for the autoregulation of renal blood flow and glomerular filtration rate, in the presence or absence of a functioning tubuloglomerular feedback mechanism, and indeed the exact nature of the effector mechanism of the tubuloglomerular feedback on glomerular filtration are still obscure. It would appear that these phenomena are related to a complex interaction of vasoconstrictory and vasodilatory substances in the juxtaglomerular apparatus (Beierwaltes *et al.*, 1980) which may be released by such stimuli as hydrostatic (Davis and Freeman, 1976) or electrochemical gradients (Wright *et al.*, 1982). It will be the precise determination of the specific stimuli for release of these substances, as well as the clarification of the interaction between the formation and release of these vasoconstrictory and vasodilatory agents that might finally provide the explanation for the phenomenon of renal autoregulation of glomerular filtration and distal tubular fluid delivery rate.

Notes

1. Normal rats eat some 2-3 mmol Na day^{-1} when fed an Altromin Standard diet, containing 0.1 mmol Na g^{-1} food, and the minimum daily requirement is in the order of 1 mmol (Cuthbertson, 1957). The 'salt-loaded' rats in this study received some 4.8 mmol Na day^{-1}, for body weights of 220-340 g, and thus the resetting or inhibition of the tubuloglomerular feedback mechanism was probably considerably less than that expected in such studies as that of Dev *et al.* (1974).

2. In this study, as in all other studies from this laboratory dealing with glomerular filtration dynamics, glomerular capillary pressure, intratubular hydrostatic pressure and nephron filtration fraction were measured in free-flowing nephrons, i.e. with the tubuloglomerular feedback mechanism

operating. Nephron filtration rates, on the other hand, were measured by quantitative proximal tubular fluid collection, i.e. with the macula densa feedback signal abolished by the blocked loop of Henle flow. Since glomerular blood flow (calculated from filtration fraction and nephron filtration rate) is required, along with the pressure gradients, to calculate the filtration coefficient and the glomerular arteriolar resistance, it is apparent that the resistances will be underestimated and the filtration coefficient overestimated compared with the true values during free flow. Furthermore, since, with the exception of one study from the same laboratory (Ichikawa, 1982a), elimination of the tubuloglomerular feedback signal at the macula densa has been shown to result in an increase in glomerular capillary pressure and filtration coefficient (Bell *et al.*, 1984; Briggs, 1984; Persson *et al.*, 1984), the resistances and filtration coefficients determined using the procedure outlined above also do not reflect the actual state of glomerular dynamics under these open-loop conditions.

Appendix

In this analysis two mathematical models of renal function are combined, and this allows, for the first time, quantitative predictions of the interactions between filtration rate, proximal tubular pressure and fluid reabsorption. The first model is that of the filtration process (Deen *et al.*, 1972), in which proximal tubular pressure appears as one of the filtration determinants. The second is a new model which permits quantitative estimation of the effect of variations in proximal fluid reabsorption on proximal tubular pressure (Figure 4.7), and hence, by combination with the filtration model, on filtration rate. A full description of this model is beyond the scope of this article and only the briefest of outlines can be given here.

In essence, the model is described by equation 1:

$$P_{\text{prox}} = P_{\text{dist}} + \text{f}\,(\dot{V}_0, \text{TF/P}_{\text{In}}^{\text{prox}}, \text{TF/P}_{\text{In}}^{\text{dist}}, r_{\text{prox}}, r_{\text{Henle}}, L_{\text{prox}}, L_{\text{Henle}}, T_{\text{prox}})\,(1)$$

That is, proximal hydrostatic pressure (P_{prox}) is assumed to be the sum of the distal tubular hydrostatic pressure (P_{dist}) and a proximal component which is, in turn, a complex function of intratubular flow rate, fluid reabsorption (defined explicitly below) and tubular geometry. The expressions describing flow profiles in a reabsorbing system of tubules were first derived by Bauer (1976) from the Navier-Stokes equations (equations 2, 3) and the equation of continuity (equation 4).

$$\frac{1}{\eta}\,\frac{\partial p}{\partial r} = \frac{\partial^2 u}{\partial r^2} + \frac{1}{r}\,\frac{\partial u}{\partial r} - \frac{u}{r^2} + \frac{\partial^2 u}{\partial z^2} \qquad (2)$$

Figure 4.7: The Parameters of Nephron Function Required for the Prediction of the Influence of Changes in Proximal Tubular Reabsorption on Proximal Tubular Pressure using the Model of Proximal Tubular Function of Bauer (1976). P_t: Proximal tubular pressure (superscripts 1 and 2 indicate early and late sites, respectively); r: radius; U: reabsorption rate (subscripts 1 and 2 indicate proximal tubule and loops of Henle, respectively)

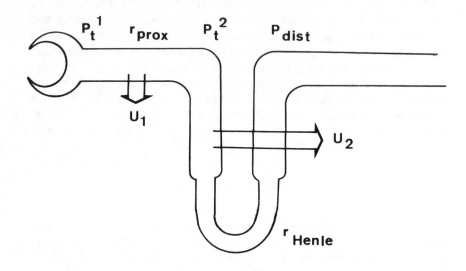

$$\frac{1}{\eta}\frac{p}{\partial z} = \frac{\partial^2 w}{\partial r^2} + \frac{1}{r}\frac{\partial w}{\partial r} + \frac{\partial^2 w}{\partial z^2} \tag{3}$$

$$\frac{\partial u}{\partial r} + \frac{u}{r} + \frac{\partial w}{\partial z} = 0 \tag{4}$$

The symbols appearing in these and following equations are defined as follows: p: local hydrostatic pressure; r: the radial coordinate ($0 \leq r \leq r_{\text{prox}}$); z: the axial coordinate ($0 \leq z \leq L_{\text{prox}}$); u, w: axial and radial flow velocities, respectively; η: viscosity, calculated from the Reynold's number, which was assumed to be 0.02.

The explicit definitions for proximal tubular reabsorption (U_1), axial tubular volume flow rate ($\dot{V}_z$), loop of Henle reabsorption (U_2) and proximal tubular radius (r_{prox}) are as follows:

$$U_1 = \dot{V}_0 - \dot{V}_z; (z = L_{\text{prox}}); \ \dot{V}_z = \dot{V}_0 / (\text{TF}/p_{\text{In}}^{\text{prox}}) \tag{5}$$

$$\dot{V}_z = \dot{V}_0 \, e^{-\lambda x}; -\lambda = (\ln P/\text{TF}_{\text{In}}^{\text{prox}})/L_{\text{prox}} \tag{6}$$

$$U_2 = \dot{V}_0 \, (\text{TF}/P_{\text{In}}^{\text{dist}} - \text{TF}/P_{\text{In}}^{\text{prox}}) \tag{7}$$

$$r_{prox} = \sqrt{\frac{\dot{V}_0 (1 - P/TF^{prox}_{In} \times T}{\ln TF/P^{prox}_{In} \times \pi \times L_{prox}}} \qquad (8)$$

The remaining definitions, assumed values and assumptions are:

P_{dist} assumed to remain constant at 7 mmHg

TF/P^{dist}_{In} the early distal tubular fluid to plasma inulin concentration ratio, assumed to remain constant at 5.0

$\dot{V}_0$ glomerular filtration rate, given literature values as shown in Figure 4.1 or allowed to vary between 12 and 48 nl min^{-1} (see below)

TF/P^{prox}_{In} the proximal tubular fluid to plasma inulin concentration ratio, either given the value 2.5, or allowed to vary between 1.5 and 3.0 (see below)

T_{prox} the proximal passage time, that is, the time for a segment of filtrate to pass through a proximal tubule of length L_{prox} and fractional fluid reabsorption$(1 - 1/TF/P^{prox}_{In})$, assumed to remain constant at 9.0 s

L_{prox} the proximal tubular length, assumed to be 0.5 cm

L_{Henle} the length of the loop of Henle, assumed to be 2×0.25 cm

r_{prox} the proximal tubular radius was calculated from an equation of Gertz and Boylan (1973), using the values listed above. It was subsequently assumed that r_{prox} remains constant along the length of the proximal tubule

r_{Henle} the radius of the loop of Henle had to be determined indirectly using the following procedure. Since P_{prox} and the other parameters necessary for the solutions to equations 1–8 were known for the literature examples in Figure 4.1, r_{Henle} could be calculated by numeric solution of these equations. From the three values thus obtained and from late proximal flow rate and loop of Henle reabsorption rates, values for r_{Henle} could be interpolated for the other hydrodynamic conditions discussed in Figure 4.1. The validity of the method for the calculation of r_{Henle}, and, indeed, the plausibility of the entire model were also checked by an additional calculation (see Figure 4.8). The above function, together with the variables and values as defined above, were used to compute proximal hydrostatic pressure for all possible combinations of $\dot{V}_0$ (varying between 12 and 48 nl min^{-1}), TF/P^{Prox}_{In} (varying between 1.5 and 3), and T_{prox} (between 7 and 14 s). From these values, the 95 per cent confidence limits for the relationship of P_{prox} as a function of $\dot{V}_0$ were calculated and compared with the data published for normal rats by Brenner and collaborators up to 1978. Figure 4.8 shows good consistency between the calculated range and the real data, implying that the totality of the above assumptions yields reasonable predictions.

Figure 4.8: Relationship between Nephron Filtration Rate (SNGFR) and Proximal Tubular Pressure (P_{tub}). The lines indicate the 95 per cent confidence limits for the relationship calculated from the model described in the text. The points are data from normal rats taken from the literature

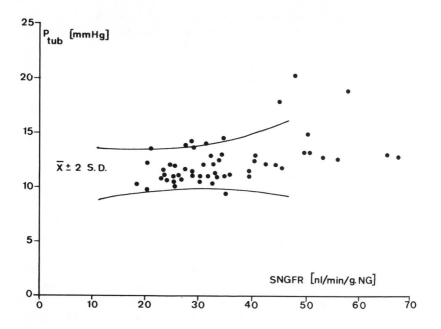

References

Andreucci, V.E., Herrera-Acosta, J., Rector, F.C. and Seldin, D.W. (1971a) 'Effective Glomerular Filtration Pressure and Single Nephron Glomerular Filtration Rate during Hydropenia, Elevated Ureteral Pressure and Acute Volume Expansion with Isolated Saline'. *J. Clin. Invest.*, *50*, 2230–4

Andreucci, V.E., Herrera-Acosta, J., Rector, F.C. and Seldin, D.W. (1971b) 'Measurement of Single-nephron Glomerular Filtration Rate by Micropuncture: Analysis of Error', *Am. J. Physiol.*, *221*, 1551–9

Bauer, H.F. (1976) 'Strömung und Resorption im renalen Tubulus', *Biomed. Tech.*, *21*, 10

Baylis, C. and Brenner, B.M. (1978) 'The Physiologic Determinants of Glomerular Ultrafiltration', *Rev. Physiol. Biochem. Pharmacol.*, *80*, 1–46

Beierwaltes, W.M., Schryver, S., Olsen, P., and Romero, J.C. (1980), 'Interaction of the Prostaglandin and Renin Angiotensin Systems in Isolated Rat Glomeruli', *Am. J. Physiol.*, *239*, F602–8

Bell, P.D., Reddington, M., Ploth, D. and Navar, LG. (1984) 'Tubuloglomerular Feedback-mediated Decreases in Glomerular Pressure in Munich-Wistar Rats', *Am. J. Physiol.*,

247, F877–80

Blantz, R.C. (1974) 'Effect of Mannitol upon Glomerular Ultrafiltration in the Hydropenic Rat', *J. Clin. Invest.*, *54*, 1135–43

Blantz, R.C. and Pelayo, J.C. (1984) 'A Functional Role for the Tubuloglomerular Feedback Mechanism', *Kidney Int.*, *25*, 739–46

Brenner, B.M., Daugharty, T.M., Ueki, I.F., and Troy, J.L. (1971) 'Quantitative Assessment of Proximal Tubule Function in Single Nephrons of the Rat Kidney', *Am. J. Physiol.*, *220*, 2058–67

Briggs, J. (1984) 'Effect of Loop of Henle Flow Rate on Glomerular Capillary Pressure', *Renal Physiol.*, *7*, 311–20

Cuthbertson, W.F.J. (1957) 'The Nutritional Requirements of Rats and Mice', *LAB*, collected papers, 5, 27

Davila, D., Davila, T., Oliw, E. and Anggard, E. (1978) 'The Influence of Dietary Sodium on Urinary Prostaglandin Excretion', *Acta Physiol. Scand.*, *103*, 100–116

Davis, J.M., Brechtelsbauer, H., Prucksunand, P., Weigl, J., Schnermann, J., and Kramer, K. (1974) 'Relationship between Salt Loading and Distribution of Nephron Filtration Rates in the Dog', *Pflügers Arch.*, *350*, 259–72

Davis, J.M., Takabatake, T. and Häberle, D.A. (1984) 'Tubuloglomerular Feedback Resetting in Acute Volume Expansion in Rats', *Pflügers Arch.*, Suppl. *400*, R21

Davis, J.O. and Freeman, R.H. (1976) 'Mechanisms Regulating Renin Release', *Physiol. Rev.*, *56*, 1–56

Deen, W., Robertson, C.R. and Brenner, B.M. (1972) 'A Model of Glomerular Ultrafiltration in the Rat', *Am. J. Physiol.*, *223*, 1178–83

DeRouffignac, C. Bonvalet, J.P. and Menard, J. (1974) 'Renin Content in Superficial and Deep Glomeruli of Normal and Salt-loaded Rats', *Am. J. Physiol.*, *226*, 150–4

Dev, B., Drescher, C. and Schnermann, J. (1974) 'Resetting Tubuloglomerular Feedback Sensitivity by Dietary Salt Intake', *Pflügers Arch.*, *346*, 263–77

Earley L.E. and Schrier, R.W. (1973) 'Intrarenal Control of Sodium Excretion by Hemodynamic and Physical Factors', in J. Orloff and R.W. Berliner (eds), *Handbook of Physiology* Section 8, American Physiological Society, Washington DC, pp. 721–62

Gertz, K.H. and Boylan, J.W. (1973) Glomerulotubular Balance', in J. Orloff, and R.W. Berliner (eds), *Handbook of Physiology, section 8*, American Physiological Society, Washington DC, pp. 763–90

Gertz, K.H., Mangos, J.A., Braun, G. and Pagel, H.D. (1966) 'Pressure in the Glomerular Capillaries of the Rat Kidney and its Relation to Arterial Blood Pressure', *Pflügers Arch.*, *288*, 369–74

Gillies, A. and Morgan, T. (1978) 'Renin Content of Individual Juxtaglomerular Apparatuses and the Effect of Diet, Changes in Nephron Flow Rate and *in vitro* Acidification on the Renin Content', *Pflügers Arch.*, *375*, 105–6

Goormaghtigh, N. (1945) 'Facts in Favour of an Endocrine Function of the Renal Arterioles', *J. Pathol. Bacteriol.*, *57*, 392–3

Gottschalk, C.W. and Mylle, M. (1956) 'Micropuncture Studies of Pressures in Proximal Tubules and Peritubular Capillaries of the Rat Kidney and their Relation to the Ureteral and Renal Venous Pressure', *Am. J. Physiol.*, *185*, 430–9

Gottschalk, C.W. and Mylle, M (1957) 'Micropuncture Study of Pressures in Proximal and Distal Tubules and Peritubular Capillaries of the Rat Kidney during Osmotic Diuresis'. *Am. J. Physiol.*, *189*, 323–8

Häberle, D.A. and Davis, J.M. (1982a) 'Interrelationship between Proximal Tubular Hydrodynamics and Tubuloglomerular Feedback in the Rat Kidney', *Kidney Int.*, *22*, Suppl. 12, S193–7

Häberle, D.A. and Davis, J.M. (1982b) 'Chronic Salt Loading: Effects on Plasma Volume and Regulation of Glomerular Filtration Rate in Wistar Rats', *Klin. Wochenschr.*, *60*, 1245–8

Häberle, D.A. and Davis, J.M. (1984) 'Resetting of Tubuloglomerular Feedback: Evidence for a Humoral Factor in Tubular Fluid', *Am. J. Physiol.*, *246*, F495–500

Hartupee, D.A., Gillies, A.H.B. and Knox, F.G. (1981) 'Measurement of Nephron Filtration in the Dog: Role of Proximal Intratubular Pressure', *Am. J. Physiol.*, *241*, F238–43

Ichikawa, I. (1982a) 'Evidence for Altered Glomerular Hemodynamics during Acute Nephron Obstruction', *Am. J. Physiol.*, *242*, F580–5

Ichikawa, I. (1982b) 'Direct Analysis of the Effector Mechanism of the Tubuloglomerular

Feedback System', *Am. J. Physiol.*, *243*, F447–55

Ichikawa, I. and Brenner, B.M. (1977) 'Evidence for Glomerular Actions of ADH and Dibutyryl cyclic AMP in the Rat', *Am. J. Physiol.*, *233*, F102–17

Kaufmann, J.S., Hamburger, R.J. and Flamenbaum, W. (1976) 'Tubuloglomerular Feedback: Effect of Dietary NaCl Intake', *Am. J. Physiol.*, *231*, 1744–9

Krause, H.H., Dume, T., Koch, K.M. and Ochwadt, B. (1967) 'Intratubulärer Druck, glomerulärer capillardruck und glomerulumfilträt nach Furosemid und Hydrochlorothiazid', *Pflügers Arch.*, *295*, 80–9

Lohfert, H., Lichtenstein, T.,Butz, M. and Hierholzer, K. (1971) 'Continuous Measurement of Renal Intratubular Pressures with Combined Pressure Transducer Microperfusion System', *Pflügers Arch.*, *327*, 191–202

Marchand, G.R., Burke, T., Haas, J.A., Romero, J.C. and Knox, F.G. (1977) 'Regulation of Filtration Rate in Sodium-depleted and -expanded Dogs', *Am. J. Physiol.*, *232*, F325–8

Mason, J., Kain, H., Shiigai, T. and Welsch, J. (1979) 'The Early Phase of Experimental Acute Renal Failure, V. The Influence of Suppressing Renin Angiotensin System', *Pflügers Arch.*, *380*, 233–43

Moore, L.C. (1984) 'Tubuloglomerular Feedback and SNGF Autoregulation in the Rat', *Am. J. Physiol.*, *247*, F267–76

Moore, L.C., Schnermann, J. and Yarimizu, S. (1979) 'Feedback Mediation of SNGFR Autoregulation in Hydropenic and DOCA- and Salt-loaded Rats', *Am. J. Physiol.*, *237*, F63

Navar, L.G. (1978) 'The Regulation of Glomerular Filtration Rate in Mammalian Kidneys', in T. Andreoli, J.E. Hoffman and D.D. Fanestil (eds), *Physiology of Membrane Disorders*, Plenum, New York, pp. 593–627

Navar, L.G., Ploth, D.W. and Bell, P.D. (1980) 'Distal Tubular Feedback Control of Renal Haemodynamics and Autoregulation', *Ann. Rev. Physiol.*, *42*, 557

Persson, A.E. Müller-Suur, R. and Selén, G. (1979) 'Capillary Oncotic Pressure as a Modifier for Tubuloglomerular Feedback', *Am. J. Physiol.*, *236*, F97–102

Persson, A.E., Gushwa, L.C. and Blantz, R.C. (1984) 'Feedback Pressure Flow Response in Normal and Angiotensin-Prostaglandin Blocked Rats', *Am. J. Physiol.*, *247*, F925–31

Ploth, D.W. and Roy, R.N. (1982) 'Renin-Angiotensin Influence on Tubuloglomerular Feedback Activity in the Rat', *Kidney Int.*, *22*, Suppl. 12, S114–21

Ploth, D.W., Dahlheim, H., Schmidmeier, E., Hermle, M. and Schnermann, J. (1978) 'Tubuloglomerular Feedback and Autoregulation of Glomerular Filtration Rate in Wistar–Kyoto Spontaneously Hypertensive Rats', *Pflügers Arch.*, *375*, 261–7

Reinhardt, H.W. and Behrenbeck, D.W. (1967) 'Untersuchungen an wachen Hunden über die Einstellung der Natriumbilanz', *Pflügers Arch.*, *295*, 266–79

Schnermann, J., Wright, F.S., Davis, J.M., Stackelberg, W.F. and Grill, G. (1970) 'Regulation of Superficial Nephron Filtration Rate by Tubuloglomerular Feedback', *Pflügers Arch.*, *318*, 147–75

Schnermann, J., Hermle, M., Schmidmeier, E. and Dahlheim, H. (1975) 'Impaired Potency for Feedback Regulation of Glomerular Filtration Rate in DOCA Escaped Rats', *Pflügers Arch.*, *358*, 325–34

Schnermann, J., Schubert, G., Hermle, M., Herbst, R., Stowe, N.T., Yarimizu, S. and Weber, P.C. (1979) 'The Effect of Inhibition of Prostaglandin Synthesis on Tubuloglomerular Feedback in the Rat Kidney', *Pflügers Arch.*, *379*, 269–79

Schnermann, J., Briggs, J., Kriz, W., Moore, L. and Wright, F.S. (1980) 'Control of Glomerular Vascular Resistance by the Tubuloglomerular Feedback Mechanism', in A. Leaf, G. Giebisch, L. Bolis and S. Gorini (eds), *Renal Pathophysiology. Recent Advances*, Raven Press, New York, pp. 165–82

Schnermann, J. and Briggs, J. (1982) 'Concentration-dependent Sodium Chloride Transport as the Signal in Feedback Control of Glomerular Filtration', *Kidney Int.*, *22*, Suppl. 12, S82–9

Schnermann, J., Briggs, J. and Weber, P.C. (1984) 'Tubuloglomerular Feedback, Prostaglandin and Angiotensin in the Regulation of Glomerular Filtration Rate', *Kidney Int.*, *25*, 52–64

Schor, N., Ichikawa, I. and Brenner, B.M. (1980) 'Glomerular Adaptations to Chronic Dietary Salt Restriction or Excess', *Am. J. Physiol.*, *238*, F428–36

Seiller, W. and Gertz, K.H. (1977) 'Single Nephron Filtration, Luminal Flow and Tubular Fluid Reabsorption along the Proximal Convolution and Pars Recta of the Rat Kidney as Influenced by Luminal Pressure Changes', *Pflügers Arch.*, *371*, 235–43

Sonnenberg, H. (1973) 'Proximal and Distal Tubular Function in Salt-deprived and in Salt-loaded Deoxycorticosterone Acetate-escaped Rats', *J. Clin. Invest.*, *52*, 263–72

Sraer, J., Siess, W., Moulonguet-Doleris, L., Oudinet, J.P., Dray, F. and Ardaillou, R. (1982) '*In vitro* Prostaglandin Synthesis by Various Rat Renal Preparations', *Biochim. Biophys. Acta*, *710*, 45–52

Steven, K. (1974) 'Influence of Nephron GFR on Proximal Reabsorption in Pentobarbital Anaesthetized Rats', *Kidney Int.*, *5*, 204–13

Steven, K. (1977) 'Glomerulotubular Balance in the Rat Kidney', *Acta Physiol. Scand. Suppl. 447*, 1–30

Thurau, K. and Schnermann, J. (1965) 'Die Natriumkonzentration an den Macula densa Zellen als regulierender Faktor für das Glomerulumfiltrat', *Klin. Wochenschr.*, *43*, 410–13

Willis, L.R., Schneider, E.G., Lynch, R.E. and Knox, F.G. (1972) 'Effect of Chronic Alteration of Sodium Balance on Reabsorption by Proximal Tubule of the Dog', *Am. J. Physiol.*, *223*, 34–9

Wright, F.S. and Briggs, J.P. (1979) 'Feedback Control of Glomerular Blood Flow, Pressure, and Filtration Rate', *Physiol. Rev.*, *59*, 958–1006

Wright, F.S., Knox, F.G., Howards, S.S. and Berliner, R.W. (1969) 'Reduced Sodium Reabsorption by Proximal Tubule of DOCA-escaped Dogs', *Am. J. Physiol.*, *216*, 869–75

Wright, F.S., Mandin, H. and Persson, A.E.G. (1982) 'Studies of the Sensing Mechanism in the Tubulo-glomerular Feedback Pathway', *Kidney Int.*, *22*, *Suppl. 12*, S90

5 RENAL PROSTAGLANDINS

C. J. Lote and J. Haylor

Introduction

The term 'prostaglandins' was coined in 1935 (von Euler, 1934, 1935) in the mistaken belief that the acidic lipid to which the name was given was derived from the prostate gland; it was almost 30 years after this 'christening' that the chemical formulae of prostaglandins (PG) E_1, E_2 and $F_{2\alpha}$ were described. However, there was a great deal of interest in the essential fatty acids in the 1930s, and Burr and Burr (1929, 1930) found that a deficiency state, in which renal degeneration occurred, could be induced in rats on a fat-free diet. In their remarkably percipient paper (1930), Burr and Burr stated 'certainly the arachidonic acid content of active tissues such as liver, pancreas, kidney, suprarenal and spleen is high, and it is natural to assume some important role for this highly unsaturated long chain acid'. As far as the kidney is concerned, it is only in the last 10 years or so that the role of arachidonic acid has become clearer.

Arachidonic acid is the precursor of renal prostaglandins (Figure 5.1). The nomenclature of prostaglandins and prostaglandin metabolites is based on the 20-carbon atom structure, prostanoic acid. They are classified by the functional groups of the cyclopentane ring, and also by the number of bonds in the side chain. Thus, PGE_2, has the ring substituents characteristic of E prostaglandins, and two double bonds in the side chain (Figure 5.1). Arachidonic acid is present in the diet (in animal tissues), and is also synthesised in the body from dietary linoleic acid (present in cereals) and dihomo-γ-linolenic acid (present in animal tissues).

Renal Prostaglandin Biosynthesis

Arachidonic acid is stored esterified in phospholipids and is released predominantly via hydrolysis by phospholipase A_2 (van den Bosch, 1980). The liberation of arachidonic acid is thought to be the rate-limiting step in prostaglandin synthesis. There are three possible routes for the metabolism of arachidonic acid within the kidney (Figure 5.2), but this chapter will concentrate on the cyclo-oxygenase pathway since relatively little is known of the importance of the mono-oxygenase and lipoxygenase routes in this organ. Once released, arachidonic acid can also be re-esterified back into phospholipid, an energy-dependent process requiring the availability of oxygen (Lands, 1979).

Figure 5.1: Molecular Structure of the Major Renal Prostaglandins and their Precursors

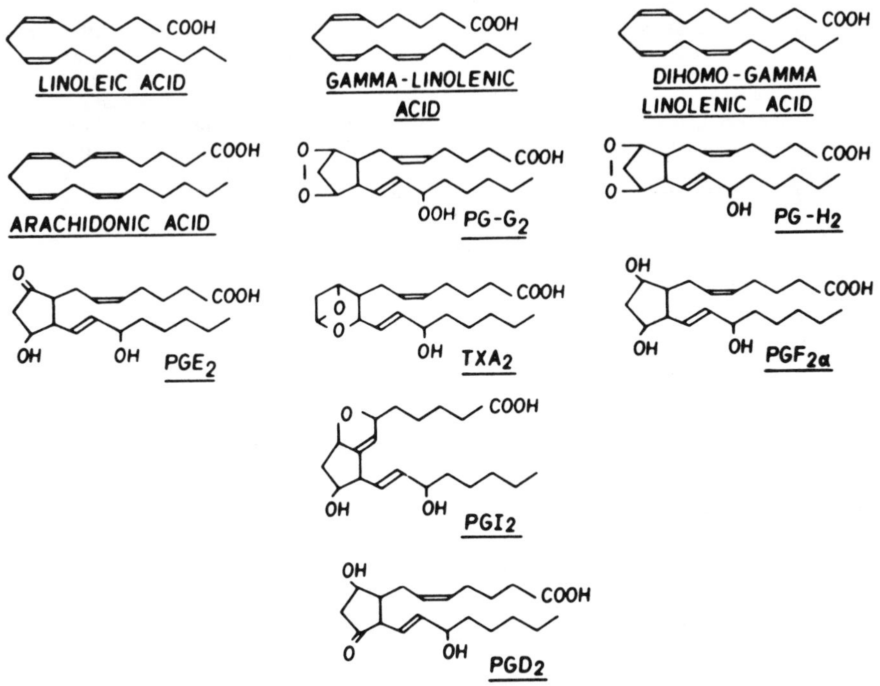

The liberation of arachidonic acid is potentially under hormonal control, its release being stimulated by vasopressin, bradykinin and angiotensin II, and inhibited by corticosteroids (Table 5.1). The hormonal stimulation of renal prostaglandin synthesis is a calcium-dependent process (Knapp *et al.*, 1977; Craven *et al.*, 1980; Zenser *et al.*, 1980) initiated by the activation of a Ca-calmodulin-sensitive phospholipase (Craven *et al.*, 1981). Studies with angiotensin II and vasopressin indicate that receptor activation may enhance calcium entry into cells through receptor-operated Ca-channels (Ausiello and Zusman, 1984) by stimulating the metabolism of phosphatidylinositol (Benabe *et al.*, 1982) through phospholipid methylation (Craven and De Rubertis, 1984). In contrast the inhibition of prostaglandin synthesis by corticosteroids (Gryglewski *et al.*, 1975; Hong and Levine, 1976) is due to the induction of an inhibitor of the activation of phospholipase A_2 (Flower and Blackwell, 1979; Hirata *et al.*, 1980). Such inhibitory activity has been described for two glycoproteins, lipomodulin and macrocortin (which may well be related to each other), in experiments performed mainly in leucocytes and the perfused lung (Flower, 1983). A similar process is thought to take place in the renal medulla (Russo-Marie *et al.*, 1983).

Arachidonic acid undergoes oxygenative cyclisation to form PGG_2, which is converted to PGH_2 by peroxidase activity. Although these endoperoxides

Figure 5.2: Routes of Arachidonic Acid Metabolism in the Kidney. Three main routes exist: to HETEs (hydroxyeicosatetraenoic acids), to HPETEs (hydroxyperoxyeicosatetraenoic acids) and, via the cyclo-oxygenase pathway, to PGE_2, $PGF_{2\alpha}$, PGD_2, PGI_2 and TXA_2. The lipoxygenase appears to be located primarily in the medulla. HPETEs inhibit the synthesis of PGI_2 (Moncada *et al.*, 1976; Ham *et al.*, 1979; Sraer *et al.*, 1982). The synthesis of HETEs is mainly cortical, via NADPH-dependent cytochrome P450 mono-oxygenase (Morrison and Pascoe, 1981; Oliw and Oates, 1981; Oliw *et al.*, 1981). It remains to be established whether lipoxygenase products have a role in the normal functioning of the kidney, as opposed to renal pathophysiology (Kuehl and Egan, 1980). The cyclo-oxygenase pathway is described in the text. TXA_2 may be important mainly in renal pathophysiology (Morrison *et al.*, 1977, 1978, 1981) rather than in the normal kidney

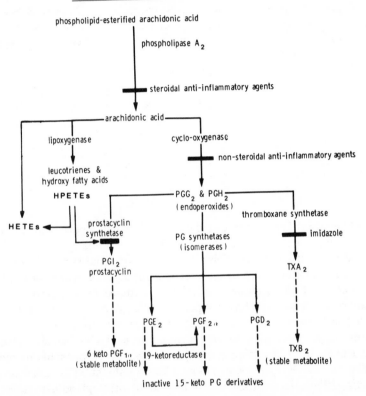

RENAL PROSTANOID SYNTHESIS

are chemically unstable, they do possess biological activity in their own right. The enzyme which may catalyse both reactions is generally termed 'cyclo-oxygenase'. However, it is strictly only a cyclo-oxygenase for the first reaction (arachidonic acid to PGG_2), and a better term for the enzyme may be endoperoxide synthetase (Yamamoto, 1983). Nevertheless, in accordance with common usage the term cyclo-oxygenase will be employed in this chapter. Prostaglandins are synthesised at several distinct sites in the kidney rather than in every cell type. Details of which arachidonate metabolites may

Table 5.1: Physiological and Pharmacological Influences on Renal Prostaglandin Synthesis. Conversion of phospholipid-esterified arachidonic acid to prostaglandins. *Note*: 25–50 per cent of released arachidonic acid is converted to prostaglandins (Needleman *et al.*, 1979; Schwarzman and Raz, 1979)

Conversion enhanced by:	*Conversion inhibited by:*
Kinins (Zusman and Keiser, 1977a)	Steroids (Zusman, 1980)
Angiotensin II, noradrenaline (Levine and Moskovitz, 1979)	
Hypertonic extracellular fluid (Danon *et al.*, 1978)	Hypotonic extracellular fluid (Danon *et al.*, 1978)
Low [K$^+$] in extracellular fluid (Zusman and Keiser, 1977b)	High [K$^+$] in extracellular fluid (Zusman and Keiser, 1977b)
	Steroidal anti-inflammatory agents (Lands and Rome, 1976)
	Mepacrine (Zusman, 1980; Vargraftig and Hai, 1972)

be produced in different renal cells are shown in Table 5.2; some of these points are still controversial. The control over the expression of the effects of arachidonate metabolites could occur at other stages in the reaction sequence, e.g. through the induction of prostaglandin-synthesising enzymes (Dunn *et al.*, 1983) or by a change in the number and/or function of membrane receptors (Limas and Limas, 1984).

In the medulla, the main sites of synthesis are the interstitial and the epithelial (collecting tubule) cells (Bohman, 1977; Zusman and Keiser, 1977a). Most reports suggest that the epithelial cells of the loop of Henle do not synthesise cyclo-oxygenase products, and although cyclo-oxygenase activity has been reported *in vitro* in the medullary thick ascending limb (Schlondorff *et al.*, 1982), Currie and Needleman (1984) have indicated that this may result from contamination by cells from the medullary collecting tubule. PGE$_2$ is thought to be the major prostaglandin synthesised in the renal medulla, although considerable amounts of PGF$_{2\alpha}$ are also produced. In the outer medulla, PGI$_2$ may be the major arachidonic acid metabolite (Sraer *et al.*, 1982).

In the cortex, the sites of synthesis include the arterioles, the glomeruli (epithelial and mesangial cells) and tubular elements (cortical collecting tubules). However, some disagreement has arisen as a result of difference in methodology of the *in vitro* techniques employed. For example, Sraer *et al.* (1983b) reported that in primary cultures of glomerular cells, the mesangial cells produced 10-fold more cyclo-oxygenase products than the epithelial cells. In cloned cells, however, this ratio appears to be reversed (Kreisberg *et al.*, 1982). In vascular elements, PGI$_2$ is the major product of arachidonic acid, and PGI$_2$ may be the main product in the cortex as a whole (Whorton *et al.*, 1978) although considerable amounts of PGE$_2$ and PGF$_{2\alpha}$ are also produced.

Table 5.2: Sites of Prostaglandin Synthesis within the Kidney

Site	Prostaglandins synthesised	References
Medulla		
interstitial cells	$PGE_2 > PGF_{2\alpha}$	Dunn *et al.* (1976)
collecting tubule	$PGE_2 > PGI_2 > PGD_2$	Grenier and Smith (1978)
thick ascending limb	$PGE_2, PGF_{2\alpha}$	Schlondorff *et al.* (1982)
Cortex		
glomerular epithelium	PGI_2, PGE_2	Kreisberg *et al.* (1982)
mesangial cells	$PGE_2 > TXB_2 > PGF_{2\alpha} > $ 6-keto $PGF_{1\alpha}$	Sraer *et al.* (1983b)
arterioles	$PGI_2 > PGF_{2\alpha} > PGE_2$	Terragno *et al.* (1978)
glomeruli	6-keto $PGF_{1\alpha}$, TXB_2, PGE_2, $PGF_{2\alpha}$	Folkert and Schlondorff (1977); Hassid *et al.* (1979); Sraer *et al.* (1979, 1982)

The glomerulus is also a site of lipoxygenase activity (Jim *et al.*, 1982; Sraer *et al.*, 1983a), and recently the leukotrienes C_4 and D_4, which were originally termed slow-reacting substance of anaphylaxis (SRS-A), have been detected in venous effluents of isolated perfused rat kidneys following stimulation with the calcium ionophore A 23187 (Pirotszky *et al.*, 1984).

In vivo, renal prostaglandin production was originally assessed either from excised tissue or from the concentration of prostaglandins in renal venous blood. Neither technique is suitable for the routine assessment of renal PG production, especially in man. The concentration of prostaglandins in peripheral plasma has also been employed, but due to prominent lung metabolism this measurement is unlikely to reflect altered renal synthesis.

Urinary Prostaglandin Excretion

Following the demonstration in the dog that two stimuli (arachidonic acid and angiotensin II), known to elevate renal PGE synthesis, could also increase urinary PGE excretion (Frolich *et al.*, 1975), the urinary excretion rate of PGE has been commonly employed as a quantitative index of prostaglandin synthesis *in vivo*. As a non-invasive technique, the measurement of PGE excretion presents many advantages, particularly in human studies. However, the possibility that changes in urinary PGE excretion do not always reflect altered renal synthesis must be considered, since, as a quantitative index, urinary PGE excretion has never been properly calibrated. For example, although Zambraski and Dunn (1980) found that exercise increased both renal venous concentration of PGE and its urinary excretion, Olsen (1981) was able to dissociate changes in papillary tissue levels of PGE from changes in urinary PGE excretion in experiments using the diuretic chlorazanil. In a recent quantitative experiment in the dog, the urinary fraction of total PGE output by the kidney was demonstrated to vary considerably, and urinary PGE excretion was therefore considered to give unreliable information concerning the synthetic rate of PGE in the kidney (Sejersted *et al.*, 1984). Important factors commonly ignored when PGE excretion is used to assess renal synthesis include the possibility that, following its synthesis, PGE is subject to metabolism and/or tubular transport prior to excretion in the urine.

Prostaglandin E excreted in the urine was originally thought to be derived from the kidney rather than the systemic circulation since, following intravenous injection in man, no whole labelled PGE_1 could be recovered in the urine (Granstrom, 1967). Glomerular filtration is not thought to be a major route for PGE present in plasma to enter the renal tubules, since filtration will be limited by protein binding (Raz, 1972); prostaglandins can, however, be synthesised in the glomerular epithelium (Hassid *et al.*, 1979), and PGE is avidly transported into the proximal tubule by the organic acid transport system (Rennick, 1977; Bito and Baroody, 1978; Irish, 1979), although proximal secretion is unlikely to contribute significantly to the amount of PGE excreted *in vivo,* since the transport inhibitors probenecid and *p*-aminohippurate did not alter the urinary excretion of PGE in the dog (Rosenblatt *et al.,* 1978). Prostaglandins may be metabolised to a considerable degree in renal tubular cells (Bito, 1976), and microinjection studies in the rat indicate a major site of reabsorption in the loop of Henle (probably the descending limb) and to a lesser extent in the distal nephron (Kauker, 1975). Stop-flow studies in the dog suggest that the loop of Henle (ascending limb) may be the major site for PGE excreted in the urine to be secreted into the renal tubular fluid (Williams *et al.,*1977; Cinotti *et al.,* 1981). The precise cellular source of PGE excreted in the urine is at present uncertain, although medullary interstitial cells (Dunn *et al.,* 1976) and the collecting tubules (Grenier and Smith, 1978) are a strong possibility. Evidence for ascending limb cells *per se* is less convincing (Currie and Needleman, 1984). The possibility that PGE synthesised in the efferent or afferent arteriole may be metabolised and hence may not reach the final urine as PGE *per se* must also be borne in mind. The transport pathways for PGE in the nephron are shown in Figure 5.3.

Figure 5.3: Transport of PGE in the Nephron. (1) Filtration limited by protein binding; (2) glomerular synthesis; (3) active secretion by organic acid pathway; (5,6) secretion probably passive; (4,7) reabsorption probably passive

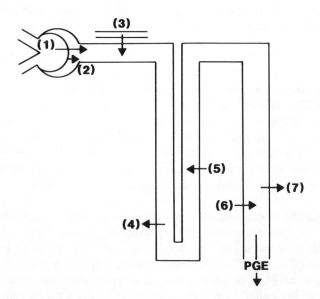

The urinary excretion rate of PGE has been measured in healthy man, frequently by techniques involving radioimmunoassay, and the values

obtained range from 10 to 60 ng h^{-1}. At urine flows exceeding about 100 ml h^{-1}, the urinary concentration of PGE remains relatively constant between 0.1 and 0.5 ng ml^{-1}. In the male, PGE excretion may be elevated due to contamination by PGE secreted from accessory sex glands (Patrono *et al.,* 1979), a problem which can be prevented by subjects abstaining from intercourse for 48 h prior to urine collection (Benzoni *et al.,* 1982). In developing children, urinary PGE excretion increases with age (Benzoni *et al.,* 1981), but no age effect could be demonstrated when values were adjusted for body surface area (Godard *et al.,* 1982). In addition, no difference in the PGE excretion rate between young and elderly adult males could be detected (Mackenzie *et al.,* 1984). In adult female subjects, urinary PGE excretion shows a marked circadian rhythm, peaking in the afternoon and paralleling changes in urine flow (Bowden *et al.,* 1977) without being appreciably influenced by posture. The urinary excretion rate of PGE has also been demonstrated to be altered by exercise (Zambraski and Dunn, 1980), urine flow (Kaye *et al.,* 1980) and urine pH (Haylor *et al.,* 1984). Since in most experiments in which urinary PGE measurements have been employed (a) there are invariably changes in urine flow, and (b) urine pH is rarely if ever measured, the influence of both of these stimuli warrants further discussion. The possible importance of these factors was highlighted in the original article by Frolich *et al.* (1975) proposing the use of PGE excretion as an index for renal synthesis, the discussion of which includes the following:

> to ascertain more precisely the extent to which urinary prostaglandins may be employed as indicators of renal prostaglandin synthesis, other parameters that influence their excretion need to be investigated. In particular, the weak acidic properties of prostaglandins suggest that their excretion could be influenced by urinary pH and flow rate.

The Flow-Dependence of Urinary PGE Excretion

There is good evidence, from both the conscious dog (Kirschenbaum and Serros, 1980; Wright *et al.,* 1981) and from man (Kaye *et al.,* 1980; Walker *et al.,* 1981) to support the concept that PGE excretion is flow-dependent. The mechanism proposed to explain this effect has been an increase in the washout of PGE synthesised in the collecting duct (Kirschenbaum and Serros, 1980). The rat has been suggested to be a species in which urinary PGE excretion is independent of urine flow (Fejes-Toth *et al.,* 1983b), and a marked negative correlation between urine flow and PGE excretion has been described in the rat (Christensen *et al.,* 1983) in the low flow range. However, PGE excretion in the conscious rat has been demonstrated to increase following an oral fluid load, and to decrease during mild water restriction (Kirschenbaum and Serros, 1980; Campbell *et al.,* 1983). In a recent series of experiments a positive linear correlation between urine flow and PGE excretion has also demonstrated following intravenous fluids in the anaesthetised rat (Haylor and Lote,

Figure 5.4: Flow-dependent and pH-dependent Urinary PGE Excretion in the Rat. (a) Relationship between PGE excretion and urine flow (at constant urine pH 6) in the anaesthetised rat infused with NH_4Cl (Haylor and Lote, 1984). Each symbol represents results obtained from a different animal ($n = 6$). Linear regression is extrapolated to the mean value obtained in the conscious rat ($n = 6$) at similar urine pH and osmolality. (b) Relationship between PGE excretion and urine pH (at constant urine flow of 1.5 ml/hr) in the conscious rat receiving oral NH_4Cl or $NaHCO_3$ (Haylor *et al.*, 1984). Vertical bars indicate SEM; the numbers refer to animals used at any one pH range

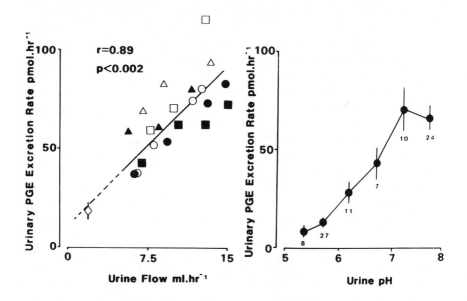

1984) performed at an acid urine pH (Figure 5.4).

Kaojarern *et al.* (1984) have proposed 'that for all experiments not addressing the contribution of, or controlling the urine flow rate, measurements of urinary PGE excretion must be interpreted with caution'. Obviously, this caution must extend to interpreting the effects of stimuli which either increase or decrease urine flow, and so encompasses much of the work performed to date on the renal PGE system in man. For example, when allowances were made for differences in urine flow, frusemide could not be demonstrated to alter PGE excretion in man (Kaojarern *et al.*, 1984).

The pH Dependence of Urinary PGE Excretion

Studies in the conscious rat have established a positive correlation between PGE excretion and urine pH (Haylor *et al.*, 1984), PGE excretion being some 10-fold higher in alkaline than in acidic urine, and the major change taking place over the pH range 6–7 (Figure 5.4). All animals in these experiments had a similar urine osmolality and flow, and sodium excretion rate, the urine being acidified with oral ammonium chloride and made alkaline with sodium bicarbonate. This relationship could also be described in rats receiving sodium chloride, where the acidification of the urine was likely to be restricted predominantly to the distal nephron (Gottschalk *et al.*, 1960). An initial attempt to confirm this finding in man proved inconclusive (Haylor *et al.*, 1985); however, when interference from changes in urine flow and from *in vitro* metabolism under alkaline conditions (Karim *et al.*, 1968) was avoided, urinary PGE excretion was found to be markedly elevated at alkaline pH in man (Haylor *et al.*, 1986). Figure 5.5 demonstrates that in healthy human subjects the effects of either elevating the urine flow or the urine pH are not additive but are mutually exclusive, which may indicate that both stimuli work to increase PGE excretion through a common mechanism. The renal tubule is not permeable to weak acids in their ionised form (Milne *et al.*, 1958); but, as shown by the Henderson equation:

$$pH = pK_a + \log \frac{\text{ionised PG–COO}^-}{\text{un-ionised PG-COOH}}$$

the ionisation of PGE_2 (pK 4.94; Uekama *et al.*, 1978), is markedly influenced by the pH of the tubular fluid, the un-ionised form of the molecule being lipid-soluble and available for reabsorption. As the urine pH increases from pH 5 to pH 8 as shown in Figure 5.4, the proportion of PGE_2 in its un-ionised, lipid soluble form decreases by 1000-fold and this is associated with a large increase in PGE excretion. If the maximum effect of alkalinising the urine on PGE excretion attained at pH 7.5–8 represents a complete absence of reabsorption, one could estimate the level of reabsorption at the usual pH values found in the rat and man (*c.* pH 6) to be some 75 per cent.

The possibility that PGE may be reabsorbed to a significant degree in the distal nephron is further supported by the lack of flow-dependent excretion at alkaline pH in man. This finding also indicates that a reduction in reabsorption may be a more plausible explanation for the flow-dependent nature of PGE excretion than the increase in passive secretion commonly proposed (Kirschenbaum and Serros, 1980). In addition, the use of alkaline urine may avoid interference from flow-dependent changes in PGE excretion when this index is employed in the assessment of renal PGE production *in vivo*.

Other possible explanations for the relationship between PGE excretion and urine pH must be borne in mind; these include problems with either the stability of PGE at different pH values (Karim *et al.*, 1968; Shaw and Ramwell, 1969) or an influence of hydrogen ions on antibody binding in the immunoassay of PGE (Granstrom and Kindahl, 1978). Neither of these possibilities is, however, consistent with the results obtained. The possibility that systemic changes in acid/base balance may also alter renal PGE synthesis would seem unlikely since:

(a) intravenous bicarbonate did not elevate renal venous PGE in the dog (Lonigro *et al.*, 1982), and

Figure 5.5: Relationship between Urinary PGE Excretion and Urine Flow in Healthy Male Subjects Following and Oral Water Load in either Acidic (pH 5.7, ○) or Alkaline (pH 7.2, ●) Urine. Vertical and horizontal bars indicate SEM (*n* = 5). (Haylor *et al.*, 1986. Reproduced with permission from *Clinical Science* © Biochemical Society 1986.)

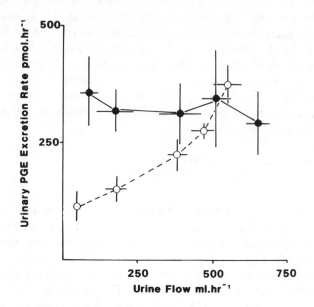

(b) two stimuli, bicarbonate and acetazolamide, both of which alkalinise the urine and elevate PGE excretion (Haylor *et al.*, 1983), produce opposite changes in plasma pH.

Recent studies proposing that renal PGE synthesis may be involved in the renal synthesis of ammonia (Jones *et al.*, 1984) have obtained a markedly different association between urine pH and urinary PGE excretion, although in these experiments the possibility that PGE might be metabolised *in vitro* was not considered, and the urine flow was not adequately controlled.

Microinjection experiments, in which labelled PGE$_2$ was injected into distal tubules in anaesthetised rats, have detected only a small degree of distal reabsorption of PGE$_2$, of 13 per cent (Kauker, 1975), or 4 per cent (Peterson *et al.*, 1984). However, the high urine flow employed in such experiments might be expected to inhibit reabsorption. Peterson *et al.* (1984) did find that distal reabsorption did not occur at alkaline urine pH values.

Whatever the mechanisms involved, it would seem probable that urine pH in addition to urine flow has been a major uncontrolled variable associated with experiments measuring urinary PGE excretion over the last 10 years.

Urinary Excretion of Arachidonate Metabolites

In healthy human subjects, the urinary excretion rate of PGF$_{2\alpha}$ has been reported to exceed that of PGE_2 by some 5 to 10-fold (Benzoni *et al.*, 1981; Ferretti *et al.*, 1981; Godard *et al.*, 1982; Ignatowska-Switalska, 1983) although others have found a ratio close to unity (Patrono *et al.*, 1979). The ratio between the excretion of $PGE_2/PGF_{2\alpha}$ in the urine has been used to assess the activity of PGE_2 9-keto reductase (an enzyme present in renal tissue which can convert PGE_2 into $PGF_{2\alpha}$), the activity of which may be influenced by salt intake or diuretic drugs (Weber *et al.*, 1977, 1979). $PGF_{2\alpha}$, however, can also be derived directly from PGH_2, the endoperoxide intermediate, and has effects on tubular reabsorption similar to those possessed by PGE_2. The renal importance of $PGF_{2\alpha}$ warrants further investigation.

The urinary excretion of 6-keto-$PGF_{1\alpha}$ (a metabolite of PGI_2) and TXB_2 (a metabolite of thromboxane A_2) is normally measured as a reflection of PGI_2 or TXA_2 synthesis. However, it is not known what proportion of such metabolites are derived from the systemic circulation in healthy human subjects. The excretion of 6-keto-$PGF_{1\alpha}$ was not influenced by elevating the urine flow (Fichman and Nadler, 1983), whereas the excretion of TXB_2 is enhanced by such elevation (Zipser and Smorlesi, 1984). The urinary excretion of TXB_2 has been used as a rejection marker following kidney transplantation (Foegh *et al.*, 1983), but blood platelets must be considered as a possible synthetic source of TXB_2 other than renal tissue (Zipser and Smorlesi, 1984).

Physiological Roles of Renal Prostaglandins

Much of the initial work on prostaglandins in relation to renal function consisted of the administration of PGE_1, PGE_2 and PGI_2 into the renal artery *in vivo* (and in some instances *in vitro*). Such studies demonstrated that these prostaglandins are potent vasodilators, which increase urine flow and sodium excretion.

The kidney produces only minute quantities of PGE_1 (Ellis *et al.*, 1979), but even if PGE_2 and PGI_2 are infused, such studies have little physiological value, since it is unlikely that prostaglandins administered in this way will act at the sites at which prostaglandins are endogenously synthesised and utilised. Studies of this kind have cast doubt on the validity of extrapolating to other species from data obtained in the rat, since it has been reported that PGE_2 produces vasoconstriction in the rat kidney *in vitro* (Malik and McGiff, 1975; Foy and Nuhu, 1984), and *in vivo* (Gerber and Nies, 1979). However, these observations depend to a great extent on the initial vascular resistance of the rat kidney, and vasodilation by PGE_2 can be readily demonstrated both in the isolated perfused kidney (Pace-Asciak and Rosenthal, 1982) and *in vivo* (Haylor and Towers, 1981, 1982), see Figure 5.6.

Figure 5.6: Renal Vasodilator Activity of PGE$_2$ in the Anaesthetised New Zealand Rat; (left) Normotensive and (right) Genetically Hypertensive. PGE$_2$ was delivered by infusion into the left renal artery, and renal blood flow was recorded using an electromagnetic flow probe. In isolated perfused rat kidneys, vasoconstrictor activity has been reported (Armstrong *et al.*, 1976) This figure is based on data from Haylor and Towers (1981, 1982)

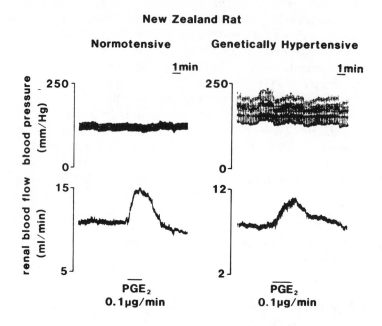

Five main renal functions of prostaglandins have emerged. These are:

(1) a role in the maintenance of renal blood flow and glomerular filtration;
(2) a role in the release of renin;
(3) a natriuretic tubular action;
(4) a water-diuretic action;
(5) a role in the regulation or maintenance of the corticomedullary solute gradient.

Roles 1 and 2 in this list are likely to depend on cortical prostaglandins, whereas 3, 4 and 5 are likely to depend on medullary prostaglandin synthesis, and are dealt with later under the general heading of 'prostaglandins and sodium homeostasis'.

Prostaglandin Synthesis and Maintenance of the Renal Blood Supply

Ischaemia is a potent stimulus for renal prostaglandin synthesis (McGiff *et al.*, 1970), and the administration of cyclo-oxygenase inhibitors to anaesthetised surgically operated animals leads to a marked reduction in renal blood flow (Kirschenbaum *et al.*, 1974; Anderson *et al.*, 1975b; Owen *et al.*, 1975; Venuto *et al.*, 1975), and glomerular filtration rate (see later). However, there are generally no effects of cyclo-oxygenase inhibitors on renal blood flow in well-hydrated healthy conscious animals or (conscious) man (Swain *et al.*, 1975; Donker *et al.*, 1976; Gullner *et al.*, 1980; Haylor, 1980; Haylor and Lote, 1980b; Gross *et al.*, 1981). Hence it is clear that the normal renal prostaglandin synthesis does not contribute to the maintenance of RBF. Stress (anaesthesia and surgery), however, increases renal prostaglandin synthesis (Terragno *et al.*, 1977; Lonigro *et al.*, 1978) and this additional PG synthesis does play a part in the maintenance of RBF.

The type of stress mentioned above would be expected to increase the adrenergically mediated neural input to the kidneys. Prostaglandin synthesis by the kidney is enhanced by vasoconstrictor stimuli, including angiotensin II, noradrenaline and vasopressin (McGiff *et al.*, 1970; Danon *et al.*, 1975; Bell and Mya, 1977; Gerber *et al.*, 1982), and may counteract the decrease in renal blood flow. Thus blockade of prostaglandin synthesis augments the vaso-constrictor response to angiotensin II (Aiken and Vane, 1973; Satoh and Zimmerman, 1975; Finn and Arendshorst, 1976) and to catecholamines (Needleman *et al.*, 1974; Swain *et al.*, 1975; Chapnick *et al.*, 1977).

Since cortical prostaglandin synthesis occurs predominantly in the vascular elements of the kidney, it seems likely that it is cortical prostaglandin synthesis (i.e. probably PGI_2) which is increased in the presence of vasoconstrictor stimuli, and helps to protect the kidney from the effects of such stimuli.

It has been proposed that renal prostaglandin synthesis mediates the autoregulation of renal blood flow (Herbaczynska-Cedro and Vane, 1973) and that increased prostaglandin synthesis leads to increases in blood flow preferentially to inner cortical regions (Larsson and Anggard, 1974; Chang *et al.*, 1975). Many studies, however, indicate that prostaglandin synthesis is not involved in the autoregulation of renal blood flow (Anderson *et al.*, 1975b; Bell *et al.*, 1975), although the ability of prostaglandins to preferentially increase blood flow to the inner cortex may contribute to the suppression of the corticomedullary gradient when vascular prostaglandin production is stimulated in addition to that at tubular sites. Arachidonic acid is also the precursor of two materials, thromboxane A_2 and leukotriene C_4, which decrease rather than increase renal blood flow (Badr *et al.*, 1984; Fitzgerald and Fitzgerald, 1984). Although these are not thought to be involved in the control of normal renal function, abnormal thromboxane synthesis has been implicated in disorders involving renal vasoconstriction (Anderson *et al.*, 1984).

Prostaglandins and Glomerular Filtration

Following their intrarenal infusion, vasodilator prostaglandins generally increase renal blood flow in the absence of changes in the glomerular filtration rate (Johnston *et al.*, 1967; Fulgraff *et al.*, 1974). In the rat, the intrarenal infusion of PGE_1 was associated with a reduction in the single nephron filtration fraction and consequently the efferent arteriolar oncotic pressure (Baylis *et al.*, 1976). Following the administration of cyclo-oxygenase inhibitors to either healthy humans or conscious animals, the glomerular filtration rate, like renal blood flow, normally remains unchanged (Schnermann and Briggs, 1981). However, the possibility that the fluid loading procedures required to accurately assess glomerular filtration may suppress renal prostaglandin production must be borne in mind (Haylor, 1980). A variety of conditions have been described in which, following cyclo-oxygenase inhibition, glomerular filtration is definitely reduced; a discussion of this is presented in an excellent review by Dunn (1984). Such conditions include some renal diseases, hepatic cirrhosis, and heart failure, and are associated with reduced renal perfusion and enhanced renal vascular resistance, which would be expected to stimulate the synthesis of prostacyclin in the afferent (and efferent) arterioles.

Arachidonate metabolites are also synthesised in the glomerular membrane (Sraer *et al.*, 1983b) and can alter the filtration coefficient (K_f) principally by influencing the tone of the mesangial cells. The influence of changes in the filtration coefficient on GFR is discussed in Chapter 2. The mechanisms by which the kidney can maintain a constant filtration rate in the face of fluctuations in arterial pressure have been extensively investigated. Recently, Schnermann *et al.* (1984) reported that over certain pressure ranges the independence of GFR from arterial blood pressure was abolished in the indomethacin-treated rat. The possibility that arachidonic acid may be involved in tubuloglomerular feedback has also been proposed (Schnermann and Briggs, 1981). However, in the rat there would appear to be some controversy over whether PGI_2 inhibits (Boberg *et al.*, 1984) or restores the feedback response.

Prostaglandins and Renin Release

Larsson *et al.* (1974) demonstrated that intra-aortic infusion of arachidonic acid (in rabbits) led to an increase in renin release, and that this increase was prevented by indomethacin. Subsequently this finding has been confirmed repeatedly in several species (Weber *et al.*, 1975, 1976; Bolger *et al.*, 1976; Whorton *et al.*, 1977; Data *et al.*, 1978a, b; Seymour and Zehr, 1979). These clear demonstrations that arachidonic acid metabolites can effect renin release have been followed by a great deal of controversy over the detailed mechanisms involved.

Renin release from the granular cells of the juxtaglomerular apparatus can occur in response to at least three different stimuli:

(1) decreases in afferent arteriolar wall tension (the 'baroreceptor' mechanism; Blaine *et al.*, 1971);

(2) a chemical signal at the macula densa (responding to changes in tubular sodium and/or chloride (Vander and Miller, 1964; see also Chapter 4).

(3) β-adrenergic receptor stimulation, either by renal sympathetic nerve activity (Taher *et al.*, 1976) or by circulating catecholamines (Assaykeen *et al.*, 1970).

The first two mechanisms are indirectly influenced by renal sympathetic nerve activity which causes α-adrenoceptor-mediated vasoconstriction, and hence, by reducing renal blood flow and glomerular filtration rate, changes the delivery of NaCl to the macula densa (and also increases renal PG synthesis). In addition, α-adrenoreceptors in the proximal tubule can alter NaCl reabsorption directly, and hence affect macula densa NaCl delivery (DiBona, 1977).

(1) *Prostaglandins and Renal 'Baroreceptor'-mediated Renin Release.* In 1978, Dunn *et al.* showed that prostaglandins E_2 and $F_{2\alpha}$ are released from the kidney in response to activation of the baroreceptor mechanism (Dunn *et al.*, 1978b). Data *et al.* (1978b), using the non-filtering canine kidney, demonstrated that indomethacin abolished the ability of the renal baroreceptor to respond to a reduced perfusion pressure with renin release, and similar findings were obtained in animals with functional kidneys (Berl *et al.*, 1979; Blackshear *et al.*, 1979). These observations have been interpreted as demonstrating that prostaglandins mediate the change in renin release induced by activating the renal baroreceptors. However, this interpretation has been criticised (Freeman and Davis, 1983), and it could be that, since low perfusion pressure activates renal prostaglandin synthesis, this is a stimulus to renin release which facilitates the direct baroreceptor stimulus to renin release, with the two mechanisms independent (Freeman *et al.*, 1982).

(2) *Prostaglandins and Macula Densa-mediated Renin Release.* Olson *et al.* (1980) have investigated the renin response to suprarenal aortic constriction in anaesthetised dogs, in which papaverine was used to block the renal baroreceptor mechanism, and renal denervation and propranolol administration were used to eliminate adrenergically mediated renin release. It was found that indomethacin blocked the (presumably macula densa controlled) increase in renin release in response to aortic constriction. Similarly, in denervated kidneys, the renin secretion in response to suprarenal aortic constriction was abolished by indomethacin or meclofenamate, indicating that renin secretion elicited by the macula densa is prostaglandin dependent (Osborn *et al.*, 1982). Francisco *et al.* (1980) have also demonstrated prostaglandin involvement in macula densa-mediated renin release.

(3) *Prostaglandins and the Neural Control of Renin Release.* Renal sympathetic nerves terminate in contact with granular cells of the juxta-glomerular apparatus and smooth-muscle cells of the afferent arterioles. Stimulation of the renal nerves increases renin release, independently of changes in arterial pressure, renal haemodynamics, or urinary sodium excretion. This direct effect of renal nerve stimulation on renin release is mediated by a β-receptor mechanism (Kopp *et al.*, 1980; Kopp and DiBona,

1984) which is independent of renal prostaglandin synthesis (Kopp *et al.*, 1981). The increase in plasma renin activity which occurs in exercise is mediated by renal sympathetic nerve activity acting via β_1-receptors, and hence is unaffected by inhibition of prostaglandin synthesis (Zambraski *et al.*, 1984). However, if α-receptors are also activated, then renin release occurs in response to the resulting vasoconstriction, and this (α-mediated) renin release *is* prostaglandin dependent (Kopp *et al.*, 1981).

Summary: Prostaglandin and Renin Release. In conclusion, it seems that renal 'baroreceptor'-induced renin release could be mediated by prostaglandins, or alternatively that renal hypoperfusion activates the baroreceptors and also enhances prostaglandin synthesis, and these then act synergistically (i.e. in parallel rather than in series) to release renin. The evidence that the macula densa-induced renin release is prostaglandin mediated is good but not conclusive, and as far as neurally mediated renin release is concerned, it seems clear that β-adrenoceptor-induced renin release does not require prostaglandin synthesis. These facts are summarised in Figure 5.7.

Figure 5.7: The Role of Renal Prostaglandin Synthesis in Renin Release. Solid lines are supported by the majority of experimental reports. Dotted lines indicate other possibilities, with some supporting experimental evidence. For further clarification, see text

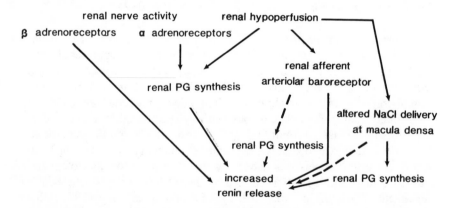

Which prostaglandins are involved in renin release? As mentioned earlier, the principal renal prostaglandins are PGE_2, $PGF_{2\alpha}$, PGI_2 and PGD_2. Which of these are (or may be) involved in renin release? Yun *et al.* (1977, 1978) demonstrated that PGE_2 stimulates renin release in the anaesthetised dog, and a similar finding has been made in isolated rat kidney cortical slices (Franco-Saenz *et al.*, 1980). However, in a similar preparation, PGI_2 also promotes renin release (Whorton *et al.*, 1977), and there are now numerous reports of PGI_2 causing renin release *in vivo*; furthermore PGI_2 appears to be more potent in this respect than PGE_2 (Gerber *et al.*, 1979; Seymour *et al.*, 1979).

Since there is considerable PGI_2 synthesised in the renal cortex (Terragno *et al.*, 1978; Whorton *et al.*, 1978), PGI_2 could be the prostaglandin primarily involved in regulating renin release, and evidence in support of this has recently been obtained from *in vitro* experiments (Schryver *et al.*, 1984).

Angiotensin–Prostaglandin Interactions. It has already been mentioned that the renal vasoconstriction elicited by angiotensin II is enhanced by the inhibition of renal prostaglandin synthesis (Aiken and Vane, 1973; McGiff, 1981), and that angiotensin II stimulates the release of both PGE_2 and PGI_2 (Needleman *et al.*, 1973, 1979; Dunn *et al.*, 1978b; Mullane and Moncada, 1980). The simultaneous activation of both vasoconstrictor (angiotensin) and vasodilator (prostaglandin) mechanisms may have important functional advantages to the kidney when its perfusion is threatened (e.g. by haemorrhage or other reduction in extracellular fluid volume). Renal prostaglandin synthesis, by protecting the kidney, could allow angiotensin II to play a part in maintaining the systemic blood pressure, without harming renal function.

Prostaglandins and Sodium Homeostasis

Following the demonstration of the natriuretic and vasodilator properties of PGE_1 in the dog (Johnston *et al.*, 1967), several attempts have been made to dissociate the increase in sodium excretion from the ability of the E-series prostaglandins to enhance renal blood flow. PGE_2 can still increase sodium excretion in the presence of a maximal vasodilator dose of acetylcholine (Shea-Donohue *et al.*, 1979), and $PGF_{2\alpha}$, a prostaglandin devoid of vasodilator activity, produces a natriuretic effect similar to that of PGE_2 (Fulgraff *et al.*, 1974). In addition, although PGE_2 and PGI_2 both increase renal blood flow, PGE_2 exerts a much greater effect on sodium output (Jones *et al.*, 1981). In the anaesthetised dog, the cyclo-oxygenase inhibitor indomethacin decreases both renal blood flow and sodium excretion (Feigen *et al.*, 1976), and attempts have been made to dissociate these two properties. In conscious animals, where renal PG synthesis is not stimulated by the surgical procedures employed (Terragno *et al.*, 1977), cyclo-oxygenase inhibitors have been demonstrated to decrease sodium and water excretion in man (Haylor, 1980), the dog (Altsheler *et al.*, 1977) and the rat (Haylor and Lote, 1980a), but in the absence of changes in either renal blood flow or glomerular filtration. Following treatment with indomethacin, conscious rats, initially in a steady state of sodium and water balance, begin to undergo volume expansion (Figure 5.8), while in man, administration of the cyclo-oxygenase inhibitor phenylbutazone in particular can result in frank oedema in some 30–40 per cent of subjects treated (Meiers and Wetzels, 1964). However, caution should be employed in directly relating the pharmacological properties of non-steroidal anti-inflammatory drugs with the physiology of cyclo-oxygenase, since such drugs can also inhibit other enzyme systems.

Recently evidence has been presented that in healthy human subjects, the

Figure 5.8: The Effect of Indomethacin (10 mg/kg Body Weight), Given Intravenously over a 15 min Period (Black Bar) to Conscious Rats at 3 h 52.5 min to 4 h 7.5 min. The control group (open symbols) received only 0.9% saline i.v. in the 6 h infusion, whereas the experimental group (solid symbols) received indomethacin in the infusate as above. (a) Urine flow; (b) urine osmolality; (c) sodium output; (d) osmolar output; (e) body fluid volume changes. The volume at 4 h is the reference point

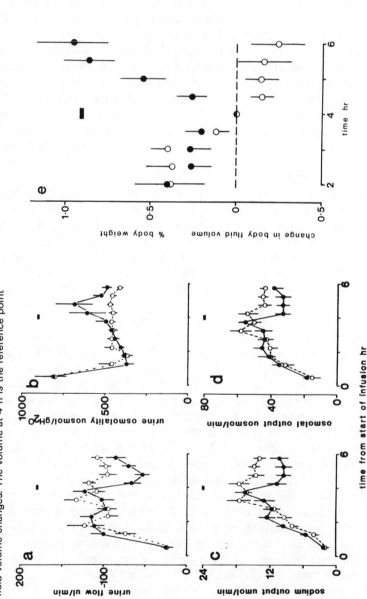

Reproduced with permission from Haylor and Lote, 1980b

anti-natriuretic properties of cyclo-oxygenase inhibitors can be divorced from their ability to reduce the urinary excretion of PGE (Critchley *et al.*, 1984; Vierhapper *et al.*, 1984). These findings, however, must be assessed in relation to the possibility that:

(a) cyclo-oxygenase inhibitors can reduce urinary PGE excretion by mechanisms other than enzyme inhibition, namely by reducing urine flow or urine pH (Lote *et al.*, 1984);

(b) The PGE excreted in the urine may not be derived from the same intrarenal source as that which modifies tubular solute transport.

What, then, is the basis of the natriuretic tubular effect of the renal prostaglandins? It seems unlikely that, in the absence of haemodynamic changes, there are any changes in proximal tubular sodium transport (Fulgraff and Meiforth, 1971; Strandhoy *et al.*, 1974; Leyssac *et al.*, 1975; Roman and Kauker, 1978; Higashihara *et al.*, 1979). Thus the natriuretic tubular action of renal prostaglandins must be attributed to effects in the loop of Henle or distal nephron. In addition to being diuretic and natriuretic, the renal prostaglandins also decrease the corticomedullary solute gradient (Ganguli *et al.*, 1977; Haylor and Lote, 1979, 1983; Passmore *et al.*, 1980) and these two effects are likely to be related.

Loop of Henle. PGE_2 is reported to inhibit NaCl absorption in the rabbit medullary thick ascending limb of Henle *in vitro* (Stokes, 1979). However, it is questionable whether this is a site of endogenous prostaglandin synthesis. Smith *et al.* (1980) and Jackson *et al.* (1980) find no prostaglandin synthesis at this site; and although Schlondorff *et al.* (1982) report cyclo-oxygenase activity in the rabbit medullary thick ascending limb *in vitro*, Currie and Needleman (1984) suggest that this could be due to the presence of medullary collecting tubule cells in their preparation.

However, since PGE_2 can elicit the inhibition of NaCl transport by acting on the luminal side of the tubule cell, it is conceivable that PGE_2 entering the loop of Henle from the medullary interstitium (Williams *et al.*, 1977) could exert this effect.

The effect itself is controversial; Fine and Trizna (1977) could find no effect of PGE_2 on medullary thick segment NaCl transport, and PGE_2 will not reduce NaCl reabsorption in this segment if the tubule is bathed in serum rather than in artificial medium (Stokes, 1979); but more recently PGE_2/ADH interactions in this segment have been defined (see later). Nevertheless, *in vivo* studies in the dog suggest that renal prostaglandins do not affect NaCl transport in the ascending limb of Henle (Work *et al.*, 1980).

The fact that cyclo-oxygenase inhibitors increase the corticomedullary solute gradient (Ganguli *et al.*, 1977; Haylor and Lote, 1979, 1983; Passmore *et al.*, 1980) could be interpreted as an effect on NaCl extrusion by the ascending limb, but alternative explanations (e.g. an effect on collecting tubule NaCl reabsorption) are also possible (see Haylor and Lote, 1983, for detailed discussion).

Prostaglandins and the Collecting Tubule

There is considerable controversy surrounding the actions of prostaglandins in the collecting tubule. The collecting tubule is a 'tight' or 'high-resistance' epithelium, similar in its transport processes to other tight epithelia such as frog skin. In this 'model' epithelium, PGE_1 and the endogenous prostaglandins (predominantly PGE_2) increase sodium transport (Lote *et al.*, 1974; Barry *et al.*, 1975; Haylor and Lote, 1976, 1977; Helman and Els, 1978), but also produce a non-specific increase in ionic permeability (Lote *et al.*, 1974; Haylor and Lote, 1976, 1977). A similar change in ionic permeability occurring in the collecting tubule, whereby prostaglandin synthesis increases the ionic permeability and inhibitors of prostaglandin synthesis reduce it, could, by altering the backflux of NaCl into the duct, account for the natriuretic tubular effect of prostaglandins. It could also explain the effects of endogenous prostaglandins on the corticomedullary solute gradient whereby prostaglandin synthesis reduces the gradient and inhibitors increase it (Ganguli *et al.*, 1977; Haylor and Lote, 1979, 1980a, 1983). Furthermore, this hypothesis could also explain some disparate observations (prostaglandins being antinatriuretic and inhibitors being natriuretic — see e.g. Kirschenbaum and Stein, 1976). These observations have been made during volume expansion and water diuresis, i.e. in circumstances in which the cortico-medullary solute gradient is reduced and hence the gradient for backflux of NaCl from interstitium to collecting tubule is also reduced. Under such circumstances the effect of prostaglandin synthesis inhibition on active sodium transport (reducing it) could outweigh the effect on permeability (also reduced) leading to increased sodium excretion.

There is some experimental support for this attractive 'unifying hypothesis' from studies using isolated collecting tubule segments. Iino and Imai (1978) have shown that, in both the cortical and medullary collecting tubules, PGE_2, acting on the peritubular membrane, reduces net sodium reabsorption and the transtubular potential difference. This was interpreted as suggesting a decrease in active sodium transport, but could equally well be explained by an increase in ionic permeability.

However, there are also experiments which cannot readily be accommodated by the hypothesis that collecting duct active Na transport and ionic permeability are both affected by prostaglandins. Stokes and Kokko (1977) showed that PGE_2 inhibited the transepithelial potential difference in rabbit cortical and outer medullary collecting tubules, but they also showed that PGE_2 inhibited net sodium transport out of the tubular lumen by inhibiting efflux but not affecting influx. Nevertheless, this experiment need not imply that *endogenous* prostaglandin biosynthesis has no effect on backflux. If prostaglandin synthesis were already high, so that ionic permeability was high, addition of PGE_2 might not elicit a further increase. Fine and Trizna (1977), however, found no effect of PGE_2 on either the transepithelial potential difference, or net sodium flux in the rabbit medullary collecting tubule, even after pretreatment with indomethacin. Thus the effects of prostaglandins on collecting-tubule epithelium must still be regarded as controversial.

Urinary PGE_2 and Sodium Homeostasis. If renal prostaglandin synthesis is necessary to excrete sodium effectively, does it follow that renal prostaglandin synthesis serves a regulatory role in maintaining sodium homeostasis? To demonstrate such a regulatory function, it would be necessary to show that renal prostaglandin biosynthesis is altered by changes in sodium balance. Studies performed to investigate this question have produced only confusion. For example, in the rabbit, chronic salt loading has been found to decrease urinary PGE_2 output (Scherer *et al.*, 1977) and salt restriction to increase it (Davila *et al.*, 1978; Stahl *et al.*, 1979). But other studies in the rabbit have indicated that there is no difference in prostaglandin E excretion between rabbits on a high NaCl diet and those on a low NaCl diet (Lifschitz *et al.*, 1980), and that prolonged prostaglandin synthesis inhibition in the rabbit has no effect on sodium balance (Davila *et al.*, 1980). In the rat, salt loading was found to increase PGE_2 excretion, but PGE_2 excretion subsequently returned to normal in spite of maintained salt loading (Tan *et al.*, 1980); but in experiments in which PGE_2 excretion was monitored over a 6 h period during either isotonic saline or dextrose infusion (at 5.8 ml/h), which produced identical urine flow rates, PGE_2 excretion was lower during the 4–6 h of saline infusion than in the corresponding period of dextrose infusion (Lote *et al.*, 1983).

In man, the findings are equally controversial. It has been reported that salt depletion increases PGE_2 excretion (Rathaus *et al.*, 1981), and a similar relationship between salt loading and PGE_2 excretion was seen by Kramer *et al.* (1980), who noted decreased PGE_2 excretion during isotonic or hypertonic saline loading, and increased PGE_2 excretion on a low-salt diet. Others, however, have not confirmed this (Hesse *et al.*, 1979), and a converse finding is suggested by the experiments of Epstein *et al.*, 1979), who reported that water immersion (which resembles volume expansion in its effects on the circulation) increased both PGE excretion and sodium excretion.

A complication of experiments which involve alterations of sodium balance is that renal sympathetic nerve activity will be altered (by baroreceptor reflexes) even when blood pressure is not measurably changed. It was recently demonstrated that sodium depletion in dogs (which greatly increased vascular resistance although it did not alter blood pressure) resulted in a two-fold increase in renal venous PGE_2 concentration (Oliver *et al.*, 1980), and the authors of this work state that 'renal synthesis of PGE_2 is significantly increased during chronic sodium depletion'. This seems a reasonable statement in view of the observations already made concerning the effects of catecholamines and renal perfusion on renal PG synthesis, but it means that we are again considering renal prostaglandins in their role as guardians of renal perfusion, rather than as agents regulating sodium excretion *per se*.

A problem of interpreting this confused literature may be due to the fact that we do not know the relative contribution, to either renal venous or urinary prostaglandins, made by the different renal sites of synthesis, and there is the possibility that prostaglandin synthesis in specific areas of the kidney (e.g. the collecting tubules) could change without necessarily altering the overall prostaglandin output. Some support for this notion is provided by *in vitro* experiments in which it has been shown that glomeruli from salt-depleted rats synthesise less PGE_2 (and more $PGF_{2\alpha}$) than those from control rats, whereas glomeruli from salt-loaded rats were not different from the controls. In contrast, papillary homogenates from salt-loaded rats had higher PGE_2 synthesis than controls, but salt depletion had no effect (Chaumet-Riffaud *et al.*, 1981).

Papillary Osmolality, Renal Prostaglandin Synthesis, and the Role of Calcium

The inhibition of prostaglandin synthesis is associated with an increase in renal medullary hypertonicity (Ganguli *et al.*, 1977; Haylor and Lote, 1979, 1983), whereas the administration of PGE_2 into the renal artery decreases medullary hypertonicity (Haylor and Lote, 1980a). Neither Ganguli *et al.* (1977) nor Haylor and Lote (1983) found evidence for a change in medullary blood flow being responsible for this effect of prostaglandin biosynthesis on papillary osmolality, although others have suggested that medullary haemodynamic changes could be responsible (Gullner *et al.*, 1980). Changes in urine flow rate along the collecting tubules can alter the corticomedullary solute gradient (Lote and Snape, 1977), but indomethacin can increase the gradient even in the absence of urine flow changes (Haylor and Lote, 1983), so an effect of prostaglandin synthesis on collecting tubule or loop of Henle net NaCl transport is the most likely explanation of the findings.

The above observations, that prostaglandin synthesis influences medullary osmolality, are rendered more intriguing by the fact that the converse also appears to be true — i.e. osmolality affects prostaglandin synthesis. Thus, prostaglandin synthesis in isolated rat renal papillae (Danon *et al.*, 1978) and in rabbit renomedullary interstitial cells in culture (Zusman and Keiser, 1980) is increased by hyperosmolality. A negative feedback control of papillary osmolality by prostaglandin synthesis (Figure 5.9) has therefore been proposed (Haylor and Lote, 1983), although clearly this represents something of an oversimplification (see, for example, Bliss and Lote, 1981).

The above reports of osmolality effects on prostaglandin synthesis involved primarily changes in NaCl concentration. Some investigators, however, have examined the effects on prostaglandin synthesis of altering other extracellular

Figure 5.9: Negative Feedback Scheme whereby Prostaglandin Synthesis in the Renal Medulla Stabilises the Osmotic Gradient

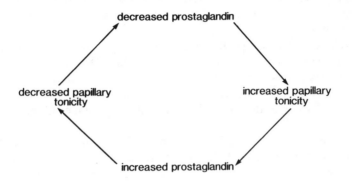

Reproduced with permission from Haylor and Lote (1983)

solutes. With potassium, the results are the opposite of those observed with NaCl. Hence, it has been shown that a decreased potassium concentration stimulates PGE biosynthesis in rabbit renomedullary interstitial cell cultures *in vitro* (Zusman and Keiser, 1977b), and in human and rabbit renal papillae (Dusing and Lee, 1980).

The ways in which altering the osmolality of the medullary extracellular fluid may influence prostaglandin synthesis appear to involve cytosolic Ca^{2+}, and its role in the activation of phospholipase A_2 (Zenser *et al.*, 1980). This view is supported by the demonstration of the calcium dependence of phospholipase A_2 activity *in vitro* (Shier, 1979), and by the finding that, in the toad bladder, hyperosmolality alters cellular Ca^{2+} homeostasis (Hardy *et al.*, 1974). The work of Craven *et al.* (1981) has indicated that renal inner medullary prostaglandin synthesis is a calcium–calmodulin-dependent process. (Evidence is accumulating which indicates that calmodulin regulates the action of Ca^{2+}, so that, in order to be physiologically active, Ca^{2+} must bind to calmodulin. Calmodulin is ubiquitously distributed in the cytosol.) Craven *et al.* (1981) found that trifluoperazine, an inhibitor of calcium–calmodulin interaction, reduces prostaglandin synthesis induced by hypertonic NaCl. Craven *et al.* (1980) showed that hypertonic urea solutions inhibit inner medullary prostaglandin synthesis, and that the addition of Ca^{2+} to Ca^{2+}-deprived inner medulla did not increase prostaglandin accumulation in the presence of a high urea concentration. These data suggest that urea inhibits Ca^{2+}-dependent prostaglandin synthesis, probably by restricting the generation of free arachidonic acid from its esterified form.

Prostaglandin–Vasopressin Interactions in the Kidney

Two major sites of prostaglandin–vasopressin interaction in the nephron have been defined: the collecting tubule, and the medullary thick ascending limb. In the former, such interactions could affect water excretion by influencing water permeability *per se*, whereas, in the latter, water excretion would be influenced by alterations of the medullary NaCl gradient and by altering the generation of free water in the tubule.

In 1965, it was observed that PGE_1 antagonises the ADH-stimulated osmotic movement of water from the toad urinary bladder (Orloff *et al.*, 1965). This antagonism was subsequently attributed to an inhibition of the rise in cyclic AMP content elicited by ADH (Omachi *et al.*, 1974), and was also found to occur in the isolated rabbit collecting tubule (Grantham and Orloff, 1968).

More recently, it has been shown that ADH enhances active NaCl extrusion from the mouse medullary thick ascending limb of Henle (Hall and Varney, 1980), and the studies of Sasaki and Imai (1980) and Hebert *et al.* (1981) confirmed these effects of ADH. Stokes (1979) had shown that PGE_2 reduces chloride extrusion from the (rabbit) medullary thick ascending limb, and Ganguli *et al.* (1977) showed that the inhibition of prostaglandin synthesis increased the medullary NaCl concentration. Hence it was logical to investigate PGE_2/ADH interactions in the medullary thick ascending limb, and such investigations have indicated an antagonistic effect of PGE_2 on the ADH-dependent component of transepithelial voltage and net chloride reabsorption in the (mouse) medullary thick ascending limb (Culpepper and Andreoli, 1983). This action of PGE_2 could be reversed by the addition of 10^{-3}M cAMP, and Torikai and Kurokawa (1983) have supported these findings with their demonstration that PGE_2 inhibits the stimulation of cAMP by ADH in the (rat) medullary thick ascending limb.

In vivo, vasopressin-prostaglandin interactions have proved more difficult to define. Observations that the administration of cyclo-oxygenase inhibitors in the rat and dog enhances the antidiuretic effect of ADH support the notion of vasopressin–prostaglandin antagonism (Anderson *et al.*, 1975a; Berl *et al.*, 1977; Fejes-Toth *et al.*, 1977; Lum *et al.*, 1977), and similar findings have been reported in man (Kramer *et al.*, 1978). However, conflicting observations have also been made. For example, in humans, indomethacin had no effect on the antidiuresis induced by the administration of incremental doses of vasopressin (Padfield and Grekin, 1981).

Vasopressin and Renal Prostaglandin Synthesis

The administration of vasopressin *in vivo* increases the urinary excretion of PGE in the rabbit (Lifschitz and Stein, 1977), in man (Zipser *et al.*, 1981a), in the dog (Fejes-Toth *et al.*, 1983c) and in the rat (Ono *et al.*, 1982). The ability of vasopressin to enhance renal PGE synthesis is not associated with the stimulation of its V_2 (antidiuretic) receptors in the collecting tubule cells (Hassid, 1981; Grenier *et al.*, 1981); however, vasopressin also stimulates V_1 (vascular) receptors, and may increase papillary osmolality, which itself is a stimulus for prostaglandin synthesis (see above). A specific antagonist of the vascular actions of vasopressin (*d*-cyclo-*o*-methyl-tyrosine arginine vasopressin) was found to inhibit the increase in PGE_2 synthesis elicited by vasopressin administration (Zipser *et al.*, 1981a; Campbell *et al.*, 1982). In addition the vasopressin analogue dDAVP, which has antidiuretic (V_2) activity but is devoid of vascular (V_1) activity, did not increase urinary PGE excretion in man (Walker *et al.*, 1981). Evidence that vasopressin does not exert its influence on papillary prostaglandin synthesis through changes in papillary osmolality has recently been obtained *in vivo* (Bouby *et al.*, 1984). This view is supported *in vitro* by experiments in both toad bladder (Zusman *et al.*, 1977) and renal medullary preparations, where vasopressin is a potent stimulator of PGE production. Vascular receptors for vasopressin present in the renal cortex may also be involved, since vasopressin-induced PGE synthesis can be demonstrated in cultured rat glomerular cells which do not respond to dDAVP (Lieberthal and Levine, 1984).

The influence of endogenous vasopressin on renal prostaglandin synthesis has been less well defined, and it is important to bear in mind that exogenous administration may not adequately mimic endogenous release. The assumption that endogenous vasopressin release may help to determine the basal level of renal PGE synthesis is based primarily on the demonstration that rats with congenital diabetes insipidus (due to a lack of vasopressin synthesis) have a lower urinary PGE excretion rate than normal (Dunn *et al.*, 1978a). However, evidence that both dDAVP and vasopressin can increase urinary PGE excretion in the Brattleboro' rat (Fejes-Toth *et al.*, 1983a) indicate that the difference could be secondary to a decrease in papillary osmolality. Severe water deprivation in the dog was associated with a marked increase in PGE excretion in the urine (Zucker *et al.*, 1983), an effect which could be attributed to a change in the secretion of other hormones or neurotransmitters in addition to vasopressin. In the rat, mild water restriction, leading to a decrease in urine flow, was associated with a decrease rather than an increase in PGE excretion (Campbell *et al.*, 1983) even though the urine osmolality exceeded some 2000 mOsmol/ kgH_2O.

Problems which are associated with the use of urinary PGE excretion as a marker for renal PGE synthesis in the presence of changes in urine flow were discussed earlier. As the urine flow alters, urinary PGE excretion may be influenced by two opposing factors, flow-dependent excretion being offset by a change in renal PGE synthesis in response to the state of hydration. Analysis of the relationship between urine flow and urinary PGE excretion in human subjects and in the anaesthetised rat indicates that a simple relationship between these two variables is not present over the lower ranges of urine flow. Such a relationship would be expected if urinary PGE excretion were only being influenced by flow-dependent excretion. In fact in the anaesthetised rat the shape of the curve was markedly biphasic (Haylor and Lote, 1984). Such results indicate that at the levels of urine flow frequently attained in conscious human subjects, the state of hydration does influence the basal level of PGE synthesis in the kidney; however, more definitive experimentation will be required before the precise contribution of endogenous vasopressin can be determined.

Prostaglandins and the Renal Kallikrein-Kinin System

The interactions of the prostaglandin and kinin systems within the kidney were recently reviewed (Nasjletti and Malik, 1981a, b), and little new information can be added to this. Kinins formed within the kidney promote the synthesis of renal prostaglandins by augmenting phospholipase activity (Antonello *et al.*, 1978), and mepacrine (phospholipase inhibitor) inhibits bradykinin-elicited PGE_2 release (Zusman and Keiser, 1977a).

Infusion of bradykinin into the renal artery leads to diuresis and natriuresis (Blasingham and Nasjletti, 1979; Carretero and Scicli, 1980), and this diuretic and natriuretic effect is reduced by indomethacin (McGiff *et al.*, 1975), suggesting that prostaglandins mediate kinin-induced natriuresis.

There is also evidence that prostaglandins can mediate kallikrein release. In Bartter's syndrome, high prostaglandin excretion is accompanied by elevated kallikrein excretion (Gill *et al.*, 1976), and both are corrected by indomethacin administration (Vinci *et al.*, 1978). In experimental animals (rats), PGE_2 and $PGF_{2\alpha}$ administration increase kallikrein excretion (Croxatto *et al.*, 1978).

Solute Excretion (Other than Sodium Chloride)

Experiments performed prior to the discovery that aspirin-like drugs inhibit cyclo-oxygenase indicated that following aspirin administration the excretion of a variety of solutes including sodium, chloride, magnesium, bicarbonate and calcium may be decreased, in the absence of any changes in GFR (Ramsay and Elliott, 1967). In addition, experiments performed using isolated frog skin have indicated that PGE_1 can increase the permeability of the epithelial tissue to potassium and calcium, as well as to sodium and chloride (Lote *et al.*, 1974). Both of these studies raise the possibility that renal arachidonate metabolism may influence the tubular handling of solutes other than sodium chloride.

Calcium. Cyclo-oxygenase inhibitors have been demonstrated to reduce calcium excretion in the rat, in the monkey, and in human subjects with hypercalciuria (Buck *et al.*, 1981, 1983; Blacklock *et al.*, 1983; Roman *et al.*, 1984). However, converse findings have also been reported in which indomethacin increased calcium excretion in normal human subjects (Colette *et al.*, 1982). The decrease in calcium excretion following cyclo-oxygenase inhibition in the conscious rat was independent of changes in GFR and was attributed to an increase in tubular reabsorption (Roman *et al.*, 1984). It was also suggested to be independent of vasopressin, since calcium excretion was reduced in both the antidiuretic and the water-diuretic animal. In isolated perfused collecting tubules, PGE_2 has been demonstrated to inhibit calcium reabsorption (Holt and Lechene, 1981). In addition, the possibility that renal arachidonate metabolites might modify the influence of parathyroid hormone on the renal handling of calcium has been proposed (Bidot-Lopez *et al.*, 1981; Dominique *et al.*, 1981).

Urea. PGE_2 and $PGF_{2\alpha}$ have both been demonstrated to decrease the stimulation of urea permeability induced by vasopressin in the toad bladder (Zook and Strandhoy, 1980). In the conscious rat, meclofenamate reduced urea excretion in the antidiuretic but not the water-diuretic animal, also suggesting an interaction between prostaglandins and the component of urea permeability sensitive to ADH (Roman *et al.*, 1984). Zook and Strandhoy (1981) proposed suppression of the corticomedullary gradient for urea as the primary mechanism by which $PGF_{2\alpha}$ exerts its diuretic and natriuretic effects. However, in the conscious rat, indomethacin could be demonstrated to enhance the osmotic gradient, including that for urea, independent of its effect on sodium and water excretion (Haylor and Lote, 1983).

Potassium. The influence of the renal prostaglandin system on potassium excretion has been studied primarily in relation to the pathophysiology of Bartter's syndrome, a condition in which hypokalaemia is a prominent feature and the urinary excretion of PGE is elevated (Gill *et al.*, 1976). Renal prostaglandins have been proposed to increase potassium excretion by several mechanisms including:

(1) the stimulation of aldosterone in response to an increased release of renin;
(2) an increase in distal K exchange in response to the depression of ascending limb function which increases distal delivery of NaCl.

The evidence that implicates either a primary or a secondary role for the renal prostaglandin system in the aetiology of Bartter's syndrome is discussed by Dunn (1981) and Stoff *et al.* (1983). Although renal prostaglandins would appear to have the potential to enhance potassium excretion, the lack of any change in potassium output following the administration of cyclo-oxygenase inhibitors to either healthy man or conscious experimental animals would suggest little involvement in the maintenance of potassium balance. In addition, the concentrating defect which can be produced by potassium depletion would also appear to be independent of the renal PGE system (Hood and Dunn, 1978; Stoff *et al.*, 1979).

Miscellaneous solutes. The excretion of ammonia can be enhanced following meclofenamate administration in the anaesthetised rat (Jones *et al.*, 1984), and a role for the prostaglandin pathway in the control of renal ammoniagenesis has been proposed. In the conscious rat, Roman *et al.* (1984) also found the excretion of phosphorus and magnesium to be reduced following meclofenamate, the effect on magnesium, like that for calcium, being present in both antidiuretic and water-diuretic animals.

Concluding Remarks

Many readers may be surprised to find no mention in this chapter of the notion that renal prostaglandins are part of an 'antipressor' mechanism which operates normally to prevent hypertension. This topic has been extensively reviewed (e.g. Spokas *et al.*, 1983). Clearly, from the foregoing, the renal prostaglandins locally affect the responses to pressor hormones, and, since prostaglandins (except TXA_2) generally have a natriuretic action, they influence the body sodium content. But is there a more direct humoral role of renal prostaglandins in the maintenance of normotension? A deficient renal synthesis of prostaglandins has been described in hypertensive humans (Tan *et al.*, 1978) but the inescapable fact remains that PGE_2 and $PGF_{2\alpha}$ are very effectively metabolised by the pulmonary circulation (Ferreira and Vane, 1967; Piper and Vane, 1977), and although PGI_2 may not be removed by the lungs (Needleman *et al.*, 1977; Moncada *et al.*, 1978), the arterial level of PGI_2 seems likely to be determined by lung and vessel synthesis (Gryglewski *et al.*, 1978) rather than by renal synthesis. Furthermore, in both normotensive and spontaneously hypertensive rats, arterial blood pressure was not affected by infusion of PGI_2-binding antibody (Pace-Asciak *et al.*, 1980). Hence the case for renal prostaglandins as circulating antihypertensive hormones seems a weak one. Of course there remains the possibility that the kidney produces vasodepressor hormones which are not prostaglandins (review, Muirhead, 1983), and the relationship of renal function to hypertension is extensively reviewed in the present volume (see Chapter 8).

Acknowledgements

The authors' work in this field since 1978 has been funded by the National Kidney Research Fund of the UK and by the United Kingdom Medical Research Council.

References

Aiken, J.W. and Vane, J.R. (1973) 'Intrarenal Prostaglandin Release Attenuates the Renal Vasoconstrictor Activity of Angiotensin', *J. Pharmacol. Exp. Ther.*, *184*, 678–87
Altsheler, P., Rosenbaum, R., Klahr, S. and Slatopolsky, E. (1977) 'Effects of Prostaglandin Synthetase Inhibitors (PSI) on the Renal Excretion of Sodium in Normal and Uremic Dogs',

Clin. Res., 25, 424A

Anderson, C.B., Tannenbaum, J.S., Sicard, G.A. and Etheredge, E.E. (1984) 'Renal Thromboxane Synthesis in Excised Kidney Distal to Renovascular Lesions', *J. Am. Med. Assoc.*, 251, 3118–20

Anderson, R.J., Berl, T., McDonald, K.M. and Schrier, R.W. (1975a) 'Evidence for an *in vivo* Antagonism between Vasopressin and Prostaglandin in the Mammalian Kidney', *J. Clin. Invest.*, 56, 420–6

Anderson, R.J., Taher, M.S., Cronin, R.E., McDonald, K.M. and Schrier, R.W. (1975b) 'Effect of β-Adrenergic Blockade and Inhibitors of Angiotensin II and Prostaglandin on Renal Autoregulation', *Am. J. Physiol.*, 229, 731–6

Antonello, A., Tremolada, C., Baggio, B., Buin, F., Favaro, S., Piccoli, A. and Borsatti, A. (1978) '*In vivo* Activation of Renal Phospholipase Activity by Bradykinin in the Rat', *Prostaglandins*, 16, 23–9

Armstrong, J.M., Blackwell, G.J., Flower, R.J., McGiff, J.C., Mullane, K.M. and Vane, J.R. (1976) 'Genetic Hypertension in Rats is Accompanied by a Defect in Renal Prostaglandin Catabolism', *Nature (Lond.)*, 260, 582–6

Assaykeen, T.A., Clayton, P.L., Goldfein, A. and Ganong, W.F. (1970) 'Effect of Alpha and Beta Adrenergic Blocking Agents on the Renin Response to Hypoglycemia and Epinephrine in Dogs', *Endocrinology*, 87, 1318–22

Ausiello, D.A. and Zusman, R.M. (1984) 'The Role of Calcium in the Stimulation of Prostaglandin Synthesis by Vasopressin in Rabbit Renal Medullary Interstitial Cells in Tissue Culture', *Biochem. J.*, 220, 139–45

Badr, K.F., Baylis, C., Pfeffer, J.M., Pfeffer, M.A., Soberman, R.J., Lewis, R.A., Austen, F., Corey, E.J. and Brenner, B.M. (1984) 'Renal and Systemic Haemodynamic Response to Intravenous Infusion of Leukotriene C4 in the Rat', *Circ. Res.*, 54, 492–9

Barry, E., Hall, W.J. and Martin, J.D.G. (1975) 'Prostaglandin E and the Movement of Salt and Water in the Frog Skin', *Gen. Pharmacol.*, 6, 141–50

Baylis, C., Deen, W.M., Myers, B.D. and Brenner, B.M. (1976) 'Effects of Some Vasodilator Drugs on Transcapillary Fluid Exchange in the Renal Cortex', *Am. J. Physiol.*, 230, 1148–56

Bell, C. and Mya, M.K.K. (1977) 'Release by Vasopressin of E-type Prostaglandins from the Rat Kidney', *Clin. Sci. Mol. Med.*, 52, 103–6

Bell, R.D., Sinclair, B.J. and Parry, W.L. (1975) 'The Effects of Indomethacin on Autoregulation and the Renal Response to Haemorrhage', *Circ. Shock*, 2, 57–63

Benabe, J.E., Spry, L.A. and Morrison, A.R. (1982) 'Effects of Angiotensin II on Phosphatidylinositol and Polyphosphoinositol Turnover in Rat Kidney. Mechanism of Prostaglandin Release', *J. Biol. Chem.*, 257, 7430–4

Benzoni, D., Vincent, M. and Sassard, J. (1981) 'Radioimmunoassay for Urinary Prostaglandin E and F$_\alpha$: Normal Values in Different Age Groups', *Clin. Chim. Acta*, 111, 9–16

Benzoni, D., Vincent, M. and Sassard, J. (1982) 'Urinary Prostaglandins and Seminal Fluid Contamination', *Prost. Leuk. Med.*, 9, 591–2

Berl, T., Raz, A., Wald, H., Horowitz, J. and Czaczkes, W. (1977) 'Prostaglandin Synthesis Inhibition and the Action of Vasopressin: Studies in Man and Rat', *Am. J. Physiol.*, 232, F529–37

Berl, T., Henrich, W.L., Erickson, A.L. and Schrier, R.W. (1979) 'Prostaglandins in the Beta-adrenergic and Baroreceptor-mediated Secretion of Renin', *Am. J. Physiol.*, 236, F472–9

Bidot-Lopez, P., Farese, R.V. and Sabir, M.A. (1981) 'Parathyroid Hormone and Adenosine 3′5′ Monophosphate Acutely Increase Phospholipids of the Phosphatidate-Polyphosphoinositol Pathway in Kidney Cortex Tubules *in vitro* by a Cycloheximide Sensitive Process', *Endocrinology*, 108, 2078–81

Bito, L.Z. (1976) 'The Dependence of Renal PG Excretion and/or Metabolism on Facilitated Transport Processes', *Prostaglandins*, 11, 472–3

Bito, L.Z. and Baroody, R.A. (1978) 'Comparison of Renal Prostaglandin and *p*-Aminohippuric Acid Transport Processes', *Am. J. Physiol.*, 234, F80–8

Blacklock, N.J., Green, R. and Greenwood, S.L. (1983) 'Effect of Indomethacin on Glomerular Filtration Rate and Calcium Excretion in the Anaesthetized Rat', *J. Physiol. (Lond.)*, 342, 77–78P

Blackshear, J.L., Spielman, W.S., Knox, F.G. and Romero, J.C. (1979) 'Dissociation of Renin Release and Renal Vasodilation by Prostaglandin Synthesis Inhibitors', *Am. J. Physiol.*, *237*, F20–4

Blaine, E.H., Davis, J.O. and Prewitt, R.L. (1971) 'Evidence for a Renal Vascular Receptor in Control of Renin Secretion', *Am. J. Physiol.*, *220*, 1593–7

Blasingham, M.C. and Nasjletti, A. (1979) 'Contributions of Renal Prostaglandins to the Natriuretic Action of Bradykinin in the Dog', *Am. J. Physiol.*, *237*, F182–7

Bliss, D.J. and Lote, C.J. (1981) 'Effect of Indomethacin on the Renal Corticomedullary Solute Gradient in Rats during the Infusion of 5% Dextrose', *J. Physiol. (Lond.)*, *320*, 47P

Boberg, U., Hahne, B. and Persson, A.E.G. (1984) 'The Effect of Intraarterial Infusion of Prostacyclin on the Tubuloglomerular Feedback Control in the Rat', *Acta Physiol. Scand.*, *121*, 65–72

Bohman, S.O. (1977) 'Demonstration of Prostaglandin Synthesis in Collecting Duct Cells and Other Cell Types of the Rabbit Renal Medulla', *Prostaglandins*, *14*, 729–44

Bolger, P.M., Eisner, G.M., Ramwell, P.W. and Slotkoff, L.M. (1976) 'Effect of Prostaglandin Synthesis on Renal Function and Renin in the Dog', *Nature (Lond.)*, *259*, 244–5

Bouby, N., Tan, M-M. T.T., Doute, M. and Bankir, L. (1984) 'Effects of Osmolality and Antidiuretic Hormone on Prostaglandin Synthesis by Renal Papilla', *Pflügers Arch.*, *400*, 96–9

Bowden, R.E., Ware, J.H., Demets, D.I. and Keiser, H.R. (1977) 'Urinary Excretion of Immunoreactive Prostaglandin E: a Circadian Rhythm, and the Effect of Posture', *Prostaglandins*, *14*, 151–61

Buck, A.C., Sampson, W.F., Lote, C.J. and Blacklock, N.J. (1981) 'The Influence of Renal Prostaglandins on Glomerular Filtration Rate and Calcium Excretion in Urolithiasis', *Brit. J. Urol.*, *53*, 485–91

Buck, A.C., Lote, C.J. and Sampson, W.F. (1983) 'The Influence of Renal Prostaglandin on Urinary Calcium Excretion in Idiopathic Urolithiasis', *J. Urol.*, *129*, 421–6

Burr, G.O. and Burr, M.M. (1929) 'A New Deficiency Disease Produced by the Rigid Exclusion of Fat from the Rat', *J. Biol. Chem.*, *82*, 345–67

Burr, G.O. and Burr, M.M. (1930) 'On the Nature and Role of the Fatty Acids Essential in Nutrition', *J. Biol. Chem.*, *86*, 587–621

Campbell, H.T., Craven, P.A. and DeRubertis, F.R. (1982) 'Evidence for Independent Actions of Vasopressin on Renal Inner Medullary Cyclic AMP and Prostaglandin E Production: Relationship of the Prostaglandin E Response to Hormone Pressor Activity', *Metabolism*, *31*, 1035–41

Campbell, H.T., Craven, P.A. and DeRubertis, F.R. (1983) 'Effects of Fluid Intake on Basal and Vasopressin-responsive Urinary Prostaglandin E', *Am. J. Physiol.*, *245*, F48–57

Carretero, G.A. and Scicli, A.G. (1980) 'The Renal Kallikrein-Kinin System', *Am. J. Physiol.*, *238*, F247–55

Chang, L.C.T., Splawinski, J.A., Oates, J.A. and Nies, A.S. (1975) 'Enhanced Renal Prostaglandin Production in the Dog. II Effects on Intrarenal Haemodynamics', *Circ. Res.*, *36*, 204–7

Chapnick, B.M., Paustian, P.W., Feigen, L.P., Joiner, P.D., Hyman, A.L. and Kadowitz, P.J. (1977) 'Influence of Inhibitors of Prostaglandin Synthesis on Renal Vascular Resistance and on Renal Vascular Responses to Vasopressor and Vasodilator Agents in the Cat', *Circ. Res.*, *40*, 348–54

Chaumet-Riffaud, P., Oudinet, J-P., Sraer, J., Lajotte, C. and Ardaillou, R. (1981) 'Altered PGE_2 and PGF_2 Production by Glomeruli and Papilla of Sodium-depleted and Sodium-loaded Rat', *Am. J. Physiol.*, *241*, F517–24

Christensen, P., Green, K. and Leyssac, P. (1983) 'The Relationship between Urinary Prostaglandin Excretion Rates and Urine Flow in Conscious Rats. Evaluation of the Radioimmunoassay by Gas Chromatography-Mass Spectometry', *Acta Physiol. Scand.*, *117*, 41–7

Cinotti, G.A., Stirati, G., Pecci, G., Pierucci, A., Pugliese, F., Simonetti, B.N., Ciabattoni, G., Valentini, F. and Patrono, C. (1981) 'Evaluation of Urinary Prostaglandin Excretion by Stop-flow Analysis in Dogs', *Minerva Nefrol.*, *28*, 203–8

Colette, C., Aguirre, L., Monnier, L. and Mimran, A. (1982) 'The Influence of Indomethacin and Possible Role of Prostaglandins on Calcium Renal Excretion', *Renal Physiol. Basel*,

5, 68–75

Craven, P.A. and DeRubertis, F.R. (1984) 'Phospholipid Methylation in the Calcium-dependent Release of Arachidonate for Prostaglandin Synthesis in the Renal Medulla', *J. Lab. Clin. Med.*, *104*, 480–93

Craven, P.A., Briggs, R. and DeRubertis, F.R. (1980) 'Calcium Dependent Action of Osmolality on Adenosine 3'5' Monophosphate Accumulation in the Rat Renal Inner Medulla. Evidence for a Relationship to Calcium Responsive Arachidonate Release and Prostaglandin Synthesis', *J. Clin. Invest.*, *65*, 524–42

Craven, P.A., Studer, R.K. and DeRubertis,F.R. (1981) 'Renal Inner Medullary Prostaglandin Synthesis. A Calcium-Calmodulin Dependent Process Suppressed by Urea', *J. Clin. Invest.*, *68*, 722–32

Critchley, J.A.J.H., Freestone,S., Marwick, K., Watson, M.L. and Prescott, L.F. (1984) 'The Acute Effects of Suprofen on Urine Volume, Sodium and PGE Excretion in Healthy Volunteers', *IUPHAR 9th Int. Congr. Pharmacol.*, 653A

Croxatto, H.R., Arriagada, R., Rojas, M., Roblero, J. and Rosas, R. (1978) 'Effects of Prostaglandin E_2 and Prostaglandin $E_{2\alpha}$ upon Urinary Kallikrein Excretion in Rats', *Clin. Sci. Mol. Med.*, *55 (Suppl. 4)*, 187S–9S

Culpepper, R.M. and Andreoli, T.E. (1983) 'Interactions among Prostaglandin E_2, Antidiuretic Hormone and Cyclic Adenosine Monophosphate in Modulation Cl⁻ Absorption in Single Mouse Medullary Thick Ascending Limbs of Henle', *J. Clin. Invest.*, *71*, 1588–1601

Currie, M.G. and Needleman, P. (1984) 'Renal Arachidonic Acid Metabolism', *Ann. Rev. Physiol.*, *46*, 327–41

Danon, A., Chang, L.C.T., Sweetman, B.J., Nies, A.S. and Oates, J.A. (1975) 'Synthesis of Prostaglandins in the Rat Renal Papilla *in vitro*. Mechanisms of Stimulation by Angiotensin II', *Biochim. Biophys. Acta*, *388*, 71–83

Danon, A., Knapp, H.R. Oelz, O. and Oates, J.A. (1978) Stimulation of Prostaglandin Biosynthesis in the Rabbit Papilla by Hypertonic Mediums', *Am. J. Physiol.*, *234*, F64–7

Data, J.L., Gerber, J.G., Crump, W.J., Frolich, J.C., Hollifield, J.W. and Nies, A.S. (1978a) 'The Prostaglandin System. A Role in Canine Baroreceptor Control of Renin Release', *Circ. Res. 42*, 454–8

Data, J.L., Rane A., Gerkens, J., Wilkinson, G.R., Nies, A.S. and Branch, R.A. (1978b) 'The Influence of Indomethacin on the Pharmacokinetics, Diuretic Response and Haemodynamics of Furosemide in the Dog', *J. Pharmacol. Exp. Ther.*, *206*, 431–8

Davila, D., Davila, T., Oliw, E. and Anggard, E. (1978) 'The Influence of Dietary Sodium on Urinary Prostaglandin Excretion', *Acta Physiol. Scand.*, *103*, 100–6

Davila, T., Davila, D., Oliw, E. and Anggard, E. (1980) 'Renal Prostaglandins and Sodium Balance in the Rabbit: Lack of Effect of Aspirin-like Drugs', *Acta Pharm. Toxicol.*, *46*, 57–61

DiBona, G.F. (1977) 'Neurogenic Regulation of Renal Tubular Sodium Reabsorption', *Am. J. Physiol.*, *233*, F73–81

Dominique, J.H., Chen, T.C., Fragola, J. and Puschett, J.B. (1981) 'Inhibition of the Renal Tubular Effects of Parathyroid Hormone on Phosphate Transport by Prostaglandin E_2', *Endocrinology*, *109*, 2267–9

Donker, A.J.M., Arisz, L., Brentjens, I.H., Van den Hem, G.K. and Hollemans, H.J.G. (1976) 'The Effect of Indomethacin on Kidney Function and Plasma Renin Activity in Man', *Nephron*, *17*, 288–96

Dunn, M.J. (1981) 'Prostaglandins and Bartter's Syndrome', *Kidney Int.*, *19*, 86–102

Dunn, M.J. (1984) 'Non-steroidal Anti-inflammatory Drugs and Renal Function', *Ann. Rev. Med.*, *35*, 411–28

Dunn, M.J., Staley, R.S. and Harrison, M. (1976) 'Characterization of Prostaglandin Production in Tissue Culture of Rat Renal Medullary Cells', *Prostaglandins*, *12*, 37–49

Dunn, M.J., Greely, H.P., Valtin, H., Kinter, L.B. and Beeuwkes, R. (1978a) 'Renal Excretion of Prostaglandin E_2 and $F_{2\alpha}$ in Diabetes Insipidus Rats', *Am. J. Physiol.*, *235*, E624–7

Dunn, M.J., Liard, J.F. and Dray, F. (1978b) 'Basal and Stimulated Rates of Renal Secretion and Excretion of Prostaglandins E_2, $F_{2\alpha}$ and 13,14 Dihydro-15 Keto F_α in the Dog', *Kidney Int.*, *13*, 136–43

Dunn, M.J., Beck, T.R., Kinter, L.B. and Hassid, A. (1983) 'The Effects of Vasopressin and Vasopressin Analogues upon Renal Synthesis of Prostaglandins', in M.J. Dunn, C. Patrono

and G.A. Cinotti (eds), *Prostaglandins and the Kidney*, Plenum, New York, pp. 151–66
Dusing, R. and Lee, J.B. (1980) 'Renomedullary Prostaglandin Biosynthesis: Dependence on Extracellular Potassium Concentrations', in A. Scriabine, A.M. Lefer and F.A. Kuehl (eds), *Prostaglandins in Cardiovascular and Renal Function*, MTP Press, Lancaster, pp. 123–37
Ellis, C.K., Whorton, R., Oelz, O., Sweetman, B.J., Wilkinson, G.R. and Oates, J.A. (1977) 'Enhanced Renal Prostaglandin Synthesis in Renal Hypertensive Rats Fed Dihomo-linolenate', *Fed. Proc.*, *36*, 703P
Ellis, C.K., Smigel, M.D., Oates, J.A., Oelz, O. and Sweetman, B.J. (1979) 'Metabolism of Prostaglandin D_2 in the Monkey', *J. Biol. Chem.*, *254*, 4152–63
Epstein, M., Lifschitz, M.D., Hoffman, D.S. and Stein, J.H. (1979) 'Relationship between Renal Prostaglandin E and Renal Sodium Handling during Water Immersion in Normal Man', *Circ. Res.*, *45*, 71–80
Feigen, L.P., Klainer, E., Chapnick, B.M. and Kadowitz, P.J. (1976) 'The Effect of Indomethacin on Renal Function in Pentobarbital Anaesthetized Dogs', *J. Pharmacol. Exp. Ther.*, *198*, 457–63
Fejes-Toth, G., Magyar, A. and Walter, J. (1977) 'Renal Response to Vasopressin after Inhibition of Prostaglandin Synthesis', *Am. J. Physiol.*, *232*, F416–23
Fejes-Toth, G., Fejes-Toth, A.N. and Frolich, J.C. (1983a) 'Acute Effects of Antidiuretic Hormone on Urinary Prostaglandin Excretion', *J. Pharmacol. Exp. Ther.*, *227*, 215–19
Fejes-Toth, G., Fejes-Toth, A.N., Rigter, B. and Frolich, J.C. (1983b) 'Urinary Prostaglandin and Kallikrein Excretion are not Flow-dependent in the Rat', *Prostaglandins*, *25*, 99–103
Fejes-Toth, G., Filep, J. and Mann, V. (1983c) 'Effect of Vasopressin on Prostaglandin Excretion in Conscious Dogs', *J. Physiol. (Lond.) 344*, 389–97
Ferreira, S.H. and Vane, F.R. (1967) 'Prostaglandins; their Disappearance from and Release into the Circulation', *Nature (Lond.)*, *216*, 868–9
Ferretti, A., Church, J.P. and Flanagan, V.P. (1981) 'Changes in Urinary PGE_2 and $PGF_{2\alpha}$ Daily Excretion Rates in Men during a Period of 4–5 Months', *Progr. Lipid Res.* *20*, 195–8
Fichman, M. and Nadler, J. (1983) 'Lack of Correlation of Urinary 6-Keto $PGF_{1\alpha}$ with Urine Volume, in Contrast to Volume Related Increases in Urinary PGE in Polyuric States', *NATO Advanced Research Workshop on Icosanoids and Ion Transport*, Paris, p. 42
Fine, L.J. and Trizna, W. (1977) 'Influence of Prostaglandins on Sodium Transport of Isolated Medullary Nephron Segments', *Am. J. Physiol.*, *232*, F383–90
Finn, W.F. and Arendshorst, W.J. (1976) 'Effect of Prostaglandin Synthetase Inhibitors on Renal Blood Flow in the Rat', *Am. J. Physiol.*, *231*, 1541–5
Fitzgerald, G.A. and Fitzgerald, D.T. (1984) 'Biosynthesis of Thromboxane A_2 in Renovascular Hypertension', *J. Am. Med. Assoc.*, *251*, 3121–2
Flower, R.J. (1983) 'The Inhibition of Prostaglandin Synthesis by the Glucocorticoids', in M. Dale and J.C. Foreman (eds), *Textbook of Immunopharmacology*, Blackwell, Oxford, pp. 289–304
Flower, R.J. and Blackwell, G.J. (1979) 'Anti-inflammatory Steroids Induce Biosynthesis of a Phospholipase A_2 Inhibitor which Prevents Prostaglandin Generation', *Nature (Lond.)*, *278*, 456–9
Foegh, M.L., Winchester, J.F., Zmudka, M., Helfrich, G.B., Ramwell, P.W. and Schreiner, G.E. (1983) 'Factors Affecting Immunoreactive Thromboxane B_2 in Kidney Transplant Patients', in M.J. Dunn, C. Patrono and G.A. Cinotti (eds), *Prostaglandins and the Kidney*, Plenum, New York, pp. 399–406
Folkert, V.W. and Schlondorff, D. (1977) 'Prostaglandin Synthesis in Isolated Glomeruli', *Prostaglandins*, *13*, 873–92
Foy, J.M. and Nuhu, S.Z. (1984) 'Effect of Bumetanide, Frusemide and Prostaglandin E_2 on the Isolated Perfused Kidney of Rat and Rabbit', *Brit. J. Pharmacol.* *82*, 165–73
Francisco, L.L., Osborn, J.L. and DiBona, G.F. (1980) 'The Role of Prostaglandins in Macula Densa Mediated Renin Release in the Rat', *Fed. Proc.*, *39*, 2952
Franco-Saenz, R., Suzuki, S., Tan, S.Y. and Mulrow, P.J. (1980) 'Prostaglandin Stimulation of Renin Release: Independence of Adrenergic Receptor Activity and Possible Mechanism of Action', *Endocrinology*, *106*, 1400–4
Freeman, R.H. and Davis, J.O. (1983) 'Factors Controlling Renin Secretion and Metabolism', in J. Genest, O. Kuchel, P. Hamet and M. Cantin (eds), *Hypertension*, 2nd ed, McGraw-Hill,

New York, pp. 225–50

Freeman, R.H., Davis, J.O., Dietz, J.R. Villareal, D., Seymour, A.A. and Echtenkamp, S.F. (1982) 'Renal Prostaglandins and the Control of Renin Release', *Hypertension, 4 (Suppl. II)*, II–106 to II–112

Frolich, J.C., Wilson, T.W., Sweetman, B.J., Smigel, M., Nies, A.S., Carr, K., Watson, J.T. and Oates, J.A. (1975) 'Urinary Prostaglandins: Identification and Origin', *J. Clin. Invest., 55*, 763–70

Fulgraff, F. and Meiforth, A. (1971) 'Effects of Prostaglandin E_2 on Excretion and Reabsorption of Sodium and Fluid in Rat Kidneys (Micropuncture Studies)', *Pflügers Arch., 330*, 243–56

Fulgraff, G., Brandenbusch, G. and Heintze, K. (1974) 'Dose Response Relation of the Renal Effects of PGA, PGE_2 and $PGF_{2\alpha}$ in Dogs', *Prostaglandins, 8*, 21–30

Ganguli, M., Tobian, L., Azar, S. and O'Donnell, M. (1977) 'Evidence that Prostaglandin Synthesis Inhibitors Increase the Concentration of Sodium and Chloride in Rat Renal Medulla', *Circ. Res., 40, Suppl. 1*, 1–135-1–139

Gerber, J.G. and Nies, A.S. (1979) 'The Haemodynamic Effects of Prostaglandins in the Rat. Evidence for Important Species Variation in Renovascular Responses', *Circ. Res., 44*, 406–10

Gerber, J.G. Keller, R.T. and Nies, A.S. (1979) 'Prostaglandins and Renin Release: the Effect of PGI_2 and PGE_2, and 13,14 Dihydro PGE_2 on the Baroreceptor Mechanism of Renin Release in the Dog', *Circ. Res., 44*, 796–9

Gerber, J.G., Anderson, R.J., Schrier, R.W. and Nies, A.S. (1982) 'Prostaglandins and the Regulation of Renal Circulation and Function', in J.A. Oates (ed.), *Prostaglandins and the Cardiovascular System*, Raven Press, New York, pp. 227–76

Gill, J.R., Frolich, J.C., Bowden, R.E., Taylor, A.A., Keiser, H.R., Seyberth, H.W., Oates, J.A. and Bartter,F.C. (1976) 'Bartter's Syndrome: A Disorder Characterized by High Urinary Prostaglandins and a Dependence of Hyperreninemia on Prostaglandin Synthesis', *Am. J. Med., 61*, 43–51

Godard, C., Valloton, M.B. and Favre, L. (1982) 'Urinary Prostaglandin, Vasopressin and Kallikrein Excretion in Healthy Children from Birth to Adolescence', *J. Paed., 100*, 898–902

Gottschalk, C.W., Lassiter, W.E. and Mylle, M. (1960) 'Localization of Urine Acidification in the Mammalian Kidney', *Am. J. Physiol., 198*, 581–5

Granstrom, E. (1967) 'On the Metabolism of Prostaglandin E_1 in Man', *Progr. Biochem. Pharmacol., 3*, 89–93

Granstrom, E. and Kindahl, H. (1978) 'Radioimmunoassay of Prostaglandins and Thromboxanes', *Adv. Prost. Thromb. Res., 5*, 119–210

Grantham, J. and Orloff, J. (1968) 'Effect of Prostaglandin E_1 on the Permeability Response of the Isolated Collecting Tubule to Vasopressin, Adenosine 3'5'-monophosphate and Theophylline', *J. Clin. Invest., 47*, 1154–61

Grenier, F.C. and Smith, W.L. (1978) Formation of 6-Keto $PGF_{1\alpha}$ by Collecting Tubule Cells Isolated From Rabbit Renal Papillae', *Prostaglandins, 16*, 759–72

Grenier, F.C., Rollins, T.E. and Smith, W.L. (1981) 'Kinin-induced Prostaglandin Synthesis by Renal Papillary Collection Tubule Cells in Culture', *Am. J. Physiol., 241*, F99–104

Gross, P.A., Schrier, R.W. and Anderson, R.J. (1981) 'Prostaglandins and Water Metabolism: a Review with Emphasis on *in vivo* Studies', *Kidney Int., 19*, 839–50

Gryglewski, R.J., Panczenko, B., Korbut, R., Grodzinska, L. and Ocetkiewicz, A. (1975) 'Corticosteroids Inhibit Prostaglandin Release from Perfused Lungs of Sensitised Guinea-pig', *Prostaglandins, 10*, 343–55

Gryglewski, R.J., Korbut, R. and Ocetkiewicz, A. (1978) 'Generation of Prostacyclin by Lungs *in vivo* and its Release into the Arterial Circulation', *Nature (Lond.), 273*, 765–7

Gullner, H.G., Gill, J.R., Bartter, F.C. and Dusing, R. (1980) 'The Role of the Prostaglandin System in the Regulation of Renal Function in Normal Women', *Am. J. Med., 69*, 718–24

Hall, D.A. and Varney, D.M. (1980) 'Effect of Vasopressin on Electrical Potential Difference and Chloride Transport in Mouse Medullary Thick Ascending Limb of Henle's Loop', *J. Clin. Invest., 66*, 792–802

Ham, E.A., Egan, R.W., Soderman, D., Gale, P.H. and Kuehl, F.A. (1979) 'Peroxidase-dependent Deactivation of Prostacyclin Synthetase', *J. Biol. Chem., 254*, 2191–4

Hardy, M.A., Balsam, P. and Bourgoignie, J.J. (1974) 'Reversible Inhibition by Lanthanum of the Hydro-osmotic Response to Serosal Hypertonicity in the Toad Bladder', *J. Membrane Biol.*, *48*, 13–19

Hassid, A. (1981) 'Transport-active Renal Tubular Epithelial Cells (MDCK and LLL-PDI) in Culture. Prostaglandin Biosynthesis and its Regulation by Peptide Hormones and Ionophore', *Prostaglandins*, *21*, 985–1001

Hassid, A., Konieczkowski, M. and Dunn, M.J. (1979) 'Prostaglandin Synthesis in Isolated Rat Kidney Glomeruli', *Proc. Natl Acad. Sci. USA*, *76*, 1155–9

Haylor, J. (1980) 'Prostaglandin Synthesis and Renal Function in Man', *J. Physiol. (Lond.)*, *298*, 383–96

Haylor, J. and Lote, C.J. (1976) 'The Role of Endogenous Prostaglandin Synthesis in the Regulation of Frog Skin Permeability', *J. Physiol. (Lond.)*, *257*, 50–51P

Haylor, J. and Lote, C.J. (1977) 'Further Evidence for a Physiological Role of Endogenous Prostaglandin Biosynthesis in the Regulation of Frog Skin Permeability', *J. Physiol. (Lond.)*, *266*, 41–2P

Haylor, J. and Lote, C.J. (1979) 'Effect of Indomethacin on Renal Tissue Composition in Conscious Saline-diuretic Rats', *J. Physiol. (Lond.)*, *296*, 90P

Haylor, J. and Lote, C.J. (1980a) 'Diuresis and Diminution of the Renal Concentration Gradient for Sodium by Prostaglandin E_2 in the Anaesthetized Rat', *J. Physiol. (Lond.)*, *320*, 48P

Haylor, J. and Lote, C.J. (1980b) 'Renal Function in Conscious Rats after Indomethacin. Evidence for a Tubular Action of Endogenous Prostaglandins', *J. Physiol. (Lond.)*, *298*, 371–81

Haylor, J. and Lote, C.J. (1983) 'The Influence of Prostaglandin E_2 and Indomethacin on the Renal Corticomedullary Solute Gradient in the Rat', *J. Pharm. Pharmacol.*, *35*, 299–305

Haylor, J. and Lote, C.J. (1984) 'Is the Urinary Excretion of PGE from the Rat Influenced by Changes in Urine Flow?', *Brit. J. Pharmacol.*, *83*, 381P

Haylor, J. and Towers, J. (1981) 'Influence of Prostaglandin E_2 on p-Aminohippuric Acid Clearance and Electromagnetically Measured Renal Blood Flow in the Rat', *J. Physiol.*, *320*, 48P

Haylor, J. and Towers, J. (1982) 'Renal Vasodilator Activity of Prostaglandin E_2 in the Rat Anaesthetized with Pentobarbitone', *Brit. J. Pharmacol.*,*76*, 131–7

Haylor, J., Lote, C.J. and Thewles, A. (1983) 'Urinary PGE_2 Excretion after Acetazolamide Administration in Rats', *J. Physiol. (Lond.)*, *338*, 62P–63P

Haylor, J., Lote, C.J. and Thewles, A. (1984) 'Urinary pH as a Determinant of PGE_2 Excretion by the Conscious Rat', *Clin. Sci.*, *66*, 675–81

Haylor, J., Toner, J.M., Jackson, P.R., Ramsay, L.E. and Lote, C.J. (1985) 'Is the Urinary Excretion of Prostaglandin E in Man Dependent on Urinary pH?', *Clin. Sci.*, *68*, 475–7

Haylor, J., Lote, C.J. and Thewles, A. (1986) 'The Influence of Sodium Bicarbonate on the Flow Dependency of Urinary PGE Excretion in Man', *Clin. Sci.*, *70*

Hebert, S.C., Culpepper, R.M. and Andreoli, T.M. (1981) 'NaCl Transport in Mouse Medullary Thick Ascending Limbs. ADH Enhancement of Transcellular NaCl Cotransport; Origin of Transepithelial Voltage', *Am. J. Physiol.*, *241*, F432–42

Helman, S.I. and Els, W.J. (1978) 'Mechanism of ADH and PGE_2 on Na Transport in Frog Skin: Studies with Microelectrodes', *Physiologist*, *21*, 52

Herbaczynska-Cedro, K. and Vane, J.R. (1973) 'Contribution of Intrarenal Generation of Prostaglandins to Autoregulation of Renal Blood Flow in the Dog', *Circ. Res.*, *33*, 428–36

Hesse, B., Christensen, P., Elmgreen, J. and Nielsen, I. (1979) 'The Relationship of Urinary Prostaglandins and Plasma Renin to Sodium Balance and Diuresis in Normal Man', *Prost. Med.*, *3*, 235–47

Higashihara, E., Stokes, J.B., Kokko, J.P., Campbell, W.B. and DuBose, T.D. (1979) 'Cortical and Capillary Micropuncture Examination of Chloride Transport in Segments of the Rat Kidney during Inhibition of Prostaglandin Production', *J. Clin. Invest.*, *64*, 1277–87

Hirata, F., Schiffmann, E., Venkatasubramanian, K., Salomon, D. and Axelrod, J. (1980) 'A Phospholipase A_2 Inhibitory Protein in Rabbit Neutrophils Induced by Glucocorticoids', *Proc. Natl Acad. Sci. USA*, *77* 2533–6

Holt, N.F. and Lechene, C. (1981) 'ADH-PGE_2 Interactions in the Cortical Collecting Tubule. II. Inhibition of Ca and P Reabsorption', *Am. J. Physiol.*, *241*, F461–7

Hong, S.C.L. and Levine, L. (1976) 'Inhibition of Arachidonic Acid Release from Cells as the

Biochemical Action on the Anti-inflammatory Steroids', *Proc. Natl Acad. Sci. USA, 73,* 1730–4

Hood, V.L. and Dunn, M.J. (1978) 'Urinary Excretion of Prostaglandin E_2 and Prostaglandin $F_{2\alpha}$ in Potassium Deficient Rats', *Prostaglandins, 15,* 273–80

Ignatowska-Switalska, H. (1983) 'Circadian Rhythm of PGE_2, $PGF_{2\alpha}$ and 6 Keto $PGF_{1\alpha}$ in Healthy Women', *Prost. Leuk. Med. 11,* 233–40

Iino, Y. and Imai, M. (1978) 'Effects of Prostaglandins on Sodium Transport in Isolated Collecting Tubules', *Pflügers Arch. 373,* 235–47

Irish, J.M. (1979) 'Secretion of Prostaglandin E_2 by Rabbit Proximal Tubules', *Am. J. Physiol., 237,* F268–73

Jackson, B.A., Edwards, R.M. and Dousa, T.P. (1980) 'Vasopressin-Prostaglandin Interactions in Isolated Tubules from Rat Outer Medulla', *J. Lab. Clin. Med., 96,* 119–28

Jim, K., Hassid, A., Sun, F. and Dunn, M.J. (1982) 'Lipoxygenase Activity in Rat Kidney Glomeruli, Glomerular Epithelial Cells and Cortical Tubules', *J. Biol. Chem., 257,* 10244–9

Johnston, H.H., Herzog, J.P. and Lauler, D.P. (1967) 'Effect of Prostaglandin E_1 on Renal Haemodynamics, Sodium and Water Excretion', *Am. J. Physiol., 213,* 939–46

Jones, E.R., Beck, T.R., Kapoor, S., Shay, R. and Narins, R.G. (1984) 'Prostaglandins Inhibit Renal Ammoniagenesis in the Rat', *J. Clin. Invest., 74,* 992–1002

Jones, R.L., Watson, M.L. and Ungar, A. (1981) 'A Comparison of the Effects of Prostaglandins E_2 and I_2 on Renal Function and Renin Release in Salt-loaded and Salt-depleted Anaesthetized Dogs', *Q. J. Exp. Physiol., 66,* 1–15

Kaojarern, S., Chennavasin, P., Burdette, A., Campbell, W.B. and Brater, D.C. (1984) 'Dependence of Urinary Prostaglandin E_2 Excretion on Urinary Volume Rather than Solute Handling or Segmental Nephron Function in Man', *Clin. Sci., 67,* 413–20

Karim, S.M.M., Devlin, J. and Hillier, K. (1968) 'The Stability of Dilute Solutions of Prostaglandins E_1, E_2, $F_{1\alpha}$ and $F_{2\alpha}$', *Eur. J. Pharmacol., 4,* 416–20

Kauker, M.L. (1975) 'Tracer Microinjection Studies of Prostaglandin E_2 Transport in the Rat Nephron', *J. Pharmacol. Exp. Ther., 193,* 274–80

Kaye, Z., Zipser, R., Hahn, J., Zia, P. and Horton, R. (1980) 'Is Urinary Flow Rate a Major Regulator of Prostaglandin E Excretion in Man ?', *Prost. Med., 4,* 303–9

Kirschenbaum, M.A. and Serros, E.R. (1980) 'Effects of Alteration in Urine Flow Rate on Prostaglandin E Excretion in Conscious Dogs', *Am. J. Physiol., 238,* F107–11

Kirschenbaum, M.A. and Stein, J.H.(1976) 'The Effect of Inhibition of Prostaglandin Synthesis on Urinary Sodium Excretion in the Conscious Dog', *J. Clin. Invest., 57,* 517–21

Kirschenbaum, M.A., White, N., Stein, J.H. and Ferris, T.F. (1974) 'Redistribution of Renal Cortical Blood Flow during Inhibition of Prostaglandin Synthesis', *Am. J. Physiol., 227,* 801–5

Knapp, H.R., Oelz, O., Roberts, L.J., Sweetman, B.J., Oates, J.A. and Reed, P.W. (1977) 'Ionophores Stimulate Prostaglandin and Thromboxane Biosynthesis', *Proc. Natl Acad. Sci. USA, 74,* 4251–5

Kopp, U. and DiBona, G.F. (1984) 'Interaction between Neural and Nonneural Mechanisms Controlling Renin Secretion Rate', *Am. J. Physiol., 246,* F620–6

Kopp, U., Aurell, M., Nilsson, I-M. and Ablad, B. (1980) 'The Role of Beta-1-adrenoceptors in the Renin Release Response to Graded Renal Sympathetic Nerve Stimulation', *Pflügers Arch., 387,* 107–13

Kopp, U., Aurell, M., Sjolander, M. and Ablad, B. (1981) 'The Role of Prostaglandins in the Alpha- and Beta-adrenoceptor Mediated Renin Release Response to Graded Renal Nerve Stimulation', *Pflügers Arch., 391,* 1–8

Kramer, H.J., Backer, A., Hinzen, S. and Dusing, R. (1978) 'Effects of Inhibition of Prostaglandin Synthesis on Renal Electrolyte Excretion and Concentrating Ability in Healthy Man', *Prost. Med., 1,* 341–9

Kramer, H.J., Prior, W., Stinnesbeck, B., Backer, A., Eden, J. and Dusing, R. (1980) 'Interaction between Renal Prostaglandin Metabolism and Salt and Water Balance in Healthy Man', *Adv. Prost. Thromb. Res., 7,* 1021–6

Kreisberg, J.I., Kurnovsky, M.J. and Levine, L. (1982) 'Prostaglandin Production by Homogenous Cultures of Rat Glomerular Epithelial and Mesangial Cells', *Kidney Int., 22,* 355–9

Kuehl, F.A. and Egan, R.W. (1980) 'Prostaglandins, Arachidonic Acid and Inflammation',

Science, 210, 978–84

Lands, E.M. (1979) 'Regulation of Prostaglandin Abundance', *Ann. Rev. Physiol., 41,* 633–52

Lands, E.M. and Rome, L.H. (1976) 'Inhibition of Prostaglandin Biosynthesis', in S.M.M. Karim (ed.), *Prostaglandins: Chemical and Biochemical Aspects,* University Park Press, Baltimore, pp. 87–138

Larsson, C. and Anggard, E. (1974) 'Increased Juxtamedullary Blood Flow on Stimulation of Intrarenal Prostaglandin Biosynthesis', *Eur. J. Pharmacol., 25,* 326–44

Larsson, C., Weber, P. and Anggard, E. (1974) 'Arachidonic Acid Increases and Indomethacin Decreases Plasma Renin Activity in the Rabbit', *Eur. J. Pharmacol., 28,* 391–4

Levine, L. and Moskovitz, M.A. (1979) 'α- and β-Adrenergic Stimulation of Arachidonic Acid Metabolism in Cells in Culture', *Proc. Natl Acad. Sci. USA, 76,* 6632–6

Leyssac P.P., Christensen, P., Hill, R. and Skinner, S.L. (1975) 'Indomethacin Blockade of Renal PGE Synthesis: Effect on Total Renal and Tubular Function and Plasma Renin Concentration in Hydropenic Rats and their Response to Isotonic Saline', *Acta Physiol. Scand., 94,* 484–96

Lieberthal, W. and Levine, L. (1984) 'Stimulation of Prostaglandin Production in Rat Glomerular Epithelial Cells by Antidiuretic Hormone', *Kidney Int., 25,* 766–70

Lifschitz, M.D. and Stein, J.H. (1977) 'Antidiuretic Hormone Stimulates Renal Prostaglandin E (PGE) Synthesis in the Rabbit', *Clin. Res., 25,* 440A

Lifschitz, M.D., Patak, R., Fadem, S., Rosenblatt, S., Burns, T., Epstein, M. and Stein, J.H. (1980) 'Factors Involved in the Regulation of Renal Prostaglandin E Production', in A. Scriabine, A.M. Lefer and F. A. Kuehl (eds), *Prostaglandins in Cardiovascular and Renal Function',* MTP Press, Lancaster, pp. 407–24

Limas, C. and Limas, C.J. (1984) 'Prostaglandin Receptors in Rat Kidney', *Arch. Biochem. Biophys., 233,* 32–42

Lonigro, A.J., Itskovitz, H.D., Crowshaw, K. and McGiff, J.C. (1978) 'Dependency of Renal Blood Flow on Prostaglandin Synthesis in the Dog', *Circ. Res., 32,* 712–17

Lonigro, A.J., Brash, D.W., Stephenson, A.H., Heitman, L.J. and Sprague, R.S. (1982) 'Effect of Ventilatory Rate on Renal Venous PGE_2 and $PGF_{2\alpha}$ Efflux in Anaesthetized Dogs', *Am. J. Physiol., 242,* F38–45

Lote, C.J. and Snape, B.M. (1977) 'Collecting Duct Flow Rate as a Determinant of Equilibration between Urine and Renal Papilla in the Rat in the Presence of a Maximal Antidiuretic Hormone Concentration', *J. Physiol. (Lond.), 270,* 533–44

Lote, C.J., Rider, J.B. and Thomas, S. (1974) 'The Effect of Prostaglandin E_1 on the Short Circuit Current and Sodium, Potassium, Chloride and Calcium Movements Across Isolated Frog (*Rana temporaria*) Skin', *Pflügers Arch., 352,* 145–53

Lote, C.J., McVicar, A.J. and Thewles, A. (1983) 'Prostaglandin E_2 Excretion, Urine Flow and Papillary Osmolality during Saline or Dextrose Infusion in the Conscious Rat', *J. Physiol. (Lond.), 336,* 39–46

Lote, C.J., Haylor J. and Towers, J.D. (1984) 'The Effect of Urine pH on the Reduction of Urinary PGE_2 Excretion by Indomethacin', *Biochem. Pharmacol., 33,* 1564–6

Lum, G., Aisenbrey, G.A., Dunn, M.J., Berl, T., Schrier, R.W. and McDonald, K.M. (1977) '*In vivo* Effect of Indomethacin to Potentiate the Renal Medullary Cyclic AMP Response to Vasopressin', *J. Clin. Invest., 59,* 8–13

Mackenzie, T., Zawada, E.T., Johnson, M.D. and Green, S. (1984) 'The Importance of Age on Prostaglandin E_2 Excretion in Normal and Hypertensive Men', *Nephron, 38,* 178–82

McGiff, J.C. (1981) 'Prostaglandins, Prostacyclin and Thromboxanes', *Ann. Rev. Pharmacol. Toxicol., 21,* 479–509

McGiff, J.C., Crowshaw, K., Terragno, N.A., Lonigro, A.J., Strand, J.C., Williamson, M.A., Lee, J.B. and Ng, K.K.F. (1970) 'Prostaglandin-like Substances Appearing in Canine Renal Venous Blood during Renal Ischaemia', *Circ. Res., 27,* 765–82

McGiff, J.C., Itskovitz, H.D. and Terragno, N.A. (1975) 'The Actions of Bradykinin and Eledoisin in the Canine Isolated Kidney: Relationships to Prostaglandins', *Clin. Sci. Mol. Med., 49,* 125–31

McGiff, J.C., Spokas, E.G. and Wong, P.Y.K. (1982) 'Stimulation of Renin Release by 6-Oxo-prostaglandin E_1 and Prostacyclin', *Brit. J. Pharmacol., 75,* 137–44

Malik, K.U. and McGiff, J.C. (1975) 'Modulation by Prostaglandins of Adrenergic Transmission in the Isolated Perfused Rabbit and Rat Kidney', *Circ. Res.*, *36*, 599–609

Meiers, H.G. and Wetzels, E. (1964) 'Phenylbutazone and Renal Function', *Arzneimittel-Forsch.* *14*, 252–8

Milne, M.D., Scribner, B.H. and Crawford, M.A. (1958) 'Non-ionic Diffusion of Weak Acids and Bases', *Am. J. Med.*, *24*, 709–29

Moncada, S., Gryglewski, R.J., Bunting, S. and Vane, J.R. (1976) 'A Lipid Peroxide Inhibits the Enzyme in Blood Vessel Microsomes that Generates from Prostacyclin Endoperoxides the Substance (Prostaglandin X) which Prevents Platelet Aggregation', *Prostaglandins*, *12*, 715–37

Moncada, S., Korbut, R., Bunting, S. and Vane, J.R. (1978) 'Prostacyclin Is a Circulating Hormone', *Nature (Lond.)*, 767–8

Morrison, A.R. and Pascoe, N. (1981) 'Metabolism of Arachidonate through NADPH-dependent Oxygenase of Renal Cortex', *Proc. Natl Acad. Sci. USA*, *78*, 7373–8

Morrison, A.R, Nishikawa, K. and Needleman, P. (1977) 'Unmasking of Thromboxane A$_2$ Synthesis by Ureteral Obstruction in the Rabbit Kidney', *Nature (Lond.)*, *267*, 259–60

Morrison, A.R., Nishikawa, K. and Needleman, P. (1978) 'Thromboxane A$_2$ Biosynthesis in the Ureter Obstructed Kidney of the Rabbit', *J. Pharmacol. Exp. Ther.*, *205*, 1–8

Morrison, A.R., Thornton, F., Blumberg, A. and Vaughan, E.D. (1981) 'Thromboxane A$_2$ is the Major Arachidonic Acid Metabolite of Human Cortical Hydronephrotic Tissue', *Prostaglandins*, *21*, 471–81

Muirhead, E. (1983) 'The Renomedullary Antihypertensive System and its Putative Hormones', in J. Genest, O. Kuchel, P. Hamet and M. Cantin (eds), *Hypertension* (2nd edn) McGraw-Hill, New York, pp. 394–407

Mullane, K.N. and Moncada, S. (1980) 'Prostacyclin Release and the Modulation of Some Vasoactive Hormones', *Prostaglandins*, *20*, 25–49

Nasjletti, K. and Malik, K.U.. (1981a) 'The Renal Kallikrein-Kinin and Prostaglandin Systems Interaction', *Ann. Rev. Physiol.*, *43*, 597–609

Nasjletti, K. and Malik, K.U. (1981b) 'Renal Kinin-Prostaglandin Relationship: Implications for Renal Function', *Kidney Int.*, *19*, 860–8

Needleman, P., Kauffman, A.H., Douglas, J.R., Johnson, E.M. and Marshall, G.R. (1973) 'Specific Stimulation and Inhibition of Renal Prostaglandin Release by Angiotensin Analogs', *Am. J. Physiol.* *224*, 1415–19

Needleman, P., Douglas, J.R. and Jakschuk, B. (1974) 'Release of Renal Prostaglandins by Catecholamines. Relationship to Renal Endocrine Function', *J. Pharmacol. Exp. Ther.*, *188*, 453–60

Needleman, P., Bronson, S.D., Wyche, A. and Sivakoff, M. (1977) 'Cardiac and Renal Prostaglandin I$_2$', *J. Clin. Invest.*, *61*, 839–49

Needleman, P., Wyche, A., Bronson, S.D., Holmberg, S. and Morrison, A.R. (1979) 'Specific Regulation of Peptide-induced Renal Prostaglandin Biosynthesis', *J. Biol. Chem.*, *254*, 9772–7

Oliver, J.A., Pinto, J., Sciacca, R.R. and Cannon, P.J. (1980) 'Increased Renal Secretion of Norepinephrine and Prostaglandin E$_2$ during Sodium Depletion in the Dog', *J. Clin. Invest.*, *66*, 748–56

Oliw, E.H. and Oates, J.A. (1981) 'Rabbit Renal Cortex Microsomes Metabolise Arachidonic Acid to Trihydroxyeicosatrienoic Acid', *Prostaglandins*, *22*, 863–71

Oliw, E.H., Lawson, J.A., Brash, A.R. and Oates, J.A. (1981) 'Arachidonic Acid Metabolism in Rabbit Renal Cortex', *J. Biol. Chem.*, *256*, 9924–31

Olsen, U.B. (1981) 'Dissociation between Renal Medullary PGE$_2$ Synthesis and Urine PGE$_2$ Excretion. Antagonism by Bumetanide of Chlorazanil Induced Urine PGE$_2$-excretion in Rats', *Prostaglandins*, *21*, 591–7

Olson, R.D., Skoglund, M.L., Nies, A.S and Gerber, J.G. (1980) 'Prostaglandins Mediate the Macula Densa Stimulated Renin Release', *Adv. Prostaglandin Thromboxane Res.*, *7*, 1135–7

Omachi, R.S., Robbie, D.E., Handler, J.S. and Orloff, J. (1974) 'Effects of ADH and Other Agents on Cyclic AMP Accumulation in Toad Bladder Epithelium', *Am. J. Physiol.*, *226*, 1152–7

Ono, M., Kogo, H. and Aizawa, Y. (1982) 'Effect of Vasopressin on Rat Urinary Prostaglandin Excretion', *J. Pharm. Dyn.*, *5*, 229–36

Orloff, J., Handler, J.S. and Bergstrom, S. (1965) 'Effect of Prostaglandin (PGE_1) on the Permeability Response of Toad Bladder to Vasopressin, Theophylline and Adenosine 3'5' Monophosphate', *Nature (Lond.), 205*, 397–8

Osborn, J.L., Thames, M.D. and DiBona, G.F. (1982) 'Neural Control of Renin Secretion', in M.J. Dunn, C. Patrono and G.A. Cinotti (eds), *Prostaglandins and the Kidney*, New York, Plenum, pp. 185–8

Owen, T.L., Ehrhart, I.C., Weidner, J.W., Scott, J.B. and Haddy, F.J. (1975) 'Effects of Indomethacin on Local Blood Flow Regulation in Canine Heart and Kidney', *Proc. Soc. Exp. Biol. Med., 149*, 871–6

Pace-Asciak, C.R. and Rosenthal, A.R. (1982) 'Constriction of the Isolated Rat Kidney by Vasopressin is Strongly Opposed by PGE_1 and PGE_2', *Progr. Lipid Res., 20*, 605–8

Pace-Asciak, C.R., Carrara, M.C., Levine, L. and Nicolaou, K.C. (1980) 'PGI_2-specific Antibodies Administered *in vivo* Suggest against a Role for Endogenous PGI_2 as a Circulating Vasodepressor Hormone in the Normotensive and Spontaneously Hypertensive Rat', *Prostaglandins, 20*, 1053–60

Padfield, P.L. and Grekin, R.J. (1981) 'The Effect of Indomethacin on Vasopressin-induced Antidiuresis in Man', *Clin. Sci., 61*, 493–6

Passmore, J.C., Rosenberg, E.M. and Hock, C.E. (1980) 'Effects of Indomethacin on Intrarenal Blood Flow and Medullary Osmolality in Dogs', *Prost. Med., 5*, 275–87

Patrono, C., Wennmalm, A., Ciabattoni, G., Nowak, J., Pugliese, F. and Cinotti, G. A. (1979) 'Evidence for an Extrarenal Origin of Urinary Prostaglandin E_2 in Healthy Men', *Prostaglandins, 18*, 623–9

Peterson, L.N., Gerber, J.G. and Nies, A.S. (1984) 'Effect of pH on the Permeability of the Distal Nephron to Prostaglandins E_2 and $F_{2\alpha}$', *Am. J. Physiol., 246*, F221–6

Piper, P. and Vane, J.R. (1977) 'The Release of Prostaglandins from Lung and Other Tissues', *Ann. NY Acad. Sci., 180*, 363

Pirotzky, E., Bidault, J., Burtin, C., Gabler, M.C. and Benveniste, J. (1984) 'Release of Platelet Activating Factor, Slow Reacting Substance and Vasoactive Amines from Isolated Rat Kidneys', *Kidney Int., 25*, 404–10

Ramsay, A.G. and Elliott, H.C. (1967) 'Effect of Acetylsalicylic Acid on Ionic Reabsorption in the Renal Tubule', *Am. J. Physiol., 213*, 323–7

Rathaus, M., Podjarny, E., Weiss, E., Weiss, R.M., Bauminger, S. and Berheim, J. (1981) 'Effect of Chronic and Acute Changes in Sodium Balance on the Urinary Excretion of Prostaglandin E_2 and $F_{2\alpha}$ in Normal Man', *Clin. Sci., 60*, 405–10

Raz, A. (1972) 'Interaction of Prostaglandins with Blood Plasma Proteins: Comparative Binding of Prostaglandins A_2, $F_{2\alpha}$ and E_2 to Human Plasma Proteins', *Biochem. J., 130*, 631–6

Rennick, B.R. (1977) 'Renal Tubular Transport of Prostaglandins: Inhibition by Probenecid and Indomethacin', *Am. J. Physiol., 233*, F133–7

Roman, R.J. and Kauker, M.L. (1978) 'Renal Effect of Prostaglandin Synthetase Inhibition in Rats, Micropuncture Studies', *Am. J. Physiol., 235*, F111–18

Roman, R.J., Skelton, M. and Lechene, C. (1984) 'Prostaglandin-Vasopressin Interactions on the Renal Handling of Calcium and Magnesium', *J. Pharm. Exp. Ther., 230*, 295–301

Rosenblatt, S.G., Patak, R.V. and Lifschitz, M.D. (1978) 'Organic Acid Secretory Pathway and Urinary Excretion of Prostaglandin E in the Dog', *Am. J Physiol., 234*, F473–9

Russo-Marie, F., Seillan, C. and Duval, D. (1983) 'Mechanism of Steroid-induced Inhibition of Prostaglandin Production by Rat Reno-medullary Cells in Culture', in M.J. Dunn, C. Patrono and G.A. Cinotti (eds), *Prostaglandins and the Kidney*, Plenum, New York, pp. 243–50

Sasaki, S. and Imai, M. (1980) 'Effects of Vasopressin on Water and NaCl Transport Across the *in vitro* Perfused Medullary Thick Ascending Limb of Henle's Loop of Mouse, Rat and Rabbit Kidney', *Pflügers Arch., 383*, 215–21

Satoh, S. and Zimmerman, B.G. (1975) 'Influence of the Renin-Angiotensin System on the Effect of Prostaglandin Synthesis Inhibitors in the Renal Vasculature', *Circ. Res., 36–7 (Suppl.)*, 189–95

Scherer, B., Siess, W. and Weber, P.C. (1977) 'Radioimmunological and Biological Measurement of Prostaglandin in Rabbit Urine: Decrease of PGE_2 Excretion at High NaCl Intake', *Prostaglandins, 13*, 1127–39

Schlondorff, D., Zanger, R., Satriano, A., Folkert, V.W. and Eveloff, J. (1982) 'Prostaglandin

Synthesis by Isolated Cells from the Outer Medulla and from the Thick Ascending Loop of Henle of Rabbit Kidney', *J. Pharmacol. Exp. Ther.*, *223*, 120–4

Schnermann, J. and Briggs, J.P. (1981) 'Participation of Renal Cortical Prostaglandins in the Regulation of Glomerular Filtration Rate', *Kidney Int.*, *19*, 802–15

Schnermann, J., Briggs, J.P. and Weber, P.C. (1984) 'Tubuloglomerular Feedback, Prostaglandins and Angiotensin in the Autoregulation of Glomerular Filtration Rate', *Kidney Int.*, *25*, 53–64

Schryver, S., Sanders, E., Bierwaltes, W.H. and Romero, J.C. (1984) 'Cortical Distribution of Prostaglandin and Renin in Isolated Dog Glomeruli', *Kidney Int.*, *25*, 512–18

Schwartzman, M. and Raz, A. (1979) 'Prostaglandin Generation in Rabbit Kidney. Hormone-activated Selective Lipolysis Coupled to Prostaglandin Biosynthesis', *Biochim. Biophys. Acta*, *572*, 363–9

Sejersted O.M., Vikse, A., Eide, I. and Kiil, F. (1984) 'Renal Venous and Urinary PGE_2 Output during Intrarenal Arachidonic Acid Infusion in Dogs', *Acta Physiol. Scand.*, *121*, 249–59

Serros, E.R. and Kirschenbaum, M.A. (1981) 'Prostaglandin-dependent Polyuria in Hypercalcaemia', *Am. J. Physiol.*, *241*, F224–30

Seymour, A.A. and Zehr, J.E. (1979) 'Influence of Renal Prostaglandin Synthesis on Renin Control Mechanisms in the Dog', *Circ. Res.*, *45*, 13–25

Seymour, A.A., Davis, J.O., Freeman, R.H., DeForrest, J.M., Rowe, B.P. and Williams, G.M (1979) 'Renin Release from Filtering and Non-Filtering Kidneys Stimulated by PGI_2 and PGD_2', *Am. J. Physiol.*, *237*, F285–90

Shaw, J.E. and Ramwell, P.W. (1969) 'Separation, Identification and Estimation of Prostaglandins', *Meth. Biochem. Anal.*, *17*, 325–71

Shea-Donohue, P.T., Bolger, P.M., Eisner, G.M. and Slotkoff, L.M. (1979) 'Effects of PGE_2 on Electrolyte and Fluid Excretion in the Canine Kidney. Evidence for a Direct Tubular Effect', *Can. J. Physiol. Pharmacol.*, *57*, 1448–52

Shier, W.T. (1979) 'Activation of High Levels of Endogenous Phospholipase A_2 in Cultured Cells', *Proc. Natl Acad. Sci. USA*, *76*, 195–9

Smith, W.L., Grenier, F.C., Bell, T.G. and Wilkin, G.P. (1980) 'Cellular Distribution of Enzymes Involved in Prostaglandin Metabolism in the Mammalian Kidney', in A. Scriabine, A.M. Lefer, and F.A. Kuehl (eds), *Prostaglandins in Cardiovascular and Renal Function*, MTP Press, Lancaster, pp. 71–91

Spokas, E.G., Quilley, J. and McGiff, J.C. (1983) 'Prostaglandins in Hypertension', in J. Genest, O. Kuchel, P. Hamet and M. Cantin (eds), *Hypertension* (2nd edn), McGraw-Hill, New York, pp. 373–93

Sraer, J., Sraer, J.D., Chansel, D., Russo-Marie, F., Kouznetzova, B. and Ardaillou, R. (1979) 'Prostaglandin Synthesis by Isolated Rat Renal Glomeruli', *Mol. Cell. Endocrinol.*, *16*, 29–37

Sraer, J., Ardaillou, N., Sraer, J.D. and Ardaillou, R. (1982) '*In vitro* Prostaglandin Synthesis by Human Glomeruli and Papillae', *Prostaglandins*, *23*, 855–64

Sraer, J., Riguad, M., Bens, M., Rabinovitch, H. and Ardaillou, R. (1983a) 'Metabolism of Arachidonic Acid via the Lipoxygenase Pathway in Human and Murine Glomeruli', *J. Biol. Chem.*, *258*, 4325–30

Sraer, J., Seiss, W., Dray, F. and Ardaillou, R. (1983b) 'Regional Differences in *in vitro* Prostaglandin Synthesis by the Rat Kidney', in M.J. Dunn, C. Patrono and G.A. Cinotti (eds), *Prostaglandins and the Kidney*, Plenum, New York, pp. 41–52

Stahl, R.A.K., Attallah, A.A., Bloch, D.L. and Lee, J.B. (1979) 'Stimulation of Rabbit Renal PGE_2 Biosynthesis by Dietary Sodium Restriction', *Am. J. Physiol.*, *237*, F344–9

Stoff, J.S., Rosa, R.M. and Epstein, F.M. (1979) 'The Concentrating Defect of Acute Potassium Depletion in Man Is Independent of Renal Prostaglandins', *Kidney Int.*, *17*, 277–83

Stoff, J.S., Clive D.M., Leone, D., MacIntyre, D.E., Brown, R.S. and Salzman, E. (1983) 'The Role of Arachidonic Acid Metabolites in the Pathophysiology of Bartter's Syndrome', in M.J. Dunn, C. Patrono and G.A. Cinotti (eds), *Prostaglandins and the Kidney*, Plenum, New York, pp. 353–64

Stokes, J.B. (1979) 'Effect of Prostaglandin E_2 on Chloride Transport across the Rabbit Thick Ascending Limb of Henle. Selective Inhibition of the Medullary Portion', *J. Clin. Invest.*, *64*, 495–502

Stokes, J.B. and Kokko, J.P. (1977) 'Inhibition of Sodium Transport by Prostaglandin E_2 across the Isolated Perfused Rabbit Collecting Tubule', *J. Clin. Invest.*, *59*, 1099–104

Strandhoy, J.W., Ott, C.E, Schneider, E.G., Willis, L.R., Beck, N.P., Davis, B.B. and Knox, F.G. (1974) 'Effects of Prostaglandin E_1 and E_2 on Renal Sodium Reabsorption and Starling Forces', *Am. J. Physiol.*, *226*, 1015–21

Swain, J.A., Heyndrickx, G.R., Boettcher, D.H. and Vatner, S.F. (1975) 'Prostaglandins: Control of Renal Circulation in the Unanaesthetized Dog and Baboon', *Am. J. Physiol.*, *229*, 826–30

Taher, M.S., McLain, L.G., McDonald, K.M. and Schrier, R.W. (1976) 'Effect of β-Adrenergic Blockade on Renin Response to Renal Nerve Stimulation', *J. Clin. Invest.*, *57*, 459–65

Tan, S.Y., Sweet, P. and Mulrow, P.J. (1978) 'Impaired Renal Production of Prostaglandin E_2: a Newly Identified Lesion in Human Essential Hypertension', *Prostaglandins*, *15*, 139–49

Tan, S.Y., Sandwisch, D.W. and Mulrow, P.J. (1980) 'Sodium Intake as a Determinant of Urinary PGE_2 Excretion', *Prost. Med.*, *4*, 53–63

Terragno, N.S., Terragno, D.A. and McGiff, J.C. (1977) 'Contribution of Prostaglandins to the Renal Circulation in Conscious, Anaesthetised and Laparotomised Dogs', *Circ. Res.*, *40*, 590–5

Terragno, N.A., Terragno, D.A., Early, J.A., Roberts, M. A. and McGiff, J.C. (1978) 'Endogenous Prostaglandin Synthesis Inhibitor in the Renal Cortex. Effects on Production of Prostacyclin by Renal Blood Vessels', *Clin. Sci.*, *55*, 1995–2025

Torikai, S. and Kurokawa, K. (1983) 'Effect of PGE_2 on Vasopressin-dependent Cell cAMP in Isolated Single Nephron Segments', *Am. J. Physiol.*, *245*, F58–66

Uekama, K., Hirayama, F., Tanaka, H. and Takematsu, K. (1978) 'Partition Behaviour and Ion Pair Formation of Some Prostaglandins', *Chem. Pharm. Bull.*, *26*, 3779–84

Van den Bosch, H. (1980) 'Intracellular Phospholipases A', *Biochim. Biophys. Acta*, *604*, 191–246

Vander, A.J. and Miller, R. (1964) 'Control of Renin Secretion in the Dog', *Am. J. Physiol.*, *207*, 537–46

Vargraftig, B.B. and Hai, N.D. (1972) 'Selective Inhibition by Mepacrine of the Release of "Rabbit Aorta Contracting Substance" Evoked by the Administration of Bradykinin', *J. Pharm. Pharmacol.*, *24*, 159–61

Venuto, R.C., O'Dorisio, T., Ferris, T.F. and Stein, J.H. (1975) 'Prostaglandin and Renal Function II. The Effect of Prostaglandin Inhibition on Autoregulation of Blood Flow in the Intact Kidney of the Dog', *Prostaglandins*, *9*, 817–28

Vierhapper, H., Jorg, J. and Waldhausl, W. (1984) 'Effect of Acetylsalicylic Acid and Indomethacin on Diuresis in Man: the Role of Cyclo-oxygenase Inhibition', *Clin. Sci.*, *67*, 579–83

Vinci, J.M., Gill, J.R., Bowden, R.E., Pisano, J.J., Izzo, J.L., Radfar, N., Taylor, A.A., Zusman, R.M., Bartter, F.C. and Keiser, H.R. (1978) 'The Kallikrein-Kinin System in Bartter's Syndrome and its Response to Prostaglandin Synthetase Inhibition', *J. Clin. Invest.*, *61*, 1671–82

Von Euler, U.S. (1934) 'Zuer Kenntnis der pharmakologischen Wirkungen Nativsekreten und extrackter mannlicher accessorischer Geschlechtsdrusen', *Arch. Exp. Pathol. Pharmakol.*, *175*, 78–84

Von Euler, U.S. (1935) 'The Specific Blood Pressure Lowering Substance in Human Prostate and Seminal Vesicle Secretions', *Klin. Wochenschr.*, *14*. 1182–3

Walker, R.M., Brown, R.S. and Stoff, J.S. (1981) 'Role of Renal Prostaglandins during Antidiuresis and Water Diuresis in Man', *Kidney Int.*, *21*, 365–70

Weber, P.C., Holzgreve, H., Stephan, R. and Herbst, R. (1975) 'PRA and Sodium and Water Excretion Following Infusion of Arachidonic Acid in Rats', *Eur. J. Pharmacol.*, *34*, 299–304

Weber, P.C., Larsson, C., Anggard, E., Hamberg, M., Corey, E.J., Nicolaou, K.C. and Samuelsson, B. (1976) 'Stimulation of Renin Release from Rabbit Renal Cortex by Arachidonic Acid and Prostaglandin Endoperoxide', *Circ. Res.*, *39*, 868–74

Weber, P.C., Larsson, C. and Scherer, B. (1977) 'Prostaglandin E_2-9-Ketoreductase as a Mediator of Salt-intake Related Prostaglandin Renin Interaction', *Nature (Lond.)*, *226*, 65–6

Weber, P.C., Scherer, B., Held, E, Seiss, W. and Stoffel, H (1979) 'Urinary Prostaglandins and Kallikrein in Essential Hypertension', *Clin. Sci.*, *57*, 2596–615

Whorton, A.R., Misono, K., Hollifield, J., Frolich, J.C., Inagami, T. and Oates, J.A. (1977) 'Prostaglandins and Renin Release I. Stimulation of Renin Release from Rabbit Renal Cortical Slices by PGI$_2$', *Prostaglandins*, *14*, 1095–104

Whorton, A.R., Smigel, M., Oates, J.A. and Frolich, J.C. (1978) 'Regional Differences in Prostacyclin Formation by the Kidney', *Biochim. Biophys. Acta*, *529*, 176–80

Williams, W.M., Frolich, J.C., Nies, A.S. and Oates, J.A. (1977) 'Urinary Prostaglandins: Site of Entry into Renal Tubular Fluid', *Kidney Int.*, *11*, 256–60

Work, J., Baehler, R.W., Kotchen, T.A., Talwalkar, R. and Luke R.G. (1980) 'Effect of Prostaglandin Inhibition on Sodium Chloride Reabsorption in the Diluting Segment of the Conscious Dog', *Kidney Int. 17*, 24–30

Wright, L.F., Rosenblatt, S.G. and Lifschitz, M.D. (1981) 'High Urine Flow Rate Increases Prostaglandin E Excretion in the Conscious Dog', *Prostaglandins*, *22*, 21–34

Yamamoto, S. (1983) 'Enzymes in the Arachidonic Acid Cascade', in C. Pace-Asciak, and E. Granstrom (eds), *Prostaglandins and Related Substances*, Elsevier, Amsterdam, pp. 171–202

Yun, J., Kelly, G., Bartter, F.C. and Smith, Jr., H. (1977) 'Role of Prostaglandins in the Control of Renin Secretion in the Dog', *Circ. Res.*, *40*, 459–64

Yun, J., Kelly, G., Bartter, F.C. and Smith, H. (1978) 'Role of Prostaglandins in the Control of Renin Secretion in the Dog', *Life Sci.*, *23*, 945–52

Zambraski, E.J. and Dunn, M.J. (1980) 'Renal Prostaglandin E$_2$ and F$_{2\alpha}$ Secretion and Excretion in Exercising Conscious Dogs', *Prost. Med.*, *4*, 311–24

Zambraski, E.J., Tucker, M.S., Lakas, C.S., Grassl, S.M. and Scannes, C.G. (1984) 'Mechanism of Renin Release in Exercising Dogs', *Am. J. Physiol.*, *246*, E71–6

Zenser, T.V., Herman, C.A. and Davis, B.B. (1980) 'Effects of Calcium and A 23187 on Renal Inner Medullary Prostaglandin E$_2$ Synthesis', *Am. J. Physiol.*, *238*, E371–6

Zipser, R.D. and Smorlesi, C. (1984) 'Regulation of Urinary Thromboxane B$_2$ in Man: Influence of Urinary Flow Rate and Tubular Transport', *Prostaglandins*, *27*, 257–71

Zipser, R.D., Myers, S.I. and Needleman, P. (1981b) 'Stimulation of Renal Prostaglandin Synthesis by the Pressor Activity of Vasopressin', *Endocrinology*, *108*, 495–9

Zipser, R.D., Little, T.E., Wilson, W. and Duke, R. (1981a) 'A Dual Effect of Antidiuretic Hormone on Urinary Prostaglandin E$_2$ Excretion in Man', *J. Clin. Endocrinol. Metab.*, *53*, 522–36

Zook, T.E. and Strandhoy, J.W. (1980) 'Inhibition of ADH-enhanced Transepithelial Urea and Water Movement by Prostaglandins', *Prostaglandins*, *20*, 1–13

Zook, T.E. and Strandhoy, J.W. (1981) 'Mechanisms of Natriuretic and Diuretic Effects of Prostaglandin F$_{2\alpha}$', *J. Pharm. Exp. Ther.*, *217*, 674–80

Zucker, A., Nasjletti, A. and Schneider, E.G. (1983) 'Effect of Water Deprivation on Urinary Excretion of PGE$_2$ in the Dog', *Am. J. Physiol.*, *245*, R329–33

Zusman, R.M. (1980) 'Regulation of Prostaglandin Biosynthesis: Studies in the Rabbit Renomedullary Interstitial Cell and the Toad Urinary Bladder *in vitro*', in A. Scriabine, A.M. Lefer and F.A. Kuehl (eds), *Prostaglandins in Cardiovascular and Renal Function*, MTP Press, Lancaster pp. 93–11

Zusman, R.M. and Keiser, H.R. (1977a) 'Prostaglandin E$_2$ Biosynthesis by Rabbit Renomedullary Interstitial Cells in Tissue Culture: Mechanisms of Stimulation by Angiotensin II, Bradykinin and Arginine Vasopressin', *J. Biol. Chem.*, *252*, 2069–71

Zusman, R.M. and Keiser, H.R. (1977b) 'Prostaglandin Biosynthesis by Rabbit Renomedullary Interstitial Cells in Tissue Culture. Stimulation by Angiotensin II, Bradykinin and Arginine Vasopressin', *J. Clin. Invest.*, *60*, 215–23

Zusman, R.M. and Keiser, H.R. (1980) 'Regulation of Prostaglandin E$_2$ Synthesis by Angiotensin II, Potassium, Osmolality and Dexamethasone', *Kidney Int.*, *17*, 277–83

Zusman, R.M., Keiser, H.R. and Handler, J.S. (1977) 'Vasopressin-stimulated Prostaglandin E Biosynthesis in the Toad Urinary Bladder: Effect on Water Flow', *J. Clin. Invest.*, *60*, 1339–47

6 HORMONAL CONTROL OF SODIUM EXCRETION

H. Sonnenberg

Introduction

In addition to changes in renal haemodynamics and in aldosterone, several intrarenal hormone systems have been implicated in the regulation of tubular transport of sodium : renin-angiotension (Leyssac, 1976), prostaglandins (Higashihara *et al.*, 1979), and kallikrein-kinin (Carretero and Scicli, 1976). Since these are in part considered in other chapters, this presentation will be restricted to discussion of 'natriuretic hormone(s)'. Although Homer W. Smith (1957) is generally credited with coining the term, he in fact postulated the existence of an antinatriuretic system in analogy to antidiuretic hormone. Apparently, one of the earliest references to 'natriuretic hormone' *per se* is by Atkins and Pearce (1959). The concept that, in addition to aldosterone, another hormone is involved in sodium homeostasis has been from the beginning a 'Cheshire cat' hypothesis (Smith, 1957); although it was advanced to explain many phenomena of sodium balance, closer examination of the evidence usually resulted in its fading away to a derisive grin. However, the need for such a system did persist, and at present the existence of one and possibly more natriuretic hormonal factors seems certain. Three separate lines of evidence lead to this conclusion: (1) mineralocorticoid escape, (2) renal response to progressive nephron loss, and (3) extracellular or intravascular fluid volume expansion.

'Natriuretic Hormone'

Evidence for Natriuretic Hormone

(1) Mineralocorticoid Escape. It has long been known that chronic injection of the sodium-retaining mineralocorticoid hormones in dog (Ragan *et al.*, 1940) and man (Clinton and Thorn, 1943) does not result in progressive salt accumulation in the body. Instead, after several days of positive sodium balance and increasing extracellular fluid volume, the kidney 'escapes' from the sodium-retaining action of the hormones, sodium intake is again balanced by renal excretion, and no further volume changes take place (August *et al.*, 1958).

The mechanism of this escape includes many factors (for review see Knox *et al.*, 1980). However, Pearce and co-workers (1969) have shown clearly that a humoral natriuretic component plays a determining role. Groups of rats were placed on either a high- or a low-salt diet. The former received, in addition, daily injections of deoxycorticosterone acetate (DOCA). After at least

4 weeks on the regimen, kidney function was studied in anaesthetised pairs of one DOCA and one salt-deprived (NaD) rat each. Urine volume and sodium excretion were measured during a 1 h control period. Blood from each animal was then allowed to mix in a common reservoir, initially primed with iso-oncotic bovine albumin solution (Figure 6.1, series 4). Isovolaemic conditions were maintained in each cross-circulated partner. After 1 h of such cross-circulation equal volumes of reservoir contents were infused intravenously into both partners. Control animals (Figure 6.1, series 5) were treated identically, except that each animal equilibrated its blood in a separate reservoir. In the control period, DOCA rats, as expected, excreted significantly more sodium than did NaD rats. Mixing of the blood during the cross-circulation period resulted in a statistically significant increase of sodium excretion in the salt-deprived partner. No such effect was observed in those NaD rats whose blood was exchanged in their own individual reservoirs. Acute intravascular expansion with the equilibrated reservoir contents demonstrated that prior mixing of blood of DOCA and NaD rats significantly increased the renal response of the latter to hypervolaemia, leaving the response of the former essentially unchanged. By contrast, the increase in sodium excretion in salt-deprived rats without prior cross-circulation with a DOCA partner was trivial. Because these results were obtained in the absence of changes in haematocrit or plasma electrolytes, they were interpreted as indicating that DOCA rats supplied a humoral natriuretic factor that allowed the NaD rats to increase renal sodium excretion both before and during acute blood volume expansion. Fractional sodium excretion in NaD rats changed from 0.05 to 0.20 and 1.30 per cent from control to cross-circulation and infusion periods, respectively. Corresponding values in the non-cross-circulated NaD group were 0.03, 0.04 and 0.18 per cent. These data show that the transferred humoral factor inhibits tubular reabsorption of sodium.

(2) Progressive Nephron Loss. Many kidney diseases result in progressive destruction of nephrons. In the face of constant intake of solutes and water, the surviving nephrons must excrete an ever-increasing amount of sodium to maintain body fluid balance (for review see Bricker and Fine, 1981). In the healthy kidney, each nephron excretes in the range of 0.5 per cent of its filtered load of sodium. In advanced renal disease, when renal function may be reduced to one-tenth normal, each remaining nephron must decrease its reabsorption of sodium ten-fold to maintain extracellular fluid volume constant. A humoral component of this adaptation is suggested by the following experiment in rats. In a cross-circulation study, Wilson and Honrath (1978) showed that reduction of nephron mass to 10–15 per cent of normal was associated with a natriuretic effect which could be transferred to a normal partner. Although a part of this influence was due to elevated urea concentration, a separate humoral natriuretic factor was also involved in the response.

Figure 6.1: Average Urine Volume and Sodium Excretion in Pairs of DOCA-treated and Salt-deprived (NaD) Rats. After a control period, circulating blood was mixed either in a common reservoir (series 4, cross-circulation), or in separate reservoirs for each rat (series 5, exchange). Equal volumes of reservoir contents were then infused intravenously into each animal

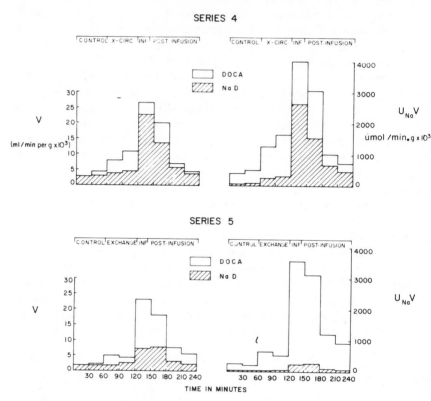

From Pearce *et al.* (1969), with permission

(3)   Body Fluid Volume Expansion. Acute intravenous infusion of isotonic or iso-oncotic solutions has been by far the most widely studied model of natriuretic hormone release. DeWardener *et al.* (1961) are generally credited with providing the first evidence for a humoral natriuretic factor. In cross-circulation experiments in dogs, both partners received large amounts of 9α-fluorocortisone and pitressin to eliminate variations in plasma levels of mineralocorticoid and antidiuretic hormones as influencing factors. Saline was then infused intravenously in one dog. A natriuresis was observed in both partners, although the response was much smaller in the non-infused animal. These results were criticised on the basis that blood dilution and/or volume changes in the non-infused dog could have been responsible for the natriuretic effect, rather than a circulating humoral factor. Lichardus and Pearce (1966) overcame these drawbacks by using iso-oncotic solution or artificial blood as

the infusate, and perfusing a kidney from a second dog at constant pressure with blood from the first one. Under these conditions a small but significant transferred natriuretic response was observed. At least a part of this effect could have been due to renal haemodynamic changes. Subsequently, other groups performed similar experiments (Bahlmann *et al.*, 1967; Blythe *et al.*, 1971; Kaloyanides and Azer, 1971). In at least one of these, haemodynamic changes did not explain the transferred natriuresis (Kaloyanides and Azer, 1971). However, in comparison with the sodium excretion by the kidneys of the volume-expanded animal, the effect due to natriuretic hormone in the perfused kidney was minor at best. Because a perfused kidney is unlikely to be able to respond normally, cross-circulation experiments in rats were designed to test for a transferred natriuresis in which there were no changes in blood composition during expansion of the donor, and in which no circumstance rendered the recipient less responsive than normal (Pearce *et al.*, 1970). Results are shown in Figure 6.2.

The technique employed equilibration of donor blood with that in the common circulation (exchange). Equilibrated blood was then infused into one cross-circulated partner (rat A) and the second was kept isovolaemic. Although rat A had a homeostatically effective natriuretic response, no transferred effect on sodium excretion was observed in the normovolaemic partner (rat B), which shared the blood circulation with the expanded animal. The possibility was considered that a humoral effector, though unable to produce a response by itself, might contribute to a response initiated by some (non-hormonal) parameter of vascular expansion. An equal volume of equilibrated blood was, therefore, infused into rat B while rat A was still volume-expanded. Although rat B now responded, no influence was seen on the pattern of the declining response of rat A. These experiments thus provided no evidence for a humoral effector mechanism of the natriuresis of intravascular volume expansion in the rat. Because other groups, using similar techniques, were also unable to transfer a natriuretic effect (Bonjour and Peters, 1970; Levinsky, 1974), the 'Cheshire-cat' hypothesis at this point seemed to be no more than a fading grin! However, it was found subsequently that if excreted urine was returned to the circulation after an infusion of blood, thereby maintaining intravascular expansion, natriuresis increased to much higher levels than if urine were not reinfused (Sonnenberg, 1971). The natriuretic response could be sustained for at least 2 h. Using this model, cross-circulation experiments demonstrated that during maintained intra-vascular volume expansion of the donor rat a humoral natriuretic effect could be detected in the normovolaemic recipient rat (Sonnenberg *et al.*, 1972). This transferred natriuresis did not depend on urine reinfusion, because when urine was not returned to the circulation, but urine losses were replaced with equal volumes of Ringer's solution, or when the expanded animal was nephrec-tomised, the humoral effect remained intact. Adrenalectomy of the donor prior to volume expansion did not prevent, although it reduced slightly, the

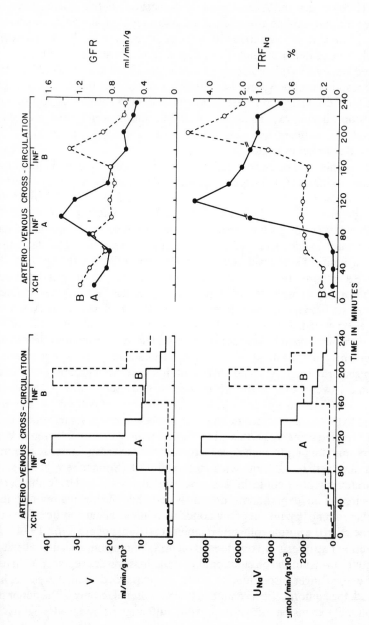

Figure 6.2: Averaged Values for Urine Volume, Sodium Excretion, Filtration Rate and Fractional Sodium Excretion in Pairs of Cross-circulated Rats (A and B), in which Aliquots of Donor Blood, Exchanged for Circulating Blood (XCH), are Infused (INF) Successively into Each Rat

From Pearce *et al.* (1970), with permission

transferred response in the recipient. To assess the physiological importance of this humoral component of volume natriuresis, the response to simple expansion (Pearce *et al.*, 1970) was compared with the recipient natriuresis when the volume-expanded donor was nephrectomised with and without prior adrenalectomy (Figure 6.3). A slight effect attributable to dilution of aldosterone in the common circulation may be inferred. However, the remaining humorally mediated natriuresis is equivalent to an appreciable fraction of the total response in simply expanded animals. The results demonstrate that the duration of the volume stimulus is important for accumulation of the natriuretic factor, suggesting a physiological role in chronic rather than acute hypervolaemia.

Nature of the Hormonal Factor

Extraction of plasma of mineralocortical-escaped dogs revealed a factor which inhibited sodium transport in the toad bladder (Buckalew and Lancaster, 1972), indicating the presence of a circulating inhibitor of sodium transport which might overcome the salt-retaining effect of DOCA administration. A small-molecular-weight factor (less than 1000 Da), which was natriuretic in the rat and inhibited short-circuit current in toad bladder, was also isolated from urine of fludrocortisone-escaped dogs (Favre *et al.*, 1975). Its concentration in the urine varied directly with the state of the sodium balance.

Patients with primary aldosteronism have in their plasma an extractable factor which inhibits short-circuit current and potential difference across frog skin preparations. Levels of this factor are elevated compared with control subjects and increased further on high-salt diet (Kramer *et al.*, 1977). This factor of less than 1000 Da may be derived from a circulating precursor larger than 10 000 Da (Kramer, 1981). A circulating humoral natriuretic factor, therefore, is a feature of both animal and human models of mineralocorticoid escape.

Bricker *et al.* (1975) extracted plasma from uraemic dogs and patients on normal sodium intake and showed that it contained a low-molecular-weight factor which inhibited sodium transport by frog skin and toad bladder. The same factor was present in the urine of uraemic patients (Bourgoignie *et al.*, 1974; Kaplan *at al.*, 1974). Accumulation of the factor was not simply the consequence of deterioration of kidney function: when dietary sodium intake of uraemic dog was reduced proportionally to the nephron loss, so that the excretory load of the ion per nephron remained constant, no increase in natriuretic substance was found in plasma (Schmidt *et al.*, 1974). The natriuretic factor has a molecular weight of less than 1000 Da, and has properties that differentiate it from prostaglandins, vasopressin, vasotocin, parathyroid hormone and angiotensin (Licht *et al.*, 1978).

Using the model of urine reinfusion, Pearce and Veress (1975) obtained plasma by an isovolaemic exchange procedure from rats undergoing

Figure 6.3: Natriuretic Response to Simple Vascular Expansion (Heavy Outline), Compared with the Transferred Natriuresis in Normovolaemic Recipients, the Cross-circulation Partners of which (Donors) were Subjected to Sustained Vascular Expansion. Broken outline: donor rats nephrectomised; thin outline: donor rats adrenalectomised. Stippled area: response due to a humoral factor of non-adrenal origin

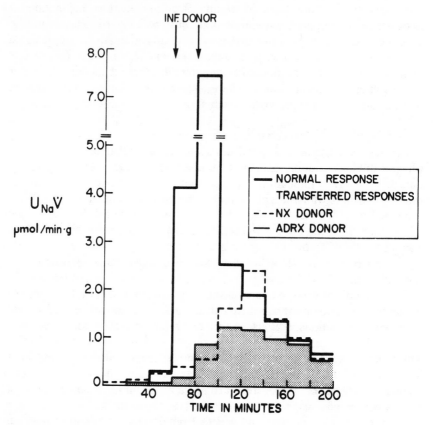

From Sonnenberg *et al.* (1972), with permission

sustained blood volume expansion, and from normovolaemic but similarly prepared controls. After gel filtration a large protein fraction (more than 30000 Da) was found to have natriuretic activity. This activity from hypervolaemic donors was significantly greater than that from the normovolaemic controls. Further fractionation (Veress *et al.*, 1980) revealed the presence of both high-molecular-weight and low-molecular-weight (less than 1500 Da) factors. These results confirm the experiments of Sealey *et al.* (1969), who found both high- and low-molecular-weight activity in plasma of sodium-loaded sheep and man.

There exist many demonstrations of natriuretic activity of extracts of urine obtained from salt-loaded human subjects (Kruck, 1967; Sealey *et al.*, 1969; Viscoper *et al.*, 1971; Clarkson and deWardener, 1972). Both high-molecular-weight and low-molecular-weight fractions were isolated (Clarkson *et al.*, 1976, 1979), and natriuretic activity was reduced if subjects were salt-deprived.

It appears, therefore, that circulating natriuretic factors are a normal component of plasma. At least two forms exist, including a high-molecular-weight substance, which may be a precursor or carrier of the low-molecular-weight hormone, as suggested by Gruber and Buckalew (1978). These factors, which are released in increased amounts when extracellular fluid volume undergoes sustained expansion, are normally excreted in the urine. The exact structure of the 'hormone' has not yet been elucidated. One group isolated a polar molecule with a molecular weight of less than 500, which was resistant to hydrolysis and proteolytic enzyme degradation (deWardener and MacGregor, 1983). This has now been shown to be identical to dopamine (H. E. deWardener, personal communication). Others purified a small-molecular-weight peptide (Gruber and Buckalew, 1978) which may share an amino acid sequence with adrenocorticotrophic hormone (Gruber *et al.*, 1982).

Source of the Hormonal Factor

No information is available on the site of production and release of the humoral factor of DOCA escape *per se*. However, when mineralocorticoid and salt administration are continued until hypertension normally develops, ablation of the anteroventral third ventricle area can prevent or reverse the increase in blood pressure (Brody *et al.*, 1978). This effect is associated with a reduction in the level of circulating transport inhibitor (Songu-Mize *et al.*, 1982), suggesting that the humoral natriuretic factor may originate from, or be influenced by, this area of the brain.

Huot *et al.* (1983) provided evidence that hypothalamic lesions in the area of the anteroventral third ventricle prevented the appearance of a ouabain-like factor in the plasma of rats with reduced renal mass. It has not yet been determined whether hypothalamic extracts from uraemic animals contain more natriuretic activity than those from normals.

The site of production of the hormone which is released during acute volume expansion is not yet known. The kidney itself has been considered a possible source. A natriuretic factor has been extracted from the kidney of the volume-expanded rats (Gonick *et al.*, 1975; Louis and Favre, 1980). Godon and Dechenne (1978) incubated kidney tissue from hypervolaemic and iso-volaemic rats; after several hours the incubation medium of the former, but not the latter, contained a large-molecular-weight natriuretic factor, which presumably was produced in those kidney cells. Cambier and Godon (1984) used isolated rat kidney perfusion to study renal release of natriuretic factor. Kidneys from a normal but not from chronically salt-deprived rats were able to release the factor into the perfusate only after addition of saline to the perfusion system. Raghavan and Gonick (1980) showed that the renal factor inhibited (Na^++K^+) ATPase.

It is unlikely, however, that the kidney is an essential source of natriuretic hormone, since prior nephrectomy of a hypervolaemic donor rat does not affect the transfer of the humoral factor to a cross circulated normovolaemic rat (Sonnenberg *et al.*, 1972). On the other hand, the brain has been a major focus of attention as the site of production and/or release. Keeler (1959) showed that lesions placed in the lateral hypothalamus of the rat resulted in an increase of urinary sodium excretion, which was not prevented by renal denervation, hypophysectomy, or adrenalectomy. Cort and Lichardus (1963) demonstrated natriuretic activity in the venous drainage from the brain during carotid occlusion. Further evidence that natriuretic hormone was a neurosecretory substance was obtained by Kaloyanides *et al.* (1977). In a study involving ablation of different endocrine organs they found that a natriuresis in an isolated kidney perfused by a hypervolaemic donor dog could be prevented only by decapitation of the donor, even though the dog's blood pressure, glomerular filtration rate, and renal blood flow were well maintained. Recently, several investigators have obtained a small-molecular-weight fraction from bovine, rat, and pig hypothalamus, which inhibits (Na^++K^+) ATPase and interacts with ouabain for binding sites on the enzyme (Fishman, 1979; Haupert and Sancho, 1979; Lichtstein and Samuelov, 1980; Whitmer *et al.*, 1982). In addition, Alaghband-Zadeh *et al.* (1981) found that the hypothalamus was the only site (of many examined) which contained a fraction that inhibited (Na^++K^+) ATPase similarly to the effect found with plasma. This inhibition increased with animals on low salt intake. Furthermore, lesions in the anterior wall of the third ventricle prevented the increase in concentration of a circulating (Na^++K^+) ATPase inhibitor, normally found during volume expansion (Pamnani *et al.*, 1981). The evidence thus favours the hypothalamus as the source of a (Na^++K^+) ATPase inhibitor related to chronic sodium balance.

Renal Mechanism of Natriuresis

Nephron Site of Action. The intrarenal site of transport inhibition during DOCA escape remains unclear. Although a decrease in the tubular fluid plasma ratio (TF/P) of inulin concentration in the proximal tubule of DOCA-escaped dogs suggested a proximal site of action (Wright *et al.*, 1969a), this result was not confirmed subsequently (Knox *et al.*, 1970). In addition, no significant difference in proximal transport was found in rats on either DOCA and high salt, or on low salt intake (Sonnenberg, 1973). Apparently, therefore, inhibition of sodium reabsorption in the superficial proximal tubule is not necessary for DOCA escape. It is, of course, possible that proximal tubules of deep nephrons not accessible to micropuncture might have responded differently.

The effect of DOCA escape on the loop of Henle is controversial. Although

Sonnenberg (1973) found a slight, but statistically significant decrease in TF/P inulin in early distal tubules of DOCA compared with NaD rats, fractional deliveries of sodium were not different. However, in DOCA rats acutely infused with saline, Haas *et al.* (1979) observed a greater sodium delivery compared with controls. It was suggested (Knox *et al.*, 1980) that superimposed volume expansion in the latter study may have unmasked a contribution of loop of Henle transport to the escape phenomenon. However, when DOCA-escaped rats were infused with blood from identically treated donors, no difference in loop function compared with corresponding NaD rats was observed (Sonnenberg, 1972). Therefore, the difference between these studies may be attributed to the type of infusate used, rather than to an unmasking of a specific transport defect in the loop of Henle of mineralocorticoid-escaped animals.

In superficial distal tubules of DOCA-escaped rats, sodium reabsorption is increased compared with NaD controls, both before (Sonnenberg, 1973) and after (Sonnenberg, 1972) acute blood volume expansion. This enhancement of distal sodium reabsorption results in reduced delivery of salt to the cortical collecting system although simultaneous natriuresis is markedly greater than in NaD rats. Thus, the distal tubule seems to remain under the salt-retaining influence of mineralocorticoid even during escape, compensating for any transport inhibition in upstream nephron segments. A homeostatically effective reduction in sodium reabsorption should, therefore, be localised downstream of the end of the superficial distal tubule.

The cortical collecting tubule has not yet been studied *in vivo*. However, *in vitro* perfusion has shown that sodium transport in this nephron segment is markedly stimulated by chronic mineralocorticoid treatment of the donor rabbit (O'Neil and Helman, 1977). It appears, therefore, that the salt-retaining influence of DOCA persists in this part of the nephron as it does in the late distal tubule. However, these results do not preclude the super-imposition of a humoral natriuretic effect, the half-life of which *in vitro* is less than that of mineralocorticoid.

Neither micropuncture of the papillary duct (Haas *et al.*, 1979) nor microcatheterisation of the whole medullary collecting system (Sonnenberg, 1976) shows a consistent effect of DOCA escape on sodium transport. Therefore, by exclusion, increased delivery of salt to the medullary collecting system by deep nephrons not accessible to micropuncture seems the most likely explanation for the natriuresis of DOCA escape.

A decrease of fractional reabsorption in the proximal tubule of uraemic kidneys has been well documented (Schultze *et al.*, 1972; Wen *et al.*, 1973; Kramp *et al.*, 1974). However, most, if not all, of this inhibition may be explained by alteration of peritubular physical factors (Maddox *et al.*, 1975). Furthermore, such inhibition does not play a determining role in the natriuresis, implicating the distal nephron as an important site of transport inhibition (Hayslett *et al.*, 1969a; Weber *et al.*, 1975). In a study on postobstructive diuresis, Sonnenberg and Wilson (1976) found that intravenous reinfusion of urine for 24 h was associated with marked increase of fractional sodium delivery to the medullary collecting duct. A similar increase was seen in volume-expanded rats with reduced nephron mass (Wilson and Sonnenberg, 1979). In rabbit cortical collecting tubules perfused *in vitro*, inhibition of transepithelial sodium transport was observed with addition of natriuretic factor to the peritubular side (Fine *et al.*, 1976a). Thus, the data are compatible with the postulate that the humoral natriuretic factor released during chronic uraemia increases salt and water delivery to the medullary collecting duct system.

In the mid-1960s, several groups showed that the diuresis and natriuresis following intravenous saline infusion in both dog (Dirks *et al.*, 1965) and rat (Cortney *et al.*, 1965; Landwehr *et al.*, 1967) was associated with decrease of fractional fluid reabsorption from the proximal tubule. These results suggested that natriuretic hormone might inhibit sodium transport in this part of the nephron. Rector *et al.* (1968) investigated the effect of plasma from saline-infused dogs on proximal tubular function. They infused plasma from non-diuretic dogs into bioassay rats during a control period, then infused plasma from a volume-expanded dog, and finally returned to non-diuretic control plasma during a recovery period. They found that infusion of plasma from the volume-expanded dog was associated with approximately 20 per cent reduction of the end-proximal TF/P ratio of inulin concentration, compared with control and recovery periods. In addition, the half-time of reabsorption of saline droplets injected into proximal tubule was prolonged by 30–40 per cent. Finally, when the reabsorptive half-times of droplets of plasma dialysate from hyper- and normovolaemic dogs were compared, the former again showed significant prolongation. Thus, the site of action of a humoral natriuretic factor seemed established. However, Hayslett *et al.* (1969b) were unable to reproduce these results. A collaborative effort by several different laboratories was therefore undertaken to clarify this question. The conclusion was as follows:

> The studies recently reported offered the first direct evidence for the existence of an inhibitory factor in plasma . . . a dialysable constituent was thought to inhibit proximal sodium reabsorption. Using the same methods, we have been unable to detect an inhibitor of proximal sodium reabsorption in the plasma or dialysates of plasma from saline-loaded animals. (Wright *et al.*, 1969b.)

Once again, 'natriuretic hormone' had proved to be elusive.

When it was shown that the inhibition of proximal transport during saline infusion could be explained on the basis of changes in hydrostatic pressure and plasma protein concentration in peritubular capillaries (Windhager *et al.*, 1969), these 'physical factors' seemed to offer an adequate explanation of volume natriuresis without resorting to a mythical hormone. However, evidence existed that proximal transport capacity was not impaired when iso-oncotic solution was infused, despite a large resultant natriuresis (Sonnenberg and Solomon, 1969). Conversely, dilution of peritubular protein concentration without extracellular fluid volume expansion did not result in natriuresis, although proximal reabsorption was inhibited (Knox *et al.*, 1968). The rat model of maintained intravascular expansion without change in blood concentration was, therefore, used in a systematic attempt to identify the nephron site(s) of inhibition of sodium transport during volume natriuresis. In the initial study (Sonnenberg, 1971) the same proximal tubules were punctured and repunctured before and during hypervolaemia. An increase of absolute fluid reabsorption, associated with elevation of single nephron filtration rate, was observed. A small and variable decrease in fractional reabsorption, which was not correlated with simultaneous urinary excretion, was ascribed to increased peritubular hydrostatic pressure. It was concluded that the natriuretic response was dependent on tubular transport alterations in nephron segments located distal to the proximal convolution. The study was therefore extended to the distal tubule, using similar techniques (Sonnenberg, 1972). Again, no inhibition of absolute fluid or sodium reabsorption as a result of expansion was observed, showing that volume natriuresis was not due to diminished transport capacity of tubular segments upstream to the distal collection site. A slight decrease in fractional reabsorption was explained by the proximal effect observed earlier, indicating that the mechanism of transport in the loop of Henle was unaffected by volume expansion. No inhibition of reabsorption along the distal tubule itself was found. Comparison of calculated end-distal tubular load of sodium with simultaneous urinary excretion showed that volume expansion resulted in decreased net reabsorption in the collecting duct system, and/or increased delivery of sodium to the system from deep nephrons inaccessible to micropuncture. Microcatheterisation of the medullary collecting system was used in an attempt to distinguished between these possibilities (Sonnenberg, 1976). During maintained intravascular volume expansion in normal rats, complete inhibition of net sodium reabsorption in the medullary duct was observed. Comparable inhibition of transport was found in DOCA-escaped and in chronically salt-deprived animals, although natriuresis was greater and lower than in control rats, respectively. These differences were due to differences in sodium delivered to the medullary collecting duct system. It was evident, therefore, that alterations both in delivery to, and reabsorption in, the medullary duct could be involved in the renal response to maintained hypervolaemia. To determine which of these changes were due to natriuretic hormone, the small-molecular-weight factor from plasma of hypervolaemic rats was injected into normovolaemic animals prepared for microcatheterisation (Sonnenberg *et al.*, 1980a). The factor enhanced the tubular load of fluid and sodium entering the medullary duct. Associated with this elevated delivery was a proportional increase in reabsorption along the duct itself. Such load dependency of transport had been found previously to be a normal feature of this nephron segment (Sonnenberg, 1978). These results explained the relatively small natriuresis due to circulating humoral factor compared with the total renal volume response (see Figure 6.3). For full expression of the excretory effect of natriuretic hormone, a simultaneous inhibition of collecting-duct reabsorption seems necessary.

Cellular Mechanism of Action. A circulating $(Na^+ + K^+)$ ATPase inhibitor was demonstrated in plasma of aldosterone-escaped man (Poston *et al.*, 1982), suggesting that the natriuresis was due to inhibition of this enzyme system found in the kidney. In addition, Pamnani *et al.* (1980) found that uninephrectomised rats given DOCA and salt until they developed hypertension showed suppression of vascular $Na^+ + K^+$ pump activity, associated with increased plasma levels of a circulating $(Na^+ + K^+)$ ATPase inhibitor.

Uraemic plasma was shown to inhibit the $(Na^+ + K^+)$ ATPase in red blood cells (Cole *et al.*, 1968). Plasma supernatants from rats with reduced renal mass showed a suppression of $Na^+ + K^+$ pump activity (Pamnani *et al.*, 1980, 1981).

Kramer *et al.* (1969) first presented evidence that circulating natriuretic hormone released during volume expansion might be an inhibitor of $(Na^+ + K^+)$ ATPase activity. Kidneys of rats subjected to 90 min of maintained extracellular fluid volume expansion showed a small but statistically significant decrease of cortical $(Na^+ + K^+)$ ATPase activity. Subsequently, these investigators (Gonick *et al.*, 1977), using the small-molecular-weight factor from hypervolaemic rat plasma, demonstrated that the net inhibition of Na^+ transport in frog skin and toad bladder was due largely to inhibition of $(Na^+ + K^+)$ ATPase. Gruber *et al.* (1980) showed that a similar factor, extracted from plasma of dogs with extracellular fluid volume expansion, was bound to two different antibodies for digoxin, and also inhibited $(Na^+ + K^+)$ ATPase activity in an *in vitro* preparation. These investigators suggested that natriuretic hormone could be an endogenous digitalis-like molecule. Using an indirect assay for ATPase activity, Fenton *et al.* (1982) found inhibitory activity in plasma and urine extracts of human subjects. Activity in plasma from subjects on a high sodium diet was approximately 20-fold greater than that in plasma from the same subjects on a low-sodium diet.

Summary: Natriuretic Hormone

The three models discussed, mineralocorticoid escape, progressive nephron loss, and maintained vascular or extracellular volume expansion, demonstrate the reality of natriuretic hormone. Although the evidence for some of the conclusions may still be controversial or lacking, the common features of the models allow the following tentative synthesis: natriuretic hormone is produced in, and released from, the hypothalamus. It is a normal constituent of plasma. It circulates in the blood as a large-molecular-weight peptide (more than 30 000 Da). This may be the precursor or carrier of a small-molecular-weight hormone (about 500 Da). Both are removed from the circulation by urinary excretion. Concentration in the plasma increases when there is a continuing need for increased renal sodium excretion. Although the exact stimulus for release of natriuretic hormone is not known, it probably involves intrathoracic hypervolaemia (deWardener and MacGregor, 1983). The hormone cross-reacts with antibodies to digitalis, interferes with $(Na^+ + K^+)$ ATPase activity *in vitro*, and functions as an endogenous inhibitor of the enzyme. Its action on the kidney is to increase delivery of sodium to the medullary collecting duct system. This may include inhibition of sodium transport in juxtamedullary nephrons and/or cortical collecting tubules.

Clinical Implications. It is not known whether a defect in the production and/or release of natriuretic hormone might be a contributory factor in disease processes. However, its possible role in the initiation and maintenance of some forms of hypertension has recently been the subject of much attention (for review see deWardener and MacGregor, 1980). This hypothesis is shown in Figure 6.4. Briefly, it is suggested that a certain proportion of the human population has an inherited defect in the renal excretion of salt. Although such a defect would be of little consequence with a low-sodium diet, high salt intake would be expected to lead to extracellular fluid volume expansion. As a result, blood levels of natriuretic hormone would rise, and renal $(Na^+ + K^+)$ ATPase inhibition would increase sodium excretion, allowing the kidney to maintain sodium balance. This beneficial adaptation has additional consequences, however. Inhibition of $(Na^+ + K^+)$ ATPase in other tissues will lead to transport abnormalities such as those demonstrated in blood cells of some models of hypertension (see also Chapter 8). At the level of the arteriole, an intracellular accumulation of sodium and, thereby, calcium would result, increasing vascular reactivity. This, in turn, would induce a gradual rise of arterial pressure.

Although hypertension has not been reported in patients as a result of chronic administration of cardiac glycosides, support for this hypothesis is given by studies in which administration of digoxin antibodies was associated with reduction of blood pressure in several experimental models of hypertension (Dietz *et al.*, 1982; Kojima *et al.*, 1982; Huang and Smith, 1984). Although it is probably not a complete explanation for essential hypertension, the hypothesis offers an attractive basis for the observed correlation between salt intake and blood pressure in human populations, and in hypervolaemic models of the disease (Haddy and Overbeck, 1976).

Unresolved Problems. The natriuresis ascribable to the circulating $(Na^+ + K^+)$ ATPase inhibitor is small compared with the renal response to acute hypervolaemia (see Figure 6.3). This is not due to inadequate plasma concentration of the inhibitor, since increasing the dose has no further effect on

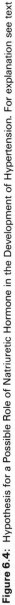
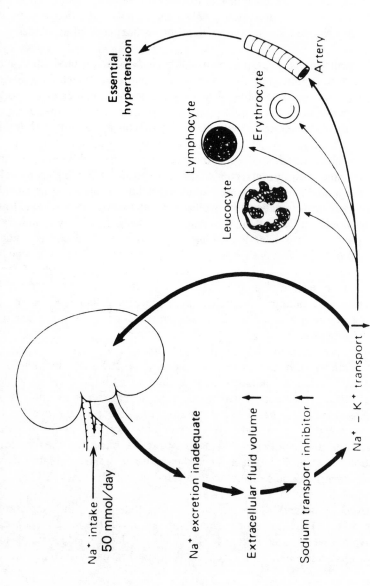

Figure 6.4: Hypothesis for a Possible Role of Natriuretic Hormone in the Development of Hypertension. For explanation see text

From deWardener and MacGregor (1980), with permission

natriuresis (Veress *et al.*, 1980). Furthermore, acute vascular (Sonnenberg, 1976) or extracellular volume expansion (Sonnenberg, 1974; Bengele *et al.*, 1980) results in complete inhibition of sodium reabsorption in the medullary collecting duct, independent of plasma levels of natriuretic hormone. Finally, the circulating factor does not affect medullary-duct transport (Sonnenberg *et al.*, 1980a). To determine whether the component of volume natriuresis which was not due to natriuretic hormone could be explained by efferent renal nerve activity, the influence of unilateral renal denervation on the response was studied (Veress *et al.*, 1982). Not unexpectedly (see Gottschalk, 1979), the denervated kidney excreted more sodium, both before and after intravascular volume expansion. However, the pattern of the renal response was identical in denervated and innervated kidneys, suggesting that efferent renal nerve activity might play a modulating, but not determining, role in the natriuresis. An investigation of possible haemodynamic influences on volume natriuresis revealed no causative effect of either renal arterial or renal venous blood pressure (Ackermann, 1975; Rudolf and Ackermann, 1984). A major component of the renal response to blood volume expansion thus could not be explained by either natriuretic hormone or by neural or haemodynamic influences on kidney function.

At this point, a resolution to the dilemma was offered by the discovery of a potent natriuretic factor in mammalian heart atria (deBold *et al.*, 1981), raising the possibility that atrial cardiocytes might be the source of the missing factor to explain fully the acute response to hypervolaemia.

Atrial Natriuretic Factor

Since the initial discovery by deBold and co-workers (Sonnenberg *et al.*, 1980b; deBold *et al.*, 1981) that myocytes from cardiac atria contain a potent natriuretic principle, development in this field has been explosive. A major reason was that this study provided at the same time a reliable source and a reproducible assay for a biologically active material. In addition, technology was poised to take advantage of this discovery, such that in less than four years progress went from purification and identification of the active principle, through cloning of cDNA for endogenous precursor, to commercial availability of synthetic peptides. Further progress seems certain to elucidate the functional significance of what appears to be a previously unsuspected hormone system.

Specific Atrial Granules

Electron micrographs of atrial cardiocytes show morphological features not seen in ventricular cells. These include a large number of Golgi cisterns and associated microvesicular elements, a high proportion of rough endoplasmic reticulum, and numerous electron-dense cytoplasmic granules. These so-called specific atrial granules were first described by Kisch (1956), and characterised by Jamieson and Palade (1964). The structural complex formed by the endoplasmic reticulum, Golgi apparatus, and electron-dense granules resembles that found in peptide-hormone-secreting cells (Kisch, 1963; Jamieson and Palade, 1964), suggesting a dual contractile and secretory role for the atrial myocytes. Such a dual role would be analogous to that of the highly differentiated smooth muscle cells of the renal juxtaglomerular apparatus, in which renin is produced and stored (Barajas and Latta, 1967; Celio and Inagami, 1981).

Chemistry. Since the specific atrial granules appeared morphologically similar to catecholamine-containing granules in adrenal medulla, Bencosme and Berger (1971) suggested that atrial granules could be a storage site for noradrenaline. However, it was shown that these granules do not contain appreciable quantities of catecholamines (deBold and Bencosme, 1973) and do not accumulate noradrenaline *in vitro* (Kuhn *et al.*, 1975). The presence of renin-like activity in rat atrial homogenates has also been reported (Rojo-Ortega *et al.*, 1979). Recently, however, Cantin *et al.* (1981) found that this activity was not localised in the specific atrial granules.

Histochemical studies indicated that the atrial granules are rich in protein (Huet and Cantin, 1974; deBold and Bencosme, 1975). The contents of the granules were selectively digested by the proteolytic enzymes pronase, pepsin and trypsin (Huet and Cantin, 1974; Cantin and Huet, 1975; Huet *et al.*, 1975; Kuhn *et al.*, 1975). These results suggest a proteinaceous nature for the granular contents.

Evidence for Secretory Nature. The morphological and biochemical data have not yet established the secretory nature of specific atrial granules. However, Theron and co-workers (1978) demonstrated occasional fragmentation of the limiting membrane of atrial granules, and diffuse accumulation of electron-dense material in the surrounding cytoplasm. They suggested that the contents of the granules were released intracellularly after lysis of the membrane. Depletion of atrial granules was observed by Saetersdal *et al.* (1979) after repeated administration of isoproterenol in gerbils. Empty granules and granules in intermediate stages of disintegration were found in the paranuclear zones of atrial myocytes. An intra- rather than extracellular release of granular contents is suggested by both of these studies, but the possibility is not excluded that the material may then diffuse into the extracellular space.

Physiological Role. Several groups of investigators have reported a relationship of atrial granules to salt and water balance. Cantin and Huet (1973) found that bilateral adrenalectomy was associated with atrial degranulation in hamsters receiving supplements of sodium chloride. Hormone replacement using DOCA and cortisol prevented this effect. Marie *et al.* (1976) demonstrated that salt administration with and without simultaneous DOCA injection resulted in a decrease in the granulation of the right atrium in rats. Conversely, water as well as sodium restriction increased atrial granularity. Using a morphometric method of assessing quantitatively the granularity of rat atria, deBold (1979) described an increase in granulation following 5 days of water deprivation, or after 3 weeks on a low-salt diet. Conversely, 3 weeks of high salt intake with daily injection of DOCA led to degranulation. In the water-deprived group a statistically significant correlation between haematocrit and granulation was observed. These results suggest a relationship between specific atrial granules and fluid and electrolyte balance.

Atrial Extract

In a study designed to assess a possible effect of atrial granule contents on kidney function, deBold *et al.* (1981) prepared saline extracts from rat atria and ventricles. Extract from 0.2 g of tissue was injected intravenously in a series of anaesthetised rats. A control group received extract from the same weight of ventricular tissue. Results are shown in Figure 6.5. Injection of atrial, but not ventricular extract caused a large and rapid increase of sodium chloride excretion. Smaller elevations of urine volume and potassium excretion were also seen. The renal response was associated with a decrease in arterial blood pressure. These results were confirmed by several different groups of investigators (Garcia *et al.*, 1982; Keeler, 1982; Pollock and Banks, 1983; Pamnani *et al.*, 1984). Natriuretic activity was found in extracts of atria from mouse, dog, pig and cow, as well as monkey and human (MacPhee *et al.*, 1982; deBold and Salerno, 1983; Nemeh and Gilmore, 1983).

The activity was found to be associated with a fraction enriched in atrial-specific granules (deBold, 1982a; Garcia *et al.*, 1982). Antibodies to partially purified atrial natriuretic factors of both high and low molecular weight were found to react with atrial-specific granules (Cantin *et al.*, 1984).

Chemistry. Following the establishment of the protein nature of atrial natriuretic factor (deBold, 1982b; Garcia *et al.*, 1982; Trippodo *et al.*, 1982) the amino acid composition of purified peptides was studied. DeBold and Flynn (1983) extracted a peptide, 'cardionatrin I', which contained 49 amino acid residues and had a molecular weight of 5499 Da. Injection in bioassay rats of 0.5 nmol induced a characteristic natriuretic response. Grammer *et al.* (1983) purified a smaller peptide which had 36 amino acid residues and a molecular weight of about 3800 Da. This material showed both natriuretic and vasorelaxant activity. Thibault *et al.* (1983) purified three factors containing 26, 31 and 33 amino acids.

The sequence of amino acids of a 28-amino acid peptide derived from 'cardionatrin I' has been determined (Flynn *et al.*, 1983). Smaller peptides of 21 and 23 amino acids, called 'atriopeptins' I and II, were also sequenced (Currie *et al.*, 1984b; Geller *et al.*, 1984a). The peptides share the same

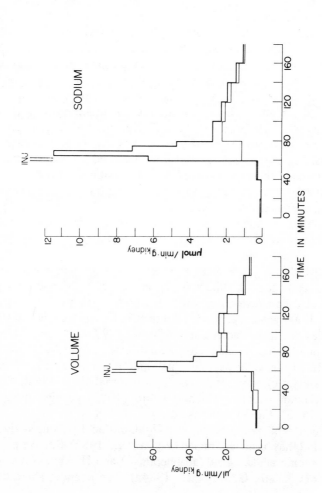

Figure 6.5: Averaged Urine Volume and Sodium Excretions in Rats before and after Injection of Atrial (Heavy Outline) or Ventricular (Light Outline) Myocardial Extracts

From deBold *et al.* (1981), with permission

sequence, with the larger one having an additional Phe-Arg extension at the carboxyl terminal. An identical sequence is also found in cardionatrin I, and is shown in Figure 6.6. Both atriopeptin I and II appear to be derived from a common high-molecular-weight precursor. The natriuretic potency of either compound was comparable to that of cardionatrin. However, their *in vitro* effects on smooth muscle were different. Atriopeptin I relaxed the cholinergic muscle of chick rectum, and did not affect the adrenergic muscle of rabbit aorta. At similar concentrations, atriopeptin II showed muscle-relaxing activity in both *in vitro* preparations. These authors also observed that synthetic analogues of the peptides exhibited the same chromatographic and biological activities as the biologically derived materials. The synthetic peptides required prior oxidation for biological activity, suggesting that a cysteine disulphide bridge is necessary for biological activity. The differences among peptides may well reflect modification by proteolysis during the extraction procedure, and the peptides may not necessarily be identical to material released *in vivo*. However, the 21- and 23-amino acid sequences may approach the minimum biologically active structures.

Almost simultaneously with these reports, other groups published analogous sequences for the small-molecular-weight factor from both rat (Atlas *et al.*, 1984; Kangawa *et al.*, 1984; Misono *et al.*, 1984; Seidah *et al.*, 1984) and human tissue (Kangawa and Matsuo, 1984), as well as for the large-molecular-weight precursor (Thibault *et al.*, 1984; Geller *et al.*, 1984b). Experiments in which DNA sequences were cloned which were comple-

Figure 6.6: Amino Acid Sequence of Rat Atrial Peptides. Solid outlines = 21 amino acid peptide, atriopeptin I; plus broken outlines = 23 amino acid peptide, atriopeptin II (Currie *et al.*, 1984b); plus dotted outlines = 28 amino acid peptide, cardionatrin I (Flynn *et al.*, 1983). Human atrial factor is identical to rat peptide with the substitution of Met for Ile as indicated (Kangawa and Matsuo, 1984)

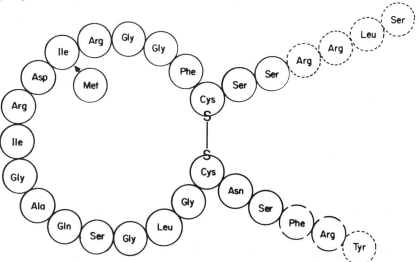

mentary to messenger RNA coding for atrial natriuretic factor (Maki *et al.*, 1984; Oikawa *et al.*, 1984; Seidman *et al.*, 1984; Yamanaka *et al.*, 1984) showed remarkably similar sequences of the precursor for natriuretic peptides. The precursor consists of 152 amino acids and contains a signal sequence with a high content of hydrophobic amino acids, a characteristic feature of precursors of secretory proteins (Kreil, 1981). These data, therefore, suggest a new function for atrial myocytes — production and release of a peptide hormone.

Effect on Renal Haemodynamics. The effect of atrial natriuretic factor on glomerular filtration rate is not yet fully established. Some investigators were unable to detect statistically significant increases in either whole kidney (deBold *et al.*, 1981; Pollock and Banks, 1983) or single nephron filtration rate (Sonnenberg *et al.*, 1981a, 1982; Briggs *et al.*, 1982). On the other hand, in the isolated perfused kidney an increase of GFR may be observed (Baines *et al.*, 1983; Camargo *et al.*, 1984). Borenstein (1982), using very short urine collection periods, was able to show that filtration doubled in the first 5 min after injection of the factor, returning to or below control values in the subsequent 5 min.

In a study of renal blood flow in the rat, Borenstein *et al.* (1983) observed that a purified atrial extract increased total blood flow and its distribution to inner cortex and medulla at the time of peak natriuretic response. These haemodynamic changes were not found with injection of ventricular extract. An increase of medullary blood flow was also reported in Dahl rats by Hirata and co-workers (1984). Both atrial extract and the 23-amino-acid peptide show dose-dependent renal vasodilatation *in vivo* (Oshima *et al.*, 1984). In isolated perfused kidneys both increase and decrease of perfusion may occur with administration of atrial natriuresis factor, depending on pre-existing vascular tone (Baines *et al.*, 1983).

Alterations in filtration rate and renal blood flow, however, cannot completely explain the natriuretic following injection of atrial factor (Baines *et al.*, 1983; Borenstein *et al.*, 1983), indicating a direct inhibitory effect on tubular sodium chloride transport.

Nephron Site of Action. To determine the site of action of atrial natriuretic factor, micropuncture and microcatheterisation were used in anaesthetised rats (Sonnenberg *et al.*, 1981a, 1982). Tubular fluid was collected from end-proximal tubules, from distal tubules, and from the outer medullary collecting duct. Samples were taken from the same sites before and after intravenous injection of either atrial or ventricular tissue extract. Results are shown in Figure 6.7. There were no differences in proximal reabsorption with the two types of injection. A small but statistically significant decrease of sodium transport was found with atrial relative to ventricular extract in the loop of Henle. However, the major inhibition of transport occurred in the medullary collecting duct. Suppression of reabsorption at this site accounted

Figure 6.7: Change in Sodium Delivery (per cent) at the Nephron Sites Indicated by (●), after Injection of Atrial (A) or Ventricular (V) Extract. For further details of protocol, see text

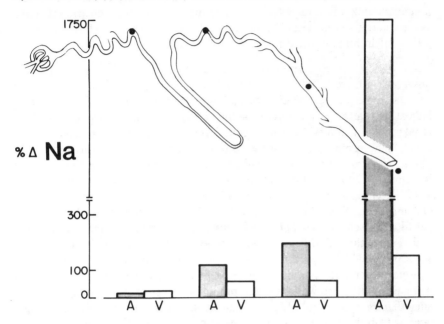

for 80 per cent of the natriuresis due to atrial factor. Briggs *et al.* (1982) also showed that the greatest effect of the factor was downstream to the distal tubule.

Mechanism of Transport Inhibition. To study the mechanism of transport inhibition, *in vitro* perfusion of thick ascending limbs of Henle's loop from rabbit and rat kidney was used. However, no effect of partially purified atrial extract was observed (Stoner and Sonnenberg, unpublished). Atrial factor also had no influence on short-circuit current in turtle bladder or frog skin (Krebs and Sonnenberg, unpublished). Other *in vitro* preparations which have been tried with negative results include red blood cell (Milojevic and Sonnenberg, unpublished), locust hindgut (Philips and Sonnenberg, unpublished) and frog cornea (Throckmorton and Gilmore, 1983). The lack of any transport effect *in vitro* suggests that the factor, as extracted from the atria, either requires activation *in vivo*, or that it releases a natriuretic agonist from some other part of the body. If the latter possibility is correct, the release is unlikely to be from brain, since the renal response to atrial factor was not impaired by decapitation of the bioassay rat (Trippodo *et al.*, 1982).

In the isolated perfused rat kidney Camargo and co-workers (1984) found that reducing the calcium concentration in, or adding verapamil to, the perfusate markedly blunted the natriuretic response to the atrial factor. These authors concluded that Ca-dependent haemodynamic changes were largely responsible for the renal effect.

In contrast to natriuretic hormone, the atrial natriuretic factor does not inhibit the enzyme $(Na^+ + K^+)$ ATPase, whether in strips of arterial blood vessels (Link *et al.*, 1981), in whole kidney homogenates (Pollock *et al.*, 1983), or in renal cortical microsomes (Pamnani *et al.*, 1984).

Smooth Muscle Effects. The decrease in arterial blood pressure first observed with crude atrial extract (deBold *et al.*, 1981) was found to persist when a single purified peptide was administered (deBold and Flynn, 1983), indicating that atrial natriuretic factor has systemic hypotensive as well as renal transport effects. *In vivo*, a reduction in total peripheral resistance and a negative inotropic effect on the hearts were observed (Ackermann *et al.*, 1982, 1984). *In vitro*, atrial extracts had potent smooth-muscle relaxing properties in strips of vascular and/or intestinal muscle (Deth *et al.*, 1982; Currie *et al.*, 1983). Synthetic peptides can mimic these actions (Currie *et al.*, 1984b; Oshima *et al.*, 1984; Garcia *et al.*, 1984). Currie and co-workers (1984a) used gel filtration chromatography to fractionate rat atrial extracts. They found high- (more than 20 000 Da) and low-molecular-weight fractions (less than 10 000 Da) which were potent natriuretic agents. Further purification of the low-molecular-weight fraction resulted in two subfractions, both of which were natriuretic, and which relaxed preferentially either vascular or intestinal smooth muscle *in vitro*. Mild proteolytic treatment of the high-molecular-weight peak with trypsin (Currie *et al.*, 1984a) or kallikrein (Currie *et al.*, 1984c) markedly enhanced smooth muscle relaxant activity, although, as reported by others (deBold, 1982b; Garcia *et al.*, 1982; Trippodo *et al.*, 1982) further proteolysis resulted in complete inactivation. It was suggested that the atria contain a high-molecular-weight peptide which is relatively inactive, but which can be converted to low-molecular-weight peptide with increased vasomotor activity. Indeed, conversion by atrial tissue of high- to low-molecular-weight peptides has been demonstrated (Trippodo *et al.*, 1984).

The mechanism of the relaxation is unknown. Hamet *et al.* (1983) have observed release of cGMP with atrial factor in both smooth-muscle strips and in kidney. Since cGMP has been implicated in muscle relaxation (Axelsson *et al.*, 1979), this might be the final effector of the vasomotor action of atrial factor. Alternatively, since the factor has recently been shown to reduce adenylate cyclase activity in homogenates of renal and mesenteric artery (Anad-Sristava *et al.*, 1984), inhibition of this enzyme may play a role in the vasorelaxation.

Role in 'Volume Natriuresis'. The natriuretic and vasodepressor actions of atrial factor are ideal properties for a regulator of blood volume. In addition, the recently reported inhibition of aldosterone release by native (Atarashi *et al.*, 1984) and synthetic (Chartier *et al.*, 1984) peptide make it seem almost too good to be true. However, extraction of a natriuretic material from atrial tissue does not prove, although it certainly suggests, a physiological role in endocrine regulation of blood volume. It has not yet been possible to identify the factor in circulating plasma.* Indirect experiments were therefore undertaken in an attempt to establish a regulatory role for this new, putative hormone system. The first (Sonnenberg *et al.*, 1981b) was predicated on the similarity of atrial natriuretic factor and the diuretic drug furosemide, both in magnitude and time course of natriuresis, and in nephron sites affected. The site of action of the drugs is the luminal membrane of the distal nephron. Secretion into luminal fluid via the proximal tubular organic acid transport system ensures delivery of high concentrations of furosemide to its distal effector site. In an effort to extend the parallelism between furosemide and atrial natriuretic factor, we studied the effect of probenecid, a blocker of proximal secretion of organic acids, on the renal response to atrial extract. It was found that probenecid indeed reduced, although it did not prevent, the renal response to the extract. To determine whether the factor could be involved in the renal regulation of blood volume, we compared the natriuresis resulting from acute hyper-volaemia in the presence and absence of probenecid. The 'volume natriuresis' following intravenous infusion of homologous blood was reduced significantly by probenecid administration. Since there were no differences in renal function which could be ascribed to probenecid *per se*, these experiments were interpreted as providing circumstantial evidence for endogenous release of atrial factor in vascular volume control.

In a second study (Sonnenberg and Veress, 1983; Veress and Sonnenberg, 1984) a classical ablation experiment was attempted. Anaesthetised rats were connected to a respirator, the chest cavity was opened, and the right atrial appendage was tied with a loop ligature and removed. The chest was then closed and, after equilibration and control renal function periods, an intravenous infusion of iso-oncotic bovine albumin solution was given. The renal response of such rats was compared with that of identically treated control animals, in which the snare was placed around the appendage but not tightened. Obviously, such right atrial appendectomy did not remove all of the 'hormone'-producing tissue of the heart. However, in the rat the content of specific atrial granules is greater in the right compared with the left atrium (Jamieson and Palade, 1964), so that a major source of factor should have been eliminated. Indeed, the 'volume natriuresis' was reduced significantly to approximately one-half of that seen in the control group (Figure 6.8). To ensure that atrial appendectomy had not compromised the circulation of experimental animals, arterial and central blood pressures, cardiac outputs, and total renal blood flows were assessed. No difference in any of the variables was found between control and experimental groups. The atria are known to be a site for receptors transmitting information regarding volume status to the brain via the vagus nerves (Gauer and Henry, 1963), suggesting the possibility

*This statement is no longer correct. 1985 has seen rapid developments in the radioimmunoassay of atrial natriuretic peptides, which have now been measured in the plasma of rats (Thibault *et al.*, 1985) and man (Larose *et al.*, 1985; see also Sugawara *et al.*, 1985) — Ed.

Figure 6.8: Time Course of Sodium Excretion before and after Iso-oncotic Infusion in Sham-operated (Heavy Lines) and Atrial Appendectomy Groups (Broken Lines). Standard errors of the means are indicated

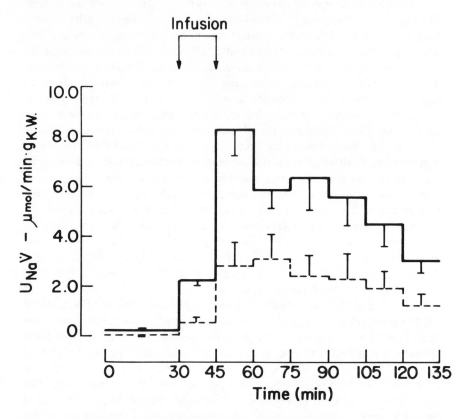

that removal of afferent receptor activity could have reduced the renal response in the experimental series. The effect of acute vagotomy was, therefore, assessed in the two groups. Again, atrial appendectomy was associated with reduction of volume natriuresis. To determine whether the kidneys of experimental rats could respond normally to natriuretic stimuli, atrial factor, as well as furosemide, was administered. No differences in renal functions from sham-operated control animals were observed. These results thus provide the first, if indirect, demonstration that natriuretic factor is released into the bloodstream during acute hypervolaemia, and indicate that atrial cardiocytes play an endocrine role in body-fluid regulation.

Cellular Release Mechanisms. To determine whether atrial myocytes could release the natriuretic factor, excised atria were incubated *in vitro*. Incubation for periods of up to 2 h did not result in measurable release of the factor into the medium, nor could release be stimulated by the β-receptor agonist isoprenaline, by the cardiac glycoside ouabain, or by complete cell depolarisation by 10-fold increase of extracellular potassium concentration. However, when acetylcholine was added to the incubation medium, natriuretic activity was found, associated with a corresponding decrease of activity in atrial tissue. This release was not due to acetylcholine-induced loss of cell integrity, since it could be blocked by the muscarinic cholinergic antagonist atropine (Sonnenberg *et al.*, 1984). These experiments suggested that stimulation of specific receptors at the cell surface could result in secretion of atrial natriuretic factor. The cellular mechanism, however, was not due to activation of adenylate cyclase, since isoprenaline, which stimulates this enzyme, elicited no release, whereas acetylcholine, with no adenylate cyclase stimulation, did cause release. A different mechanism must, therefore, be responsible for stimulation-secretion coupling in atrial myocytes. One such mechanism is activation of the polyphosphoinositide system, which has been receiving increasing attention as a mediator of cellular responses to receptor activation (for review see Michell and Kirk, 1981). Since muscarinic cholinergic, α-adrenergic, and vascular-type vasopressin receptors (V_1) receptors all share the ability to stimulate this system, the effect of adrenaline and vasopressin on atrial release of natriuretic factor was evaluated (Sonnenberg and Veress, 1984). Addition of adrenaline to incubated atria again caused release of the factor, an effect which was blocked by the α-receptor antagonist phentolamine. Similarly, vasopressin (AVP) addition was associated with release of atrial natriuretic factor. However, deamino-8-D-arginine vasopressin (dDAVP), which is equipotent to AVP in activating adenylate cyclase, but does not affect V_1 receptors (Manning *et al.*, 1976), was without effect. It was concluded, therefore, that activation of the poly-phosphoinositide system is the cellular mechanism resulting in secretion of atrial natriuretic factor.

Regulation of Release

The physiological regulation of this cellular release mechanism is still unknown. Since acute intravascular or extracellular fluid volume expansion is associated with increased central venous pressure, an attractive hypothesis is that atrial stretch *per se* causes release of the factor. However, it is not obvious how stretch would stimulate the cellular receptors regulating the polyphospho-inositol system. In addition, it has long been known that chronic high spinal section (Pearce and Sonnenberg, 1965) or cardiac denervation (Gilmore and Daggett, 1966) interfere with the renal volume response to iso-oncotic hypervolaemia although increases in central venous pressure were normal. Since atrial natriuretic factor is involved in the response (Veress and Sonnenberg, 1984), it may be inferred that release of the factor requires the integrity of cardiac nervous pathways.

As reviewed by Gauer and Henry (1963), atrial stretch receptors are involved in body-fluid volume regulation. Activation of such receptors caused natriuresis in both anaesthetised dogs (Linden, 1976) and unanaesthetised dogs (Reinhardt *et al.*, 1977). Associated with such activation was a reflex decrease in sympathetic tone to the kidney (Karim *et al.*, 1972), and a reduction of renin release (Reinhardt *et al.*, 1980a). However, the natriuresis could not be explained by decreased activity of the renin-angiotensin-aldosterone system (Reinhardt *et al.*, 1980b), nor by haemodynamic changes (Reinhardt *et al.*, 1980c) and was, therefore, ascribed to release of an unknown circulating natriuretic substance. That this might be atrial natriuretic factor is suggested by the following consideration. Activation of atrial stretch receptors results in a reflex increase of activity in efferent cardiac sympathetic nerves (Karim *et al.*, 1972). This, in turn, could stimulate α-receptors of atrial myocytes, activating the cellular release mechanism for atrial natriuretic factor, with consequent 'volume natriuresis'. The finding by Reinhardt and associates (Kaczmarczyk *et al.*, 1981) that cardiac denervation prevented the natriuretic response to atrial stretch is in agreement with such a reflex.

Afferent information from atrial stretch receptors reaches the central nervous system via the vagus nerves (Kappagoda *et al.*, 1979). However, sectioning of the vagus nerves did not materially influence the release of atrial natriuretic factor (Veress and Sonnenberg, 1984), or the renal response to iso-oncotic blood volume expansion (Veress and Pearce, 1972). These results indicate that atrial stretch receptor activity is not essential for release of natriuretic factor, and suggest that hypervolaemia may also cause stimulation of cardiac sympathetic nerves by other means. Further investigation of regulation of atrial factor release is obviously required.

Summary: Atrial Natriuretic Factor

The data considered above strongly suggest that, in analogy to the juxtaglomerular apparatus of the kidney, modified myocytes from cardiac atria fulfil dual contractile and secretory roles. Atrial natriuretic factor appears to be the efferent limb of a previously unsuspected regulatory system for body-fluid homeostasis, which may not only play a role in normal sodium balance, but may also be involved in the pathogenesis of, or compensation for, altered salt and water regulation in disease states.

Clinical Implications. At present, discussion of a possible involvement of atrial natriuretic factor in disease states is speculative. Since the factor has hypotensive as well as natriuretic properties, it seemed reasonable to investigate its relationship to animal models of hypertension. Sonnenberg and co-workers (1983a) found that atria from spontaneously hypertensive rats of the Okamoto strain contained significantly less natriuretic factor than those of Wistar-Kyoto control rats of the same age and weight. The observation could be explained either by reduced production of the factor by atrial cardiocytes, or by increased release into the bloodstream, thus depleting tissue stores. In the former case, the difficulty of sodium elimination in these hypertensive rats (Kawabe *et al.*, 1979) could be due to an inadequate stimulus affecting essentially normal kidneys, whereas in the latter case a primary defect in kidney function would be compensated by an increased stimulus for sodium excretion. To distinguish between these possibilities, identical doses of atrial factor were administered to hypertensive and control bioassay rats (Sonnenberg *et al.*, 1983b). No renal defect relative to control animals was observed, suggesting that, in this model, production of the natriuretic factor was impaired.

Hirata *et al.* (1984), on the other hand, found that salt-sensitive Dahl rats had a higher content of atrial natriuretic factor than salt-resistant rats, even before the former developed hypertension. In addition, kidneys of salt-sensitive rats were less responsive to a standard dose of the factor, indicating that in this model a renal defect was associated with compensatory hyperproduction of atrial factor. No information is yet available on the possible role of atrial natriuretic factor in human hypertension.

Recently, Chimoskey *et al.* (1984) have shown a decrease in atrial content of natriuretic factor in a strain of myopathic hamsters, compared with control animals. They suggest that this deficiency may be the cause of the venous congestion and the oedema of this experimental model.

Comparison with the Natriuretic Hormone. Based on both morphological and physiological considerations, natriuretic hormone and atrial natriuretic factor are two different entities. Although both seem to be peptides, the former has a molecular weight in the range of 500 Da, whereas the minimum biologically active size of the latter appears to be above 2000 Da. Natriuretic hormone inhibits short-circuit current and potential difference across frog skin, whereas atrial natriuretic factor shows no such transport effects *in vitro*. The sites from which the materials can be extracted are different (brain, heart), as are their effects on kidney function. Natriuresis elicited by atrial factor is of higher magnitude and shorter duration than that obtainable by natriuretic hormone (Veress *et al.*, 1980; deBold *et al.*, 1981). Sites of transport inhibition in the nephron are also different (Sonnenberg *et al.*, 1980a, 1981a, 1982). Their effects on arterial blood pressure also indicate different compounds: whereas natriuretic hormone may cause chronic vasoconstriction (deWardener and MacGregor, 1983), atrial factor induces acute vasodilatation. Finally, the former appears to be an endogenous $(Na^+ + K^+)$ ATPase inhibitor, whereas the latter does not inhibit this enzyme system (Pamnani *et al.*, 1984).

The results on nephron sites of action suggest a synergism of the renal effects of natriuretic hormone and atrial natriuretic factor: whereas the former increases delivery of salt and water to the medullary collecting duct, in the absence of transport inhibition at this site tubular reabsorption would rise proportionally, resulting in only a minor increase of natriuresis. Conversely, atrial natriuretic factor, acting in isolation, would suppress sodium reabsorption in the medullary duct, resulting in quantitative excretion of an unchanged delivered load. Maximal natriuresis would result when delivery to the duct system is increased and reabsorption in the duct is inhibited. One may speculate that circulating natriuretic hormone levels are sufficient to compensate for small, chronic alterations in body sodium content, but that atrial natriuretic factor is required when large acute changes occur, or when release and/or renal action of natriuretic hormone is insufficient to maintain salt balance. Such reasoning would explain the increased sensitivity of uraemic kidneys to natriuretic hormone (Fine *et al.*, 1976b), if it is assumed that in these animals increased blood levels of atrial natriuretic factor are necessary to help to excrete the required amount of sodium per remaining nephron.

If atrial factor is indeed a second natriuretic hormone, why were we and others unable to detect it in cross-circulation experiments? To answer this question we injected a maximally effective dose of atrial extract into one of a pair of cross-circulated rats (Veress and Sonnenburg, unpublished). Rats receiving the extract responded with the expected natriuresis. However, their partners sharing the common circulation showed no alteration of sodium excretion, despite a blood exchange of approximately one-tenth of cardiac output per minute. These results suggest that endogenously released factor in a hypervolaemic animal is quickly destroyed in the circulation, so that renally effective concentrations are not built up in a cross-circulated partner. This may also be the reason for the short duration of action of the extract.

Conclusion

Although the concept that a salt-losing hormone is an essential feature of fluid volume regulation has been controversial, the sum of the evidence for its existence now appears conclusive. Its role in chronic salt balance is being elucidated, and understanding of its mechanism of action offers new insights into the cause of certain pathological conditions. In addition, the recent discovery of the atrial natriuretic factor opens the possibility that this is a second hormone system allowing the heart to regulate its workload on a short-term or emergency basis. Although the interaction between these two entities is still unknown, further investigations into regulation of release, and of renal as well as extrarenal action, seem certain to advance our understanding of fluid volume regulation.

References

Ackermann, U. (1975) 'On the Regulation of the Renal Response to Blood Volume Expansion by Vascular Parameters in the Rat', *Pflügers Arch.*, *355*, 151–64

Ackermann, U., Irizawa, T. and Sonnenberg, H (1982) 'Cardiovascular Effects of Atrial Natriuretic Factor (ANF) in Anesthetized Rats', *Fed. Proc.*, *41*, 1353 (abstract)

Ackermann, U., Irizawa, T.G., Milojevic, S. and Sonnenberg, H. (1984) 'Cardiovascular Effects of Atrial Extracts in Anesthetized Rats', *Can. J. Physiol. Pharmacol.*, *62*, 819–26

Alaghband-Zadeh, J., Fenton, S., Millett, J., Hancock, K. and deWardener, H.E. (1981) 'The Effect of Sodium Intake on the Content of a Substance in the Rat Hypothalamus which Stimulates Glucose 6-Phosphate Dehydrogenase (G6PD) *in vitro*', *Clin. Sci.*, *61*, 43p (abstract)

Anad-Sristava, M.B., Franks, D.J., Cantin, M. and Genest, J. (1984) 'Atrial Natriuretic Factor Inhibits Adenylate Cyclase Activity', *Biochem. Biophys. Res. Comm.*,*121*, 855–62

Atarashi, K., Mulrow, P.J., Franco-Saenz, R., Snadjar, R. and Rapp, J. (1984) 'Inhibition of Aldosterone Production by an Atrial Extract', *Science, 224*, 992-4

Atkins, E.L. and Pearce, J.W. (1959) 'Mechanism of the Renal Response to Plasma Volume Expansion', *Can. J. Biochem. Physiol.*, *37*, 91–102

Atlas, S.A., Kleinert, H.D., Camargo, M.J., Januszewicz, A., Sealey, J.E., Laragh, J.H., Schilling, J.W., Lewicki, J.A., Johnson, L.K. and Maack, T. (1984) 'Purification, Sequencing and Synthesis of Natriuretic and Vasoactive Rat Atrial Peptide', *Nature (Lond.)*, *309*, 717–19

August, J.L., Nelson, D.H. and Thorn, G.W. (1958) 'Response of Normal Subjects to Large Amounts of Aldosterone', *J. Clin. Invest.*, *37*, 1549–55

Axelsson, K.L., Wikberg, J.E.S. and Anderssen, R.G.G. (1979) 'Relationship between Nitroglycerine, Cyclic GMP, and Relaxation of Vascular Smooth Muscle', *Life Sci.*, *24*, 1779–86

Bahlmann, J., McDonald, S.J., Ventom, M.G. and deWardener, H.E. (1967) 'The Effect on Urinary Sodium Excretion of Blood Volume Expansion without Changing the Composition of Blood in the Dog', *Clin. Sci.*, *32*, 403–13

Baines, A.D., deBold, A.J. and Sonnenberg, H. (1983) 'Natriuretic Effect of Atrial Extract on Isolated Perfused Rat Kidney', *Can. J. Physiol. Pharmacol.*, *61*, 1462–6

Barajas, L. and Latta, H. (1967) 'Structure of the Juxtaglomerular Apparatus', *Circ. Res., 21* (Suppl. II), 1115–28

Bencosme, S.A. and Berger, J.M. (1971) 'Specific Granules in Mammalian and Non-mammalian Vertebrate Cardiocytes', in E. Bajusz and G. Jasmin (eds) *Methods and Achievements in Experimental Pathology, vol. 5: Functional Morphology of the Heart*, Karger, Basel, pp. 173–213

Bengele, H.H., Lechene, C. and Alexander, E.A. (1980) 'Sodium and Chloride Transport along the Inner Medullary Collecting Duct: Effect of Saline Expansion', *Am. J. Physiol.*, *238*, F504–8

Blythe, W.B., D'Avila, D., Gitelman, H.J. and Welt, L.G. (1971) 'Further Evidence for a Humoral Natriuretic Factor', *Circ. Res.*, *28*, Suppl. II, 21–31

Bonjour, J.P. and Peters, G. (1970) 'Non-occurrence of a Natriuretic Factor in Circulating Blood of Rats after Expansion of the Extracellular or the Intravascular Space', *Pflügers Arch.*, *318*, 21–34

Borenstein, H.B. (1982) 'The Renal Hemodynamic Effects of Atrial Natriuretic Factor in Rats', MSc Thesis, University of Toronto, Canada

Borenstein, H.B., Cupples, W.A., Sonnenberg, H. and Veress, A.T. (1983) 'The Effect of a Natriuretic Atrial Extract on Renal Haemodynamics and Urinary Excretion in Rats', *J. Physiol. (Lond.)*, *334*, 133–40

Bourgoignie, J.J., Hwang, K.H., Ipakchi, E. and Bricker, N.S. (1974) 'The Presence of a Natriuretic Factor in Urine of Patients with Chronic Uremia. The Absence of the Factor in Nephrotic Uremic Patients', *J. Clin. Invest.*, *53*, 1559–67

Bricker, N.S. and Fine, L.G. (1981) 'The Renal Response to Progressive Nephron Loss', in B.M. Brenner and F.C. Rector, Jr (eds), *The Kidney*, W.B. Saunders, Philadelphia, pp. 1056–96

Bricker, N.S., Schmidt, R.W., Favre, H., Fine, L. and Bourgoignie, J.J. (1975) 'On the Biology of Sodium Excretion: the Search for a Natriuretic Hormone', *Yale J. Biol. Med.*, *48*, 293–303

Briggs, J.P., Steipe, B., Schubert, G. and Schnermann, J. (1982) 'Micropuncture Studies of the Renal Effects of Atrial Natriuretic Substance', *Pflügers Arch.*, *395*, 271–6

Brody, M.J., Fink, G.D., Buggy, J., Haywood, J.R., Gordon, F.J. and Johnson, A.K. (1978) 'The Role of Anteroventral Third Ventricle (AV3V) Region in Experimental Hypertension', *Circ. Res.*, *43* (Suppl. I), I2–13

Buckalew, V.M. and Lancaster, C.D. (1972) 'The Association of a Humoral Sodium Transport Inhibitory Activity with Renal Escape from Chronic Mineralocorticoid Administration in the Dog', *Clin. Sci.*, *42*, 69–78

Camargo, M.J.F., Kleinert, H.D., Atlas, S.A., Sealey, J.E., Laragh, J.H. and Maack, T. (1984) 'Ca-dependent Hemodynamic and Natriuretic Effects of Atrial Extract in Isolated Rat Kidney', *Am. J. Physiol.*, *246*, F447–56

Cambier, P. and Godon, J.P. (1984) 'Role of Prostaglandins in the Production of Natriuretic Factor by the Isolated Kidney', *Renal Physiol.*, *7*, 163–75

Cantin, M. and Huet, M. (1973) 'Corticoid Dependence of Atrial Specific Granules in the Hamster', *Fed. Proc.*, *32*, 876a (abstract)

Cantin, M. and Huet, M. (1975) 'Chemical Nature of Atrial Specific Granules', in A. Fleckenstein and G. Rona (eds), *Recent Advances in Studies on Cardiac Structure and Metabolism*, *vol. 6*, *Pathophysiology and Morphology of Myocardial Cell Alterations*, University Park Press, Baltimore, pp. 313–22

Cantin, M., Michelakis, A.M. and Genest, J. (1981) 'Renin Activity of the Myocardium. Relationship with Atrial Specific Granules', *Fed. Proc.*, *40*, 437 (abstract)

Cantin, M., Gutkowska, J., Thibault, G., Milne, R.W., Ledoux, S., MinLi, S., Chapeau, C., Garcia, R., Hamet, P. and Genest, J. (1984) 'Immunocytochemical Localization of Atrial Natriuretic Factor in the Heart and Salivary Glands', *Histochemistry*, *80*, 113–27

Carretero, O.A. and Scicli, A.G. (1976) 'Renal Kallikrein: its Localization and Possible Role in Renal Function', *Fed. Proc.*, *35*, 194–8

Celio, M.R. and Inagami, T. (1981) 'Renin in the Human Kidney. Immunohistochemical Localization', *Histochemistry*, *72*, 1–10

Chartier, L., Schiffrin, E., Thibault, G. and Garcia, R. (1984) 'Atrial Natriuretic Factor Inhibits the Stimulation of Aldosterone Secretion by Angiotensin II, ACTH, and Potassium *in vivo* and *in vitro*', *Endocrinology*, *115*, 2026–8

Chimoskey, J.E., Spielman, W.S., Brant, M.A. and Heidemann, S.R. (1984) 'Cardiac Atria of B10 14.6 Hamsters are Deficient in Natriuretic Factor', *Science*, *223*, 820–2

Clarkson, E.M. and deWardener, H.E. (1972) 'Inhibition of Sodium and Potassium Transport in Separated Renal Tubule Fragments Incubated in Extracts of Urine Obtained from Salt-loaded Individuals', *Clin. Sci.*, *42*, 607–17

Clarkson, E.M., Raw, S.M. and deWardener, H.E. (1976) 'Two Natriuretic Substances in Extracts of Urine from Normal Man when Salt-depleted and Salt-loaded', *Kidney Int.*, *10*, 387–92

Clarkson, E.M., Raw, S.M. and deWardener, H.E. (1979) 'Further Observations on a Low Molecular Weight Natriuretic Substance in the Urine of Normal Man', *Kidney Int.*, *16*, 710–21

Clinton, M. and Thorn, G.W. (1943) 'Effect of Desoxycorticosterone Acetate Administration on Plasma Volume and Electrolyte Balance of Normal Human Subjects', *Bull. Johns Hopkins Hosp.*, *72* 255–64

Cole, C.H., Balfe, J.W. and Welt, L.G. (1968) 'Induction of a Ouabain-sensitive ATPase Defect by Uremic Plasma', *Trans. Assoc. Am. Phys.*, *81*, 213–20

Cort, J.H. and Lichardus, B. (1963) 'The Natriuretic Activity of Jugular Vein Blood during Cartoid Occlusion', *Physiol. Bohemoslov.*, *12*, 497–501

Cortney, M.A., Mylle, M., Lassiter, W.E. and Gottschalk, C.W. (1965) 'Renal Tubular *120*, 461–6

Currie, M.G., Geller, D.M., Cole, B.R., Boylan, J.G., Wu, Y.S., Holmberg, S.W. and Needleman, P. (1983) 'Bioactive Cardiac Substances: Potent Vasorelaxant Activity in Mammalian Atria', *Science*, *221*, 71–3

Currie, M.G., Geller, D.M., Cole, B.R. and Needleman, P. (1984a) 'Proteolytic Activation of a Bioactive Cardiac Peptide by *in vitro* Trypsin Cleavage', *Proc. Natl Acad. Sci. USA*, *81*, 1230–6

Currie, M.G., Geller, D.M., Cole, B.R., Siegel, N.R., Fok, K.F., Adams, S.P. Eubanks, S.P., Galluppi, G.R. and Needleman, P. (1984b) 'Purification and Sequence Analysis of Bioactive Atrial Peptides (Atriopeptins)', *Science*, *223*, 67–9

Currie, M.G., Geller, D.M., Chao, J., Margolius, H.S., and Needleman, P. (1984c) 'Kallikrein Activation of a High Molecular Weight Atrial Peptide', *Biochem. Biophys. Res, Comm.*, *119*, 685–8

DeBold, A.J. (1979) 'Heart Atria Granularity: Effects of Changes in Water-Electrolyte Balance', *Proc. Soc. Exp. Biol. Med.*, *161*, 508–11

DeBold, A.J. (1982a) 'Tissue Fractionation Studies on the Relationship between Atrial Natriuretic Factor and Specific Atrial Granules', *Can. J. Physiol. Pharmacol.*, *60*, 324–30

DeBold, A.J. (1982b) 'Atrial Natriuretic Factor of the Rat Heart. Studies on Isolation and Properties', *Proc, Soc. Exp. Biol. Med.*, *170*, 133–8

DeBold, A.J. and Bencosme, S.A. (1973) 'Studies on the Relationship between the Catecholamine Distribution in the Atrium and the Specific Granules Present in Atrial Muscle Cells. 2. Studies on the Sedimentation Pattern of Atrial Noradrenaline and Adrenaline'. *Cardiovasc. Res.*, *7*, 364–9

DeBold, A.J. and Bencosme, S.A. (1975) 'Selective Light Microscopic Demonstration of the Specific Granulation of the Rat Atrial Myocardium by Lead-Hematoxylin-Tartrazine', *Stain Technol.*, *50*, 203–5

DeBold, A.J. and Flynn, T.G. (1983) 'Cardionatrin I — a Novel Heart Peptide with Potent Diuretic and Natriuretic Properties', *Life Sci.*, *3*, 297–302

DeBold, A.J. and Salerno, T.A. (1983) 'Natriuretic Activity of Extracts obtained from Hearts of Different Species and from Various Rat Tissues', *Can. J. Physiol. Pharmacol.*, *61*, 127–30

DeBold, A.J., Borenstein, H.B., Veress, A.T. and Sonnenberg, H. (1981) 'A Rapid and Potent Natriuretic Response to Intravenous Injection of Atrial Myocardial Extract in Rats', *Life Sci.*, *28*, 89–94

Deth, R.C., Wong, K., Fukozawa, S., Rocco, R., Smart, J.L., Lynch, C.J. and Awad, R. (1982) 'Inhibition of Rat Aorta Contractile Response by Natriuresis-inducing Extract of Rat Atrium', *Fed. Proc.*, *41*, 983 (abstract)

DeWardener, H.E. and MacGregor, G.A. (1980) 'Dahl's Hypothesis that a Saluretic Substance may be Responsible for a Sustained Rise in Arterial Pressure: its Possible Role in Essential Hypertension', *Kidney Int.*, *18*, 1–9

DeWardener, H.E. and MacGregor, G.A. (1983) 'The Relation of a Circulating Transport Inhibitor (the Natriuretic Hormone?) to Hypertension', *Medicine*, *62*, 310–26

DeWardener, H.E., Mills, I.H., Clapham, W.F. and Hayter, C.J. (1961) 'Studies on the Efferent Mechanism of the Sodium Diuresis which Follows the Administration of Intravenous Saline in the Dog', *Clin. Sci.*, *21*, 249–58

Dietz, R., Rascher, W., Schomig, A., Strasser, R. and Kubler, W. (1982) 'Lowering of Blood Pressure in Sodium Loaded Rats by Administration of Digoxin Antibodies', *Am. J. Cardiol.*, *49*, 912 (abstract)

Dirks, J.H., Cirksena, W.J. and Berliner, R.W. (1965) 'The Effect of Saline Infusion on Sodium Reabsorption by the Proximal Tubule of the Dog', *J. Clin. Invest.*, *44*, 1160–70

Favre, H., Hwang, K.H., Schmidt, R.W., Bricker, N.S. and Bourgoignie, J.J. (1975) 'An Inhibitor of Sodium Transport in the Urine of Dogs with Normal Renal Function', *J. Clin. Invest.*, *56*, 1302–11

Fenton, S., Clarkson, E., MacGregor, G., Alaghband-Zadeh, J. and DeWardener, H.E. (1982) 'An Assay of the Capacity of Biological Fluids to Stimulate Renal Glucose-6-phosphate Dehydrogenase Activity *in vitro* as a Marker of their Ability to Inhibit Sodium Potassium-dependent Adenosine Triphosphatase Activity', *J. Endocrinol.*, *94*, 99–110

Fine, L., Bourgoignie, J.J., Hwang, K.H. and Bricker, N.S. (1976a) 'On the Influence of the Natriuretic Factor from Uremic Patients on Bioelectric Properties and Sodium Transport of the Isolated Mammalian Collecting Tubule', *J. Clin. Invest.*, *58*, 590–7

Fine, L.G., Bourgoignie, J.J., Weber, H. and Bricker, N.S. (1976b) 'Enhanced End-organ Responsiveness of the Uremic Kidney to the Natriuretic Factor', *Kidney Int.*, *10*, 364–72

Fishman, M.C. (1979) 'Endogenous Digitalis-like Activity in Mammalian Brain', *Proc. Natl Acad. Sci. USA*, 4661–3

Flynn, T.G., DeBold, M. and DeBold, A.J. (1983) 'The Amino Acid Sequence of an Atrial Peptide with Potent Diuretic and Natriuretic Properties', *Biochem. Biophys. Res. Comm.*, *117*, 859–65

Garcia, R., Cantin, M., Thibault, G., Ong, H. and Genest, J. (1982) 'Relationship of Specific Granules to the Natriuretic and Diuretic Activity of Rat Atria', *Experientia*, *38*, 1071–3

Garcia, R., Thibault, G., Nutt, R.F., Cantin, M. and Genest, J. (1984) 'Comparative Vasoactive Effects of Native and Synthetic Atrial Natriuretic Factor (ANF)', *Biochem. Biophys. Res. Transport of Water, Solute, and PAH in Rats Loaded with Isotonic Saline', *Am. J. Physiol.*, *209*, 1199–1205

Gauer, O.H. and Henry, J.P. (1963) 'Circulating Basis of Fluid Volume Control', *Physiol. Rev.*, *43*, 423–81

Geller, D.M., Currie, M.G., Wakitani, K., Cole, B.R., Adams, S.P., Fok, K.F., Siegel, N.R., Eubanks, S.R., Galluppi, G.R. and Needleman, P. (1984a) 'Atriopeptins: a Family of Potent

Biologically Active Peptides Derived from Mammalian Atria', *Biochem. Biophys. Res. Comm.*, *120*, 333–8

Geller, D.M., Currie, M.G., Siegel, N.R., Fok, K.F., Adams, S.P. and Needleman, P,. (1984b) 'The Sequence of an Atriopeptigen: a Precursor of the Bioactive Atrial Peptides', *Biochem. Biophys. Res. Comm.*, *121*, 802–7

Gilmore, J.P. and Daggett, W.M. (1966) 'Response of the Chronic Cardiac Denervated Dog to Acute Volume Expansion', *Am. J. Physiol.*, *210*, 509–12

Godon, J.P. and Dechenne, C. (1978) '*In vitro* Production of a Natriuretic Material of Renal Origin', *Renal Physiol.*, *1*, 201–10

Gonick, H.C.,Saldanha, L.F. and Lu, E. (1975) 'A Natriuretic Principle Derived from Kidney Tissue of Volume-expanded Rats', *J. Clin. Invest.*, *56*, 247–55

Gonick, H.C., Kramer, H.J., Paul, W. and Lu, E. (1977) 'Circulating Inhibitor of Sodium-Potassium-activated Adenosine Triphosphatase after Expansion of Extracellular Fluid Volume in Rats', *Clin. Sci.*, *53*, 329–34

Gottschalk, C.W. (1979) 'Renal Nerves and Sodium Excretion', *Ann. Rev. Physiol.*, *41*, 229–40

Grammer, R.T., Fukumi, H., Inagami, T. and Misono, K.S. (1983) 'Rat Atrial Natriuretic Factor. Purification and Vasorelaxant Activity', *Biochem. Biophys. Res. Comm.*, *116*, 696–703

Gruber, K.A. and Buckalew, V.M., Jr (1978) 'Further Characterization and Evidence for a Precursor in the Formation of Plasma Antinatriferic Factor', *Proc. Soc. Exp. Biol. Med.*, *159*, 463–7

Gruber, K.A., Whitaker, J.M. and Buckalew, V.M., Jr. (1980) 'Endogenous Digitalis-like Substance in Plasma of Volume-expanded Dogs', *Nature (Lond.)*, *287*, 743–5

Gruber, K.A., Hennessy, J.F., Buckalew, V.M., Jr and Lymangrover, J.R. (1982) 'Identification of a Heptapeptide with Digitalis and Natriuretic Hormone Like Properties', *Abstracts, Am. Soc. Nephrol.*, *77A* (abstract)

Haas, J.A., Berndt, T. and Knox, F.G. (1979) 'Collecting Duct Function in Desoxy-corticosterone-treated Rats', *J. Clin. Invest.*, *63*, 211–14

Haddy, F.J. and Overbeck, H.W. (1976) 'The Role of Humoral Agents in Volume-expanded Hypertension', *Life Sci.*, *19*, 935–48

Hamet, P., Cantin, M., Garcia, R., St-Louis, J., Tremblay, J., Thibault, G., and Genest, J. (1983) 'Study of the Mechanism of the Action of Atrial Natriuretic Factor', *Proc. Can. Fed. Biol. Soc.*, *26*, 112 (abstract)

Haupert, G.T., Jr and Sancho, J.M. (1979) 'Sodium Transport Inhibitor from Bovine Hypothalamus', *Proc. Natl Acad. Sci. USA*, *76*, 4658–60

Hayslett, J.P.,Kashgarian, M. and Epstein, F.H. (1969a) 'Mechanism of Change in the Sodium per Nephron when Renal Mass is Reduced', *J. Clin. Invest.*, *48*, 1002–6

Hayslett, J.P. Weinstein, E, Kashgarian, M. and Epstein, F.H. (1969b) 'Attempts to Demonstrate a Hormonal Natriuretic Factor by Micropuncture Techniques', *Yale J. Biol. Med.*, *41*, 415–21

Higashihara, E., Stokes, J.B., Kokko, J.P., Campbell, W.B. and DuBose, T.D. Jr (1979) 'Cortical and Papillary Micropuncture Examination of Chloride Transport in Segments of the Rat Kidney during Inhibition of Prostaglandin Production', *J. Clin. Invest.*, *64*, 1277–87

Hirata, V., Ganguli, M., Tobian L. and Iwai, J. (1984) 'Dahl-S Rats Have Increased Natriuretic Factor in Atria but are Markedly Hyporesponsive to it', *Hypertension*, *6*, I148–55

Huang, C.T. and Smith, R.M. (1984) 'Lowering of Blood Pressure in Chronic Aortic Coarctate Hypertensive Rats with Antidigoxin Antiserum', *Life Sci.*, *35*, 115–18

Huet, M. and Cantin, M. (1974) 'Ultrastructural Cytochemistry of Atrial Muscle Cells. II. Characterization of the Protein Content of Specific Granules', *Lab. Invest.*, *30*, 525–32

Huet, M., Benchimol, S., Castonguay, Y. and Cantin, M. (1975) 'The Chemical Nature of Human Atrial Specific Granules', in P.-E. Roy and P. Harris (eds), *Recent Advances in Studies on Cardiac Structure and Metabolism, vol. 8, The Cardiac Sarcoplasm*, University Park Press, Baltimore, pp. 59–76

Huet, S.J., Pamnani, M.B.,Clough, D.L., Buggy, J., Bryant, H.J., Harder, D.R. and Haddy, F.J. (1983) 'Sodium-Potassium Pump Activity in Reduced Renal-mass Hypertension', *Hypertension*, *5*, (Suppl.*I*), 194–100

Jamieson, J.D. and Palade, G.E. (1964) 'Specific Granules in Atrial Muscle Cells', *J. Cell Biol.*,

23, 151–72

Kaczmarczyk, G., Drake, A., Eisele, R., Mohnhaupt, R., Noble, M.I.M., Simgen, B., Stubbs, J. and Reinhardt, H.W. (1981) 'The Role of the Cardiac Nerves in the Regulation of Sodium Excretion in Conscious Dogs', *Pflügers Arch.*, *390*, 125–30

Kaloyanides, G.J. and Azer, M. (1971) 'Evidence for a Humoral Mechanism in Volume Expansion Natriuresis', *J. Clin. Invest.*, *50*, 1603–12

Kaloyanides, G.J., Cohen, L. and DiBona, G.F. (1977) 'Failure of Selected Endocrine Organ Ablation to Modify the Natriuresis of Blood Volume Expansion in the Dog', *Clin. Sci.*, *52*, 351–6

Kangawa, K. and Matsuo, H. (1984) 'Purification and Complete Amino Acid Sequence of γ-human Atrial Natriuretic Peptide (γ-hANP)', *Biochem. Biophys. Res. Comm.*, *48*, 131–9

Kangawa, K., Fukuda, A., Kubota, I., Hayashi, Y. and Matsuo, H. (1984) 'Identification in Rat Atrial Tissue of Multiple Forms of Natriuretic Polypeptides of about 3000 Daltons', *Biochem. Biophys. Res. Comm.*, *121*, 585–91

Kaplan, M.A., Bourgoignie, J.J., Rosecan, J. and Bricker, N.S. (1974) 'The Effects of the Natriuretic Factor from Uremic Urine on Sodium Transport, Water and Electrolyte Content, and Pyruvate Oxidation by the Isolated Toad Bladder', *J. Clin. Invest.*, *53*, 1568–77

Kappagoda, C.T., Linden, R.J. and Sivananthan, N. (1979) 'The Nature of the Atrial Receptor Responsible for a Reflex Increase in Heart Rate in the Dog', *J. Physiol.*, *291*, 393–412

Karim, F., Kidd, C., Malpus, C.M. and Penna, P.E. (1972) 'The Effects of Stimulation of the Left Atrial Receptors on Sympathetic Efferent Nerve Activity', *J. Physiol.*, *227*, 243–60

Kawabe, K., Watanabe, T.X., Shiono, K. and Sokabe, H. (1979) 'Role of the Kidney in the Pathogenesis of SHR, and Other Hypertensive Rats Determined by Renal Allografts', *Jap. Heart J.*, *20 (Suppl. 1)*, 87–9

Keeler, R. (1959) 'Effect of Hypothalamic Lesions on Renal Excretion of Sodium', *Am. J. Physiol.*, *197*, 847–9

Keeler, R. (1982) 'Atrial Natriuretic Factor Has a Direct Prostaglandin-independent Action on Kidneys', *Can. J. Physiol. Pharmacol.*, *60*, 1078–82

Kisch, B. (1956) 'Electron Microscopy of the Atrium of the Heart. I. Guinea Pig', *Exp. Med. Surg.*, *14*, 99–112

Kisch, B. (1963) 'A Significant Electron Microscopic Difference between the Atria and the Ventricles of the Mammalian Heart', *Exp. Med. Surg.*, *21*, 193–221

Knox, F.G., Howards, S.S., Wright, F.S., Davis, B.B. and Berliner, R.W. (1968) 'Effect of Dilution and Expansion of Blood Volume on Proximal Sodium Reabsorption', *Am. J. Physiol.*, *215*, 1041–8

Knox, F.G., Howards, S.S., Wright, F.S., Davis, B.B. and Berliner, R.W. (1968) 'Effect of Dilution and Expansion of Blood Volume on Proximal Sodium Reabsorption', *Am. J.Physiol.*, *215*, 1041–8

Knox, F.G., Schneider, E.G., Dresser, T.P. and Lynch, RE. (1970) 'Natriuretic Effect of Increased Proximal Delivery in Dogs with Salt Retention', *Am. J. Physiol.*, *219*, 904–10

Knox, F.G., Burnett, F.C. Jr, Kohan, D.E., Spielman, W.S. and Strand, J.C. (1980) 'Escape from the Sodium-retaining Effects of Mineralocorticoids', *Kidney Int.*, *17*, 263–76

Kojima, I., Yoshihara, S. and Ogata, E. (1982) 'Involvement of Endogenous Digitalis-like Substance in Genesis of Deoxycorticosterone-Salt Hypertension', *Life Sci.*, *30*, 1775–82

Kramer, H.J. (1981) 'Natriuretic Hormone — a Circulating Inhibitor of Sodium- and Potassium-activated Adenosine Triphosphatase. Its Potential Role in Body Fluid and Blood Pressure Regulation', *Klin. Wochenschr.*, *59*, 1225–30

Kramer, H.J., Gonick, H.C., Paul, W. and Lu, E. (1969) 'Third Factor: Inhibitor of Na-K-ATPase? *Abstracts, 4th Int. Congr. Nephrol.*, p. 373 (abstract)

Kramer, H.J., Backer, A. and Kruck, F. (1977) 'Antinatriferic Activity in Human Plasma Following Acute and Chronic Salt-loading', *Kidney Int.*, *12*, 214–22

Kramp, R.A., MacDowell, M., Gottschalk, C.W. and Oliver, J.R. (1974) 'A Study by Microdissection and Micropuncture of the Structure and the Function of the Kidneys and the Nephrons of Rats with Chronic Renal Damage', *Kidney Int.*, *5*, 147–76

Kreil, G. (1981) 'Transfer of Proteins across Membranes', *Ann. Rev. Biochem.*, *50*, 317–48

Kruck, F. (1967) 'Biologischer Nachweis eines humoralen natriuretischen Prinzips im Urin gesunder Menschen', *Klin. Wochenschr.*, *45*, 30–4

Kuhn, H., Richards, J.G. and Tranzer, J.P. (1975) 'The Nature of Rat "Specific Heart Granules" with Regard to Catecholamines: an Investigation of Ultrastructural Cytochemistry', *J. Ultrastruct. Res.*, *50*, 159–66

Landwehr, D.M., Klose, R.M. and Giebisch, G. (1967) 'Renal Tubular Sodium and Water Reabsorption in the Isotonic Sodium Chloride-loaded Rat', *Am. J. Physiol.*, *212*, 1327–33

Larose, P., Meleche, S., Souiche, P., du Deléan, A. and Ong, H. 'Radioimmunoassay of Atrial Natriuretic Factor: Human Plasma Levels', *Biochem. Biophys. Res. Commun.*, *130*, 553–8

Levinsky, N.G. (1974) 'Natriuretic Hormones', *Adv. Metabl. Disord.*, *7*, 37–71

Leyssac, P.P. (1976) 'The Renin Angiotensin System and Kidney Function: a Review of Contributions to a New Theory', *Acta Physiol. Scand. Suppl.* 422

Lichardus, B. and Pearce, J.W. (1966) 'Evidence for a Humoral Natriuretic Factor Released by Blood Volume Expansion', *Nature (Lond.)*, *209*, 407–9

Licht, A., Stein, S. and Bricker, N.S. (1978) 'Hormonal Changes and Transport Adaptation in Chronic Renal Failure: the Possible Role of a Natriuretic Hormone', *Biochem. Soc. Trans. (Lond.)*, *6* 837–9

Lichtstein, D. and Samuelov, S. (1980) 'Endogenous "Ouabain Like" Activity in Rat Brain', *Biochem. Biophys. Res. Comm.*, *96*, 1518–23

Linden, R.J. (1976) 'Reflexes from Receptors in the Heart', *Cardiology*, *61*, 7–30

Link, W.T., Pamnani, M.B., Huot, S.J. and Haddy, F.J. (1981) 'Effect of Atrial Extract on Vascular Na^+, K^+ Pump Activity', *Physiologist*, *24*, 59 (abstract)

Louis, F. and Favre, H. (1980) 'Natriuretic Factor in Rats Acutely Expanded by Ringer's versus Albumin Solution', *Kidney Int.*, *18*, 20–8

MacPhee, A.A., Trippodo, N.C. and Cole, F.E. (1982) 'Natriuretic Activity in Extracts of the Human Atrium', *64th Ann. Meeting Endocrin. Soc.*, p.191 (abstract)

Maddox, D.A., Bennett, C.M., Deen, W.M., Glassock, R.J., Knutson, D. and Brenner, B.M. (1975) 'Control of Proximal Tubule Fluid Reabsorption in Experimental Glomerulo-nephritis', *J. Clin. Invest.*, *55*, 1315–25

Maki, M., Takayanagi, R., Misono, K.S., Pandey, K.N., Tibbetts, C. and Inagami, T. (1984) 'Structure of Rat Atrial Natriuretic Factor Precursor Deduced from cDNA Sequence', *Nature (Lond.)*, *309*, 722–4

Manning, M., Balaspiri, L., Moehring, J., Halda, J. and Sawyer, W.H. (1976) 'Synthesis and Some Pharmacological Properties of Deamino (4-Threonine, 8-D-Arginine) Vasopressin and Deamino (8-D-Arginine) Vasopressin, Highly Potent and Specific Antidiuretic Peptides, and (8-D-Arginine) Vasopressin and Deamino-Arginine Vasopressin', *J. Med. Chem.*, *19*, 842–5

Marie, J.-P., Guillemot, H. and Hatt, P.-Y. (1976) 'Degree of Granularity of the Atrial Cardiocytes. Morphometric Study in Rats Subjected to Different Types of Water and Sodium Load', *Pathol. Biol.*, *24*, 549–54

Michell, R.H. and Kirk, C.J.(1981) 'Why is Phosphatidylinositol Degraded in Response to Stimulation of Certain Receptors?', *Trends Pharmacol. Sci.*, *2*, 86–9

Misono, K.S., Fukumi, H., Grammer, R.T. and Inagami, T. (1984) 'Rat Atrial Natriuretic Factor: Complete Amino Acid Sequence and Disulfide Linkage Essential for Biologic Activity', *Biochem. Biophys. Res. Comm.*, *119*, 524–9

Nemeh, M.N. and Gilmore, J.P. (1983) 'Natriuretic Activity of Human and Monkey Atria', *Circ. Res.*, *53*, 420–3

Oikawa, S., Imai, M., Ueno, A., Tanaka, S., Noguchi, T., Nakazato, H., Kangawa, K., Fukuda, A. and Matsuo, H. (1984) 'Cloning and Sequence Analysis of cDNA Encoding a Precursor for Human Atrial Natriuretic Polypeptide', *Nature (Lond.)*, *309*, 724–6

O'Neil, R.G. and Helman, S.I. (1977) 'Transport Characteristics of Renal Collecting Tubules: Influences of DOCA and Diet', *Am. J. Physiol.*, *233*, F544–58

Oshima, T., Currie, M.G., Geller, D.M. and Needleman, P. (1984) 'An Atrial Peptide is a Potent Renal Vasodilator Substance', *Circ. Res.*, *54*, 612–16

Pamnani, M.B., Clough, D.L., Huot, S.J. and Haddy, F.J. (1980) 'Vascular Sodium-Potassium Pump Activity in Various Models of Experimental Hypertension', *Clin. Sci.*, *59*, 179s–81s

Pamnani, M.B., Buggy, J., Huot, S.J. and Haddy, F.J. (1981) 'Studies on the Role of a Humoral Sodium-transport Inhibitor and the Anteroventral Third Ventricle (AV3V) in Experimental Low-renin Hypertension', *Clin. Sci.*, *61*, 57s–60s

Pamnani, M.B., Clough, D.L., Chen, J.S., Link, W.T. and Haddy, F.J. (1984) 'Effects of Rat Atrial Extract on Sodium Transport and Blood Pressure in the Rat', *Proc. Soc. Exp. Biol. Med.*, *176*, 123–31

Pearce, J.W. and Sonnenberg, H. (1965) 'Effects of Spinal Section and Renal Denervation on the Renal Response to Blood Volume Expansion', *Can. J. Physiol. Pharmacol.*, *43*, 211–24

Pearce, J.W. and Veress, A.T. (1975) 'Concentration and Bioassay of a Natriuretic Factor in Plasma of Volume Expanded Rats', *Can. J. Physiol. Pharmacol.*, *53*, 742–7

Pearce, J.W., Sonnenberg, H., Veress, A.T. and Ackermann, U. (1969) 'Evidence for a Humoral Factor Modifying the Renal Response to Blood Volume Expansion in the Rat', *Can. J. Physiol. Pharmacol.*, *47*, 377–86

Pearce, J.W., Sonnenberg, H., Lichardus, B. and Veress, A.T. (1970) 'Interaction of Extrarenal and Intrarenal Factors in "Volume Natriuresis"', in *Regulation of Body Fluid Volumes by the Kidney*, J.H. Cort and B. Lichardus (eds), Karger, Basel, pp. 72–92

Pollock, D.M. and Banks, R.O. (1983) 'Effect of Atrial Extract on Renal Function in the Rat', *Clin. Sci*, *65*, 47–55

Pollock, D.M., Mullins, M.M. and Banks, R.O. (1983) 'Failure of Atrial Myocardial Extract to Inhibit Renal Na+, K+-ATPase', *Renal Physiol.*, *6*, 295–9

Poston, L., Wilkinson, S., Sewell, R.B. and Williams, R. (1982) 'Sodium Transport during the Natriuresis of Volume Expansion; a Study Using Peripheral Blood Leucocytes', *Clin. Sci.*, *63*, 243–9

Ragan, C., Ferrebee, J.W., Phyfe, P., Atchley, D.W. and Loeb, R.F. (1940) 'A Syndrome of Polydipsia and Polyuria Induced in Normal Animals by Desoxycorticosterone Acetate', *Am. J. Physiol.*, *131*, 73–8

Raghavan, S.R.V. and Gonick, H.C. (1980) 'Partial Purification and Characterization of Natriuretic Factor from Rat Kidney', *Proc. Soc. Exp. Biol. Med.*, *164*, 101–4

Rector, F.C., Jr, Martinez-Maldonado, M., Kurtzman, N.A., Sellman, J.C., Oerther, F. and Seldin, D.W. (1968) 'Demonstration of a Hormonal Inhibitor of Proximal Tubular Reabsorption during Expansion of Extracellular Volume with Isotonic Saline', *J. Clin. Invest.*, *47*, 761–73

Reinhardt, H.W., Kaczmarczyk, G., Eisele, R., Arnold, B., Eigenheer, F. and Kuhl, U. (1977) 'Left Atrial Pressure and Sodium Balance in Conscious Dogs on a Low Sodium Intake', *Pflügers Arch.*, *370*, 59–66

Reinhardt, H.W., Eisele, R., Kaczmarczyk, G., Mohnhaupt, R., Oelkers, W. and Schimmrich, B. (1980a) 'The Control of Sodium Excretion by Reflexes from the Low Pressure System Independent of Adrenal Activity', *Pflügers Arch.*, *384*, 171–6

Reinhardt, H.W., Kaczmarczyk, G., Mohnhaupt, R. and Simgen, B. (1980b) 'The Possible Mechanism of Atrial Natriuresis — Experiments on Chronically Instrumented Dogs', in B. Lichardus, R.W. Schrier and J. Ponec (eds), *Hormonal Regulation of Sodium Excretion*, Elsevier/North-Holland and Biomedical Press, Amsterdam, pp. 63–72

Reinhardt, H.W., Kaczmarczyk, G., Mohnhaupt, R. and Simgen, B. (1980c) 'Atrial Natriuresis under the Condition of a Constant Renal Perfusion Pressure', *Pflügers Arch.*, *389*, 9–15

Rojo-Ortega, J.M., DeBold, A.J. and Bencosme, S.A. (1979) 'Renin-like Activity in the Rat Heart Atria', *J. Mol. Cell. Cardiol.*, *11*, S1, 52 (abstract)

Rudolf, J.R. and Ackermann, U. (1984) 'Renal Venous Pressure and Volume Natriuresis in the Rat', *Can. J. Physiol. Pharmacol.*, *62*, 80–3

Saetersdal, T., Jodalen, H., Lie, R., Rotevatn, S., Engedal, H. and Myklebust, R. (1979) 'Effects of Isoproterenol on the Dense Core and Perigranular Membrane of Atrial Specific Granules', *Cell Tissue Res.*, *119*, 213–24

Schmidt, R.W., Bourgoignie, J.J. and Bricker, N.S. (1974) 'On the Adaptation of Sodium Excretion in Chronic Uremia. The Effects of Proportional Reduction of Sodium Intake', *J. Clin. Invest.*, *53*, 1736–41

Schultze, R.G., Weisser, F. and Bricker, N.S. (1972) 'The Influence of Uremia on Fractional Sodium Reabsorption by the Proximal Tubule of Rats', *Kidney Int.*, *2*, 59–65

Sealey, J.E., Kirschmann, J.D. and Laragh, J.H. (1969) 'Natriuretic Activity in Plasma and Urine of Salt-loaded Sheep and Man', *J. Clin. Invest.*, *48*, 2210–24

Seidah, N.G., Lazure, C., Chretien, M., Thibault, G., Garcia, R., Cantin, M., Genest, J., Nutt, R.F., Brady, S.F., Lyle, T.A., Paleveda, W.J., Colton, C.D., Ciccarone, T.M. and Veber, D.F. (1984) 'Amino Acid Sequence of Homologous Rat Atrial Peptides: Natriuretic Activity of Native and Synthetic Forms', *Proc. Natl Acad. Sci. USA*, *81*, 2640–4

Seidman, C.E., Duby, A.D., Choi, E., Graham, R.M., Haber, E., Homcy, C., Smith, J.A. and Seidman, J.G. (1984) 'The Structure of Rat Preproatrial Natriuretic Factor as Defined by a Complementary DNA Clone', *Science*, *225*, 324–6

Smith, H.W. (1957) 'Salt and Water Receptors — an Exercise in Physiologic Apologetics', *Am. J. Med.*, *23*, 623–52

Songu-Mize, E., Bealer, S.L. and Caldwell, R.W. (1982) 'Effect of AV3V Lesions on Development of DOCA-salt Hypertension and Vascular Na$^+$ Pump Activity', *Hypertension*, *4*, 575–80

Sonnenberg, H. (1971) 'The Renal Response to Blood Volume Expansion in the Rat: Proximal Tubular Function and Urinary Excretion', *Can. J. Physiol. Pharmacol.*, *49*, 525–35

Sonnenberg, H. (1972) 'Renal Response to Blood Volume Expansion: Distal Tubular Function and Urinary Excretion', *Am. J. Physiol.*, *223*, 916–24

Sonnenberg, H. (1973) 'Proximal and Distal Tubular Function in Salt-Deprived and in Salt-loaded Deoxycorticosterone Acetate-escaped Rats', *J. Clin. Invest.*, *52*, 263–72

Sonnenberg, H. (1974) 'Medullary Collecting-duct Function in Antidiuretic and in Salt- or Water-diuretic Rats', *Am. J. Physiol.*, *226*, 501–6

Sonnenberg, H. (1976) 'Collecting Duct Function in Deoxycorticosterone Acetate-escaped, Normal, and Salt-deprived Rats: Response to Hypervolemia', *Circ. Res.*, *39*, 282–8

Sonnenberg, H. (1978) 'Microcatheterization Studies of Medullary Collecting Duct Function in the Rat Kidney', in H.G. Vogel and K.J. Ullrich (eds), *New Aspects of Renal Function*, Excerpta Medica, Amsterdam, pp. 175–80

Sonnenberg, H. and Solomon, S. (1969) 'Mechanism of Natriuresis following Intravascular and Extracellular Volume Expansion', *Can. J. Physiol. Pharmacol.*, *47*, 153–9

Sonnenberg, H. and Veress, A.T. (1983) 'Atrial Natriuretic Factor Mediates the Renal Response to Acute Hypervolemia', *Proc. 16th Ann. Meet. Am. Soc. Nephrol.*, A180 (abstract)

Sonnenberg, H. and Veress, A.T. (1984) 'Cellular Mechanism of Release of Atrial Natriuretic Factor', *Biochem. Biophys. Res. Comm.*, *124*, 443–9

Sonnenberg, H. and Wilson, D.R. (1976) 'The Role of the Medullary Collecting Ducts in Postobstructive Diuresis', *J. Clin. Invest.*, *57*, 1564–74

Sonnenberg, H., Veress, A.T. and Pearce, J.W. (1972) 'A Humoral Component of the Natriuretic Mechanism in Sustained Blood Volume Expansion', *J. Clin. Invest.*, *51*, 2631–44

Sonnenberg, H., Chong, C.K., Milojevic, S. and Veress, A.T. (1980a) 'Site of Action of Plasma Natriuretic Factor in the Rat Kidney', in B. Lichardus, R.W. Schreir and J. Ponec (eds), *Hormonal Regulation of Sodium Excretion*, Elsevier/North-Holland Biomedical Press, Amsterdam, pp.357–63

Sonnenberg, H., Veress, A.T., Borenstein, H.B. and DeBold, A.J. (1980b). 'Rapid and Potent Natriuretic Response to Intravenous Injection of Atrial Myocardial Extract in Rats', *The Physiologist*, *23*, 13 (abstract)

Sonnenberg, H., Cupples, W.A., DeBold, A.J. and Veress, A.T. (1981a) 'Intrarenal Localization of the Natriuretic Effect of Cardiac Atrial Extract', *Ann. NY Acad. Sci.*, *372*, 213–14

Sonnenberg, H., Chong, C.K. and Veress, A.T. (1981b) 'Cardiac Atrial Factor — An Endogenous Diuretic?', *Can. J. Physiol. Pharmacol.*, *59*, 1278–9

Sonnenberg, H., Cupples, W.A., DeBold, A.J. and Veress, A.T. (1982) 'Intrarenal Localization of the Natriuretic Effect of Cardiac Atrial Extract', *Can. J. Physiol. Pharmacol.*, *60*, 1149–52

Sonnenberg, H., Molojevic, S., Chong, C.K. and Veress, A.T. (1983a) 'Atrial Natriuretic Factor: Reduced Cardiac Content in Spontaneously Hypertensive Rats', *Hypertension*, *5*, 672–5

Sonnenberg, H., Veress, A.T. Milojevic, S. and Chong, C.K. (1983b) 'Atrial Natriuretic Factor in Spontaneously Hypertensive and Wistar-Kyoto Rats', *Fed. Proc.*, *42*, 523 (abstract)

Sonnenberg, and H., Krebs, R.F. and Veress, A.T. (1984) 'Release of Atrial Natriuretic Factor from Incubated Rat Heart Atria', *IRCS Physiol.*, in press

Sugawara, A., Nakao, K., Morii, N., Sakamoto, M. *et al.* 'α-Hematin Atrial Natriuretic Polypeptide is Released from the Heart and Circulates in the Body', *Biochem. Biophys. Res. Commun.*, *129*, 439–46

Theron, J.J., Biagio, R., Meyer, A.C. and Boekkooi, S. (1978) 'Ultrasonic Observations on the Maturation and Secretion of Granules in Atrial Myocardium', *J. Mol. Cell. Cardiol.*, *10*, 561–72

Thibault, G., Garcia, R., Seidah, N.G., Lazure, C., Cantin, M., Chretien, M. and Genest, J. (1983) 'Purification of Three Rat Atrial Natriuretic Factors and their Amino Acid Composition', *FEBS Lett.*, *164*, 286–90

Thibault, G., Garcia, R., Cantin, M., Genest, J., Lazure, C., Seidah, N.G., and Chretien, M.

(1984) 'Primary Structure of a High M_r Form of Rat Atrial Natriuretic Factor', *FEBS Lett.*, *167*, 352–6

Thibault, G., Lazure, C., Schiffrin, E.L., Gukkowska, J. *et al.*, 'Identification of a Biologically Active Circulating Form of Rat Atrial Natriuretic Factor', *Biochem. Biophys. Res. Commun.*, *130*, 981–6

Throckmorton, D.C. and Gilmore, J.P. (1983) 'Effect of Atrial Natriuretic Factor on Frog Cornea', *Fed. Proc.*, *42*, 475 (abstract)

Trippodo, N.C., MacPhee, A.A., Cole, F.E. and Blakesley, H.L. (1982) 'Partial Chemical Characterization of a Natriuretic Substance in Rat Atrial Heart Tissue', *Proc. Soc. Exp. Biol. Med.*, *170*, 502–8

Trippodo, N.C., Ghai, R.D., MacPhee, A.A. and Cole, F.E. (1984) 'Atrial Natriuretic Factor: Atrial Conversion of High to Low Molecular Weight Forms', *Biochem. Biophys. Res. Comm.*, *119*, 282–8

Veress, A.T. and Pearce, J.W. (1972) 'Effect of Vagotomy on the Renal Response to Blood Volume Expansion in the Rat', *Can. J. Physiol. Pharmacol.*, *50*, 463–6

Veress, A.T. and Sonnenberg, H. (1984) 'Right Atrial Appendectomy Reduces the Renal Response to Acute Hypervolemia in the Rat', *Am. J. Physiol.*, *247*, R610–13

Veress, A.T., Milojevic, S. and Sonnenberg, H. (1980) 'Characterization of the Natriuretic Activity in the Plasma of Hypervolaemic Rats', *Clin. Sci.*, *59*, 183–9

Veress, A.T., Chong, C.K. and Sonnenberg, H. (1982) 'Effect of Acute Unilateral Renal Denervation on Intrarenal Haemodynamics and Urinary Excretion in Rats before and during Hypervolaemia', *Clin. Sci.*, *62*, 457–64

Viscoper, R.J., Czaczkes, J.W., Schwartz, N. and Ullmann, T.D. (1971) 'Natriuretic Activity of a Substance Isolated from Human Urine During the Excretion of a Salt Load. Comparison of Hypertensive and Normotensive Subjects', *Nephron*, *8*, 540–8

Weber, H., Lin, K.-Y. and Bricker, N.S. (1975) 'Effect of Sodium Intake on Single Nephron Glomerular Filtration Rate and Sodium Reabsorption in Experimental Uremia', *Kidney Int.*, *8*, 14–20

Wen, S.F., Wong, N.L.M., Evanson, R.L., Lockhart, E.A. and Dirks, J.H. (1973) 'Micropuncture Studies of Sodium Transport in the Remnant Kidney of the Dog. The Effect of Graded Volume Expansion', *J. Clin. Invest.*, *52*, 386–97

Whitmer, K.R., Wallick, E.T., Epps, D.E., Lane, L.K., Collins, J.H. and Schwartz, A. (1982) 'Effects of Extracts of Rat Brain on the Digitalis Receptor', *Life Sci.*, *30*, 2261–75

Wilson, D.R. and Honrath, U. (1978) 'Cross-circulation Study of Natriuretic Factors in Rats with Reduced Nephron Mass', *Am. J. Physiol.*, *235*, F465–72

Wilson, D.R. and Sonnenberg, H. (1979) 'Medullary Collecting Duct Function in the Remnant Kidney before and after Volume Expansion', *Kidney Int.*, *15*, 487–501

Windhager, E.E., Lewy, J.E. and Spitzer, A. (1969) 'Intrarenal Control of Proximal Tubular Reabsorption of Sodium and Water', *Nephron*, *6*, 247–59

Wright, F.S., Knox, F.G., Howards, S.S. and Berliner, R.W. (1969a) 'Reduced Sodium Reabsorption by the Proximal Tubule of DOCA-escaped Dogs', *Am. J. Physiol.*, *216*, 869–75

Wright, F.S., Brenner, B.M., Bennett, C.M., Keimowitz, R.I., Berliner, R.W., Schreir, R.W., Verroust, P.J., DeWardener, H.E. and Holzgreve, H. (1969b) 'Failure to Demonstrate a Hormonal Inhibitor of Proximal Sodium Reabsorption', *J. Clin. Invest.*, *48*, 1107–13

Yamanaka, M., Greenberg, B., Johnson, L., Seilhamer, J., Brewer, M., Freidemann, T., Miller, J., Atlas, S., Laragh, J., Lewicki, J. and Fiddes, J. (1984) 'Cloning and Sequence Analysis of the cDNA for the Rat Atrial Natriuretic Factor Precursor', *Nature (Lond.)*, *309*, 719–22

7 DOPAMINE AND THE KIDNEY

M.R. Lee

Introduction

In the last few years it has become apparent that dopamine has an important part to play in the physiological regulation of renal function. It has also become evident that dopamine is formed in the kidney, probably largely in the renal tubules, and acts locally to produce natriuresis and vasodilatation. Very recently abnormalities of dopamine mobilisation by the kidney have been identified in hypertensive disorders and, perhaps most exciting of all, several renally specific dopaminergic agonists have been developed which may correct these abnormalities without serious systemic side-effects.

Action of Infused Dopamine on the Kidney

McDonald et al. (1964) reported that intravenous infusion of dopamine in seven normal subjects at dose levels of 2.6 to 7.1 μg kg^{-1} min^{-1} increased renal plasma flow from a mean of 507 ml min^{-1} to a mean of 798 ml min^{-1}; inulin clearance from 109 to 136 ml min^{-1} and sodium excretion from 171 to 575 μmol min^{-1}. These changes were accompanied by marked increases in cardiac output but no change in heart rate or arterial blood pressure. Other sympathomimetic amines such as noradrenaline, adrenaline and isoprenaline do not share this effect on renal function.

McNay et al. (1965) then went on to apply the same experimental design to the dog, when they gave 6 μg kg^{-1} min^{-1} intravenously to both the anaesthetised and unanaesthetised animal. The increase in sodium excretion was similar to that previously observed in man but the increments in glomerular filtration rate and renal blood flow were smaller (on a percentage basis). When dopamine was administered into the renal artery, the changes in RBF, GFR and $U_{Na}V$ were greater on the infused side, suggesting that the effects were not secondary to the systemic haemodynamic effects of the catecholamine.

A major point of contention is whether the natriuresis observed in such studies results from a direct action of dopamine on renal tubular receptors or depends upon an increase in glomerular filtration rate. Under certain circumstances a dissociation can be observed between the natriuresis and the increments in renal blood flow. For example, Brotzu (1970) reported that chlorpromazine could reduce the increase in renal blood flow without affecting the natriuresis, whereas McGiff and Burns (1967), by administering

218

phentolamine, or by renal nerve stimulation, abolished the natriuresis without damping the effect on renal blood flow.

The likely answer to this problem is that there are both vascular and tubular receptors for dopamine (see below). The argument is strongly reminiscent of that concerning the effects of angiotensin II on the kidney, where it has now been accepted that there are multiple receptors, both vascular and tubular.

The Renal Vascular Receptor for Dopamine

Goldberg *et al.* (1968) then went on to investigate the structural requirements of the renal vascular receptor by studying the effect on renal blood flow of a large group of related phenylethylamines of the general structure:

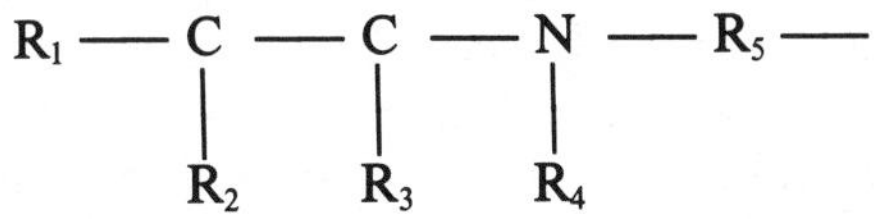

$$R_1 - \underset{\underset{R_2}{|}}{C} - \underset{\underset{R_3}{|}}{C} - \underset{\underset{R_4}{|}}{N} - R_5 -$$

Only one amine, epinine (N-methyldopamine; Figure 7.1) produced clear-cut renal vasodilatation, in a manner similar to dopamine, i.e. the effect was unaffected by the β-adrenoceptor antagonist, propranolol. Generally epinine was approximately 50 per cent as effective as dopamine in increasing renal blood flow.

Figure 7.1: The Molecular Structure of Dopamine and Epinine (N-methyldopamine)

R = H Dopamine
R = CH₃ Epinine

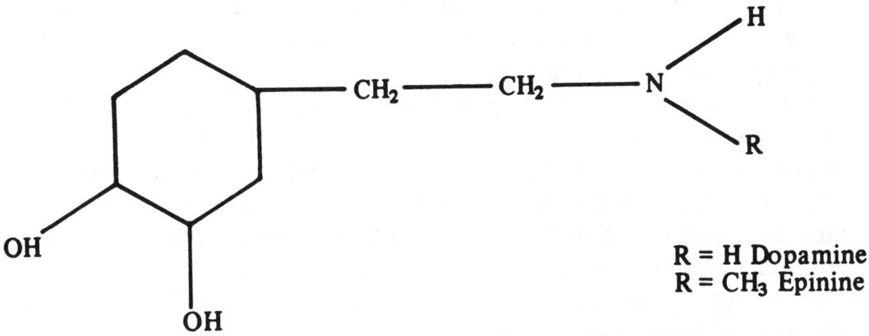

Epinine possesses more α-adrenoreceptor-agonist activity than dopamine, and full vasodilatation in the dog, equivalent to that produced by dopamine, is seen only after the administration of phenoxybenzamine to block the α-agonist effect. Hornykiewicz (1958) reported that, in the guinea pig, epinine produced an initial pressor effect followed by a longer hypotensive effect, whereas dopamine produced only the depressor (vasodilator) effect in this species.

Similar vasodilatation can be produced in the renal vascular bed by apomorphine (Goldberg *et al.*, 1968) and in the mesenteric vascular beds of the cat and dog by dopamine (Eble, 1964). Originally Rossum (1966) suggested that haloperidol was a dopamine blocking agent. Accordingly, Yeh *et al.* (1969) then went on to demonstrate that the renal vasodilatation produced by dopamine (and epinine) could be specifically antagonised by haloperidol, a member of the butyrophenone series of drugs.

More recently Kotake *et al.* (1981) have studied the glomerular receptors for dopamine in the rat. Having identified a dopamine-sensitive adenylate cyclase in the glomeruli, they compared the ability of dopamine, isoprenaline and the dopamine analogues 2-amino-6,7-dihydroxy-1,2,2,4-tetrahydronaphthalene (A-6,7-DTN), 2-amino-5,6-dihydroxy-1,2,3,4-tetrahydronaphthalene (A-5,6-DTN), and N,N-di-*n*-propyl dopamine, to stimulate cyclic AMP production in intact cell preparations and homogenates of rat glomeruli and corpus striatum. All of the agonists increased cyclic AMP production in glomeruli. By employing the dopamine antagonist fluphenazine (a phenothiazine) and the β-receptor antagonist propranolol, it was possible to show that the former blocked the effects of A-6,7-DTN and dopamine, whereas the latter blocked the effects of isoprenaline and A-5,6-DTN and also attenuated the response to dopamine. The profile of activity observed was similar in both the glomeruli and the corpus striatum.

These findings suggest that there are two types of vascular receptor in the rat glomerulus, β-adrenergic and dopaminergic, and that dopamine can activate both types depending on its concentration. Dopamine in the β-rotameric conformation, as typified by A-6,7-DTN, will activate the dopaminergic receptors, whereas in the α-rotameric conformation (as in A-5,6-DTN) it will activate the β-receptors. The potency series for the dopaminergic receptor, in both glomerulus and striatum, was dopamine equivalent to A-6,7-DTN; both are greater than dipropyldopamine.

Chapman *et al.* (1980) investigated the effects of dopamine and sulpiride on the rat kidney, particularly in relation to cortical and medullary blood flow, and confirmed that sulpiride is a selective dopaminergic blocking agent. The actions of the compound on the cortical and medullary circulation were different; sulpiride produced a small vasodilatation in the renal medulla but a definite cortical vasoconstriction. The authors suggested that this effect of sulpiride could be explained by the presence of dopamine-containing neurones in the renal cortex (Bell *et al.*, 1978; Dinerstein *et al.*, 1978), so that sulpiride would prevent neurogenically induced renal-cortical vasodilatation. This may be so, but, as pointed out in a later section, most of the cortical dopamine appears to be generated in the tubules from L-dopa filtered at the glomerulus. The experiments on the antagonist sulpiride should therefore be repeated on the kidneys of rats, acutely and chronically denervated, to establish what contribution, if any, renal dopaminergic vasodilator nerves make to the control of the cortical circulation.

Chapman *et al.* (1980) observed that a subpressor dose of dopamine had greater vasodilator action on renal medullary blood flow than on cortical blood flow, and they propose that this effect could contribute to the diuretic and natriuretic actions of the catecholamine. However, although an increased medullary blood flow could contribute to a washout of this usually hyperosmolar area, it is highly likely that there are specific tubular receptors for dopamine which mediate, at least in part, the natriuretic effect (see below).

It will be convenient at this point to give a description of the dopamine receptors, an extremely controversial subject. Recently Goldberg and Kohli (1983) have attempted to overcome some of the difficulties in this area and have updated the classification of Kebabian and Calne (1979). The DA_1 receptor is present in the vascular smooth muscle and is activated by dopamine, whereas the DA_2 receptor is present in neurones such as the caudate nucleus and is activated by dipropyldopamine or apomorphine. In contrast to the DA_2 receptor, where all analogues are equally potent, dopamine is more active than its analogues on the DA_1 receptor. Moreover only the β-rotamer is active at the DA_1 receptor, whereas both α- and β-rotamers are active at the DA_2 receptor. Ergot derivatives are active at the DA_2 receptor but not at the DA_1, whereas apomorphine is a full agonist at the DA_2 receptor but only a weak partial agonist at the DA_1 receptor.

In terms of antagonists the enantiomers of sulpiride play a crucial role in delineation, the R enantiomer being up to four times more active at the DA_1 receptor, whereas S is more than 100 times more active than R at the DA_2 receptor. Domperidone is a potent antagonist at the DA_2 receptor but not at the DA_1 receptor.

The DA_2 receptors seem to mediate inhibition in the postganglionic sympathetic nerve and also to be responsible for prolactin release, emesis and many behavioural responses.

Renal Tubular Actions and Receptors for Dopamine

Early studies on this subject did not support a specific tubular action for dopamine. May and Carter (1970) injected the catecholamine into the renal portal system of the chicken and failed to produce a natriuresis, although others have proposed that dopamine can act at the proximal tubule (Seely and Dirks, 1967) or distal convoluted tubule (Morimoto, 1968).

Recent evidence on γ-glutamyl-L-dopa in man (see below) would suggest a proximal tubular action, but further work is required on this point. Isolated tubular preparations should also be studied in an attempt to locate the site and category of the presumed dopamine receptors. Deis and Alonso (1970) found that dopamine increased urine volume in rats, and similar findings have been reported more recently (Cadnapaphornchai *et al.*, 1977). This might suggest that dopamine has the capacity to antagonise the effect of antidiuretic hormone at the distal tubule and collecting duct. Further work is needed to establish the site and nature of the interaction with arginine vasopressin (ADH).

Renal Tubular Transport of Dopamine

In the chicken the leg veins drain directly to the renal portal vein, and it has been demonstrated that dopamine, injected into the leg vein, finds its way rapidly into the urine. Small doses of dopamine can be given which do not produce cardiovascular changes (Sanner, 1963). Rennick (1968) was also able to show that in the dog, dopamine, given into the renal artery, was excreted in the urine; tubular secretion contributed about 80 per cent and glomerular filtration about 20 per cent of the total catecholamine found. No attempt was made to determine whether dopamine was secreted into the urine in the free or conjugated forms (see below).

Dopamine in the Urine out of Proportion to the other Catecholamines

When the first reliable fluorimetric methods for the analysis of catecholamines in urine became available, based on their extraction by alumina (Anton and Sayre, 1964), it soon became apparent that the amount of dopamine was five to twenty times that of noradrenaline (Crout, 1963). The initial assumption was made that the increased levels of dopamine reflected the load filtered at the glomerulus and were derived directly from the plasma dopamine.

More recently, sensitive radiokinetic assays for dopamine have become available, most of which depend upon the conversion of dopamine to labelled 3-methoxytyramine (Da Prada and Zurcher, 1976). This has extended the range of sensitivity of the assay into the picomole or femtomole range. These workers reported mean plasma catecholamine levels in man as follows: noradrenaline 1.05 ± 0.12 nmol litre^{-1}, adrenaline 0.45 ± 0.06 nmol litre^{-1} and dopamine 0.74 ± 0.03 nmol litre^{-1}. Assuming an average glomerular filtration rate of 120 ml min^{-1}, this should result in a dopamine excretion rate of approximately 130 nmol per 24 h. In fact Crout (1963) found values in man of 650–2285 nmol per 24 h.

In order to examine this problem further, Ball *et al.* (1978) determined plasma and urine levels of free dopamine simultaneously (in man) and were able to calculate an apparent renal clearance for dopamine of 1996 ± 453 ml min^{-1} (range 402–3844 ml min^{-1}), greatly in excess of glomerular filtration rate, and, in most individuals, greater than calculated renal plasma flow.

More recently, Ball *et al.* (1982) have studied the renal handling of L-dopa, dopamine, noradrenaline and adrenaline in the dog. In the anaesthetised greyhound, blood samples were taken from the aorta at the origin of the renal artery and from the renal vein during a timed urine collection. Arterial plasma dopa and adrenaline were consistently higher than the renal venous levels of these substances, suggesting extraction by the kidney. In contrast, noradrenaline and dopamine appeared to be added to the renal venous blood, and both of these catecholamines must therefore be presumed to be formed in the kidney. The dopa extracted by the kidney did not appear as free dopa in the urine but was presumably metabolised to dopamine within the kidney, some of the catecholamine finding its way into the renal venous effluent and some into the urine. The L-dopa removed by the kidney could be taken up by dopaminergic neurones or by the proximal convoluted tubule (see below).

Possible Sources for the Excess Dopamine in the Urine

Three main proposals have been put forward in an attempt to explain the large amounts of dopamine found in animal and human urine:

(1) that the kidney deconjugates dopamine compounds reaching the kidney and free dopamine is then secreted into the urine;
(2) that dopamine is released from renal dopaminergic nerves in the cortex of the kidney and spills over into the urine;
(3) that dopamine is formed in the renal tubular cells, particularly those of the proximal tubule, by the action of L-amino acid decarboxylase (L-dopa decarboxylase) and the catecholamine is then secreted into the tubular lumen.

(1) The Deconjugation Hypothesis

Unger *et al.* (1980) have proposed that dopamine, derived largely from the adrenal gland, is rapidly conjugated both to the 3-orthosulphate and to the glucuronide. These compounds circulate to the kidney, where deconjugase enzymes, e.g. β-D-glucuronidase and arylsulphatase, act on the conjugates to release free dopamine, first into the renal tissue and then, after secretion, into the urine. This hypothesis, once compelling, has now become very unlikely for a number of reasons.

(a) Carbidopa, when given orally to man (Ball and Lee, 1977), reduced the urine output of dopamine at least temporarily. As carbidopa can inhibit dopa decarboxylase activity in the kidney, this renal enzyme must be necessary for the intrarenal production of dopamine (suggesting L-dopa as the renal source).
(b) Studies in the rat by Ball (1978) showed that free dopamine and the conjugates increased in parallel in animals subjected to salt loading. If the deconjugation hypothesis was correct, then, as free catecholamine in the urine rose, there should have been a corresponding fall in the conjugates.

This evidence suggests that the sulphate and glucuronide act simply as an overspill for dopamine formed both in the kidney and elsewhere in the body.

(c) Akpaffiong (1981) has shown that when the adrenal glands are removed from rats, it is still possible to elicit a marked increase in urine dopamine by oral salt loading. This evidence strongly suggests that the adrenal gland, though a major source for circulating dopamine, does not contribute in any important way to the renal production of dopamine.

(d) Studies on the renal prodrugs γ-glutamyl-L-dopa and γ-glutamyl dopamine suggest that the former is a more effective source of urine dopamine and indeed in turn a more effective renal dopaminergic agonist (see below). This evidence once again suggests that L-dopa rather than dopamine (or its conjugates) is the most important source of renal (and urine) dopamine.

(2) The Renal Dopaminergic Nerves

This aspect of work on dopamine in the kidney stems from the work of Bell and Lang (1973) who stimulated the midbrain and hypothalamus in anaesthetised guanethidine-treated dogs and produced renal vasodilatation. This effect could be blocked by haloperidol, a known dopamine antagonist. The work suggested that there was a dopaminergic pathway from the midbrain to the renal cortical blood vessels. Subsequently the same group were able to demonstrate dopamine-containing neuronal elements in the dog kidney (Bell *et al.*, 1978).

Using histofluorescence techniques for noradrenaline and dopamine, Dinerstein *et al.* (1979) were able to demonstrate fluorescent material on the arcuate and interlobular arteries and on the glomerular vascular pole in the dog kidney. As the location moved towards the glomerular tuft, so the fluorescence changed in character, from that typical of noradrenaline to that characteristic of dopamine. The distinction between noradrenaline and dopamine was made on the basis of the rapidity with which hydrochloric acid faded the fluorescence, dopamine being relatively more resistant than noradrenaline. They also denervated a kidney in the dog, by the technique of iliac-artery transplantation. Two weeks following the operation all fluorescent material had disappeared from the kidney, whether derived from noradrenaline or dopamine.

The importance of this direct dopaminergic innervation of the vascular pole of the renal glomerulus, including presumably the juxtaglomerular apparatus, cannot be overemphasised. A possible role for dopamine in the control of renin release will be described in a later section. It is sufficient to mention here that stimulation of the renal dopaminergic nerves may have a bidirectional effect on renin release, being a balance between interlobular artery and afferent arteriolar vasodilatation (renin stimulated) and nerve endings terminating directly on the juxtaglomerular cells (renin release inhibited).

Whether dopamine released from the cortical dopaminergic endings can contribute in a material way to the excess dopamine present in the urine is doubtful. At most sites in the body, when neurotransmitter is released into the synaptic cleft, rapid and effective mechanisms exist for re-uptake of the catecholamine. Indeed, to demonstrate the catecholamine in overflow experiments, these re-uptake mechanisms must be blocked by compounds such as cocaine and imipramine (Axelrod, 1973). However, further studies are required on the urine output of dopamine from the kidneys of animals, acutely and chronically denervated, to make further progress in this matter.

(3) Tubular Production of Dopamine from L-Dopa

The normal biosynthetic pathway for dopamine is shown in Figure 7.2. Two important enzymes are usually concerned with synthesis, tyrosine hydroxylase (EC 1.14.3.a; Nagatsu, 1973) and aromatic L-amino acid decarboxylase (dopa decarboxylase; EC 4.1.1.26; Nagatsu, 1973). There is no evidence that tyrosine hydroxylase, the rate-limiting enzyme for catecholamine synthesis in neuronal tissue, is present in any significant concentration in the kidney. Dopa decarboxylase is in high concentration in the kidney and appears to be located both in the proximal and distal convoluted tubules (Goldstein *et al.*, 1972). Ball and Lee (1977) therefore proposed the idea that L-dopa, filtered at the glomerulus and then taken up into the proximal tubular cell, was the major source of renal and urinary dopamine.

Important evidence in support of this hypothesis has been gathered by Chan (1976). He studied the proximal tubular transport of L-dopa (and its derivatives) by microperfusion and capillary perfusion techniques. L-dopa, L-tyrosine and L-phenylalanine were rapidly reabsorbed, but L-α-methyldopa and dopamine were not. The transport of L-dopa was not inhibited by either a dopa decarboxylase inhibitor (MK-486) or by a monoamine oxidase inhibitor (peniprazine), suggesting that intratubular metabolism of the absorbed L-dopa did not play a major part in this process. Cyanide did block absorption of the amino acid. Chan concluded that the reabsorption of L-dopa in the proximal convoluted tubule of the rat was an active process with great structural specificity.

Others have demonstrated that the reabsorption of amino acids from the proximal tubule of mammalian kidney is a carrier-mediated process stimulated by the sodium ion (Fox *et al.*, 1964; Ullrich *et al.*, 1974). This could be one of the mechanisms whereby an increase in the filtered load of sodium might stimulate the uptake of L-dopa into the proximal tubule and its onward conversion to dopamine (see below).

Further striking evidence comes from the work of Baines and Chan (1980). These investigators injected ³H-L-dopa into the proximal tubule, or peritubular space, in both innervated and denervated rat kidneys. L-Dopa was converted rapidly into dopamine in the urine and there was no definite difference between innervated and denervated kidneys. It was estimated that at

Figure 7.2: The Biosynthetic Pathway for the Catecholamines

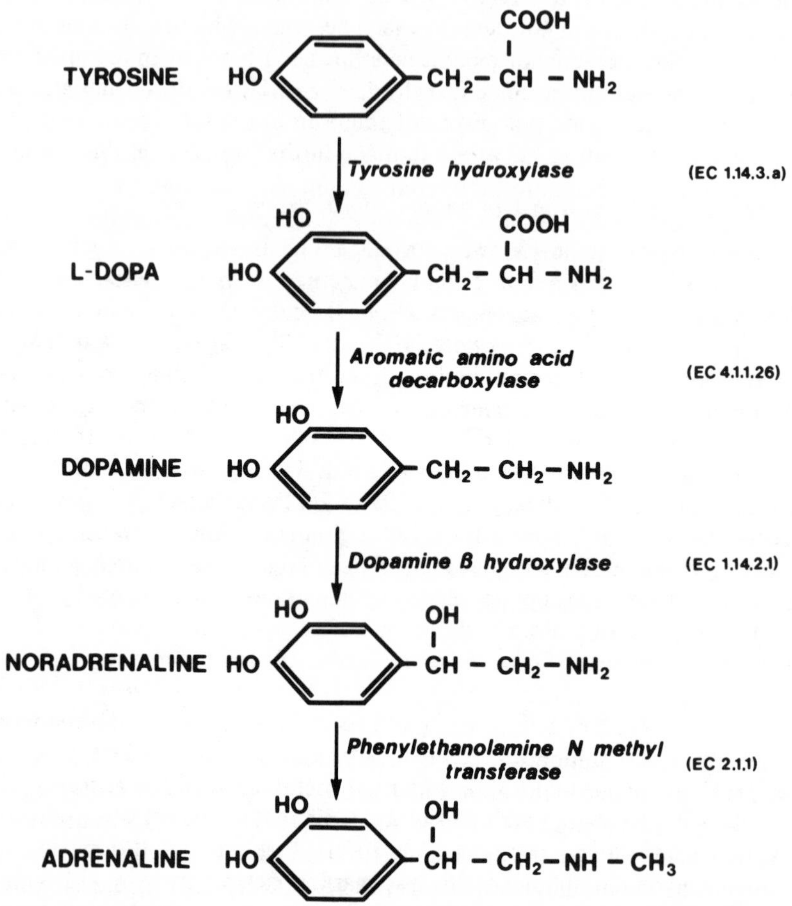

least 30 per cent of urine-free dopamine was derived from circulating L-dopa. This is a minimum estimate for conversion and does not make allowance for the tubular conversion of dipeptides of L-dopa, for example γ-glutamyl-L-dopa, which may also act as a source of renal and urinary dopamine (see next section). When labelled L-tyrosine was injected into the tubule, there was little conversion to urinary dopamine, suggesting once again that there is little tyrosine hydroxylase activity in the kidney, even when innervated.

Support for the hypothesis that circulating L-dopa is the major source of renal (and urinary) dopamine also comes from the work of Brown and Allison (1981) who gave 250 mg L-dopa orally to normal volunteers. Plasma L-dopa and urine dopamine increased in parallel, but plasma dopamine concentration rose little. The increase in plasma L-dopa, but not in plasma dopamine, could have accounted for the increase in urine dopamine and gave rise to a calculated renal clearance for L-dopa of 114 ± 20 ml min^{-1}. The kidney appeared to have sufficient decarboxylase activity to deal with the increased L-dopa reaching it in the blood supply, establishing that conversion to dopamine in the tubules was rate limited not by the enzyme but by the availability of the substrate (L-dopa). This would add weight to the suggestion made above that it is the rate of uptake of the precursor into the proximal tubular cell that determines the overall production rate for renal dopamine. The rate of this uptake may well depend on the filtered sodium chloride load.

It could be argued that there are two alternative possibilities for the production of extra dopamine in the tubules on salt loading:

(1) increased activity of L-dopa decarboxylase;
(2) decreased activity of tubular amine oxidase. However, Ball (1978), in experiments on salt-loaded rats, found no support for a change in either of these two enzymic mechanisms.

This evidence, taken together with that from the gludopa studies (given in the next section), is overwhelmingly in favour of the view that the major source of renal and urine dopamine is circulating L-dopa. The final piece of evidence required to complete the jigsaw is to prove that this rate of uptake of L-dopa by the kidney increases when the animal (or man) is given extra salt.

(4) Evidence Derived from Studies with γ-L-Glutamyl-L-Dopa (Gludopa)

Incontrovertible evidence for L-dopa as an intrarenal source for the synthesis of dopamine comes from studies with the dipeptide γ-L-glutamyl-L-dopa. The kidney is highly active in the uptake and metabolism of γ-glutamyl derivatives of amino acids and peptides (Orlowski and Wilk, 1976, 1978). This activity is probably dependent on the high concentration of the enzyme γ-glutamyl transpeptidase (γ-glutamyl transferase, γGT; EC 2.3.2.2) in the proximal tubule and possibly in the loop of Henle also (Albert *et al.*, 1961; Glenner *et al.*, 1962). The enzyme catalyses the transfer of a γ-glutamyl group, either to another amino acid, or to water (reactions 1 and 2):

$$\gamma\text{-glutamyl amino acid}_\text{I} + \text{amino acid}_\text{II} \rightarrow \gamma\text{-glutamyl amino acid}_\text{II} + \text{amino acid}_\text{I} \tag{1}$$

or

$$\gamma\text{-glutamyl amino acid}_\text{I} + H_2O \rightarrow \text{glutamate} + \text{amino acid}_\text{I} \tag{2}$$

Wilk and his colleagues (1978) therefore synthesised γ-L-glutamyl-L-dopa as a potentially renally specific dopaminergic prodrug. They hoped that this dipeptide would be selectively accumulated in the kidney and there converted sequentially by γGT and L-dopa decarboxylase to dopamine (see Figure 7.3). From the work of Lovenberg *et al.* (1962) it was known already that L-amino acid decarboxylase (dopa decarboxylase) was abundant in the kidney.

Figure 7.3: The Renal Conversion of γ-L-Glutamyl-L-dopa to Dopamine

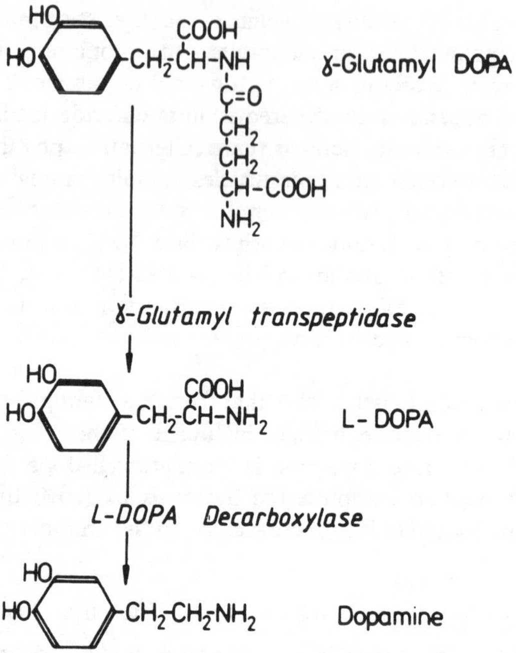

Wilk *et al.* (1978) administered gludopa to rats and noted that there was a marked accumulation of dopamine in the kidney, in contrast to L-dopa itself where tissue distribution was much more uniform. High levels of dopamine in the kidney were more persistently maintained by gludopa than by L-dopa. Moreover, gludopa significantly elevated renal plasma flow (by 60 per cent) at a dose of 10 nmol/g per 30 min, at which dose level L-dopa had no effect on blood flow. The ratio between the renal and pressor thresholds for gludopa was greater than that for L-dopa, emphasising once again the relative renal specificity of the dipeptide. Stimulated by Wilk's results with this compound on renal blood flow, Casson *et al.* attempted to use gludopa as a protective agent in the rat against acute renal failure produced by subcutaneous injection of glycerol. At a total dose of 107.2 mg kg^{-1}, gludopa gave the rats substantial protection against the biochemical and histological sequelae of glycerol damage (Casson *et al.*, 1982, 1983a).

More recently we have infused the dipeptide into man. When normal volunteers were given gludopa intravenously at a rate of 12.5 μg kg^{-1} min^{-1}

for 2 h, there was a significant natriuresis but no change in pulse rate or blood pressure. Surprisingly, plasma renin activity fell both during and after the natriuresis, presumably due to a direct action of intrarenally generated dopamine on the renal juxtaglomerular cells (Worth *et al.*, 1984).

In summary the evidence based on the studies with γ-glutamyl-L-dopa would support the view:

(1) that L-dopa is an important source of renal dopamine, at least in the rat and man;
(2) that when dopamine is generated within the kidney it acts there under normal circumstances to depress renin release from the juxtaglomerular cells. Studies on renin release in which dopamine is given intravenously (or intrarenal arterially) should therefore be interpreted with caution (see section below) as dopamine may be reaching the juxtaglomerular cells by a non-physiological route through the circulation.

The presumed sequence of events is as follows. Gludopa is actively transported into the proximal tubular cells; converted intracellularly to dopamine, which acts either directly (or after secretion) on the tubular membrane transport systems with a resulting increased sodium loss in the urine. How tubular dopamine gains access to the juxtaglomerular cells is unknown, but it might be transported by the macula densa to the renin control systems in the juxtaglomerular cells.

Control of Renal Dopamine Production

Since it has become apparent that dopamine is produced in the kidney, several groups of investigators have examined the factors that could influence output of dopamine in the urine. As dopamine infusion can cause a natriuresis in several species, it was logical to examine the obverse situation. Could sodium administration affect renal production and urine output of dopamine? Alexander *et al.* (1974) studied normal volunteers in which dietary sodium intake had been increased from 9 mmol per 24 h to more than 200 mmol per 24 h. Urine dopamine output increased from a mean of 130 μg to a mean of 195 μg per 24 h.

When sodium chloride was infused intravenously, urine dopamine output increased by about 30 per cent over the basal output of the catecholamine. At the time these experiments were carried out, it was not appreciated that the source of the additional dopamine might be renal, and the authors interpreted the results as being a result of a change in the discharge rate from the renal nerves. The same type of interpretation was also placed on the fall in urine dopamine on standing (Cuche *et al.*, 1972). However, as has been pointed out in an earlier part of this chapter, it would seem unlikely that renal dopaminergic nerves make any major contribution to renal and urine dopamine.

Our group at Leeds therefore decided to examine, in the rat, the response of urinary dopamine to changes in the diet (Ball *et al.*, 1978). Groups of rats were maintained on a low sodium diet under metabolic balance conditions. Equimolar dietary supplements of sodium chloride, sodium bicarbonate, potassium chloride and ammonium chloride were given, to study the specificity of the previously observed increase in dopamine excretion following dietary sodium chloride supplementation. Mean dopamine excretion increased significantly in rats given the chlorides of sodium, potassium and ammonium, but fell in rats given sodium bicarbonate. The fall in urine dopamine in rats given bicarbonate may be spurious as the catecholamine might have been destroyed in the urine, since dopamine is unstable in alkaline media.

Oates (1979) went on to study the renal tissue dopamine concentrations in rats given equimolar quantities of the same dietary electrolytes as above. The chlorides of sodium, potassium and ammonium increased renal tissue dopamine content but had no effect on liver and brain dopamine. There was no change in renal tissue dopamine after sodium bicarbonate, suggesting that in the urine experiments dopamine had indeed been destroyed in the alkaline urine, at least to some extent.

These results were of interest for two principal reasons; first, the chloride ion seemed to be important in the generation of the dopamine response; and secondly the effects of the chloride and bicarbonate ions resembled the effects of these ions on renin release from the juxtaglomerular cells, i.e. chloride seems to be a more efficient suppressor for renin release than bicarbonate (Kotchen *et al.*, 1976). There may be a direct inhibitory link between dopamine and renin at the intrarenal level, and this may be one explanation of the chloride/bicarbonate effect. Another possibility is that the kidney has a common sensing mechanism for electrolyte variation, controlling both dopamine and renin release, conceivably through the macula densa mechanism of the distal convoluted tubule.

Oates *et al.* (1979) then went on to study urinary and plasma dopamine in six normal subjects who had their dietary sodium increased from 20 to 220 mmol per 24 h. Plasma dopamine changed little but urine dopamine increased from a mean of 1.2 μmol per 24 h to a mean of 1.8 μmol per 24 h on the second day of salt load. The peak of urine dopamine led the highest urine sodium output by one day, suggesting that in this situation dopamine mobilisation leads sodium excretion and does not follow it (Figure 7.4). In contrast, when fludrocortisone is given to normal volunteers (0.2 mg twice daily for 5 days) urine dopamine excretion falls and then gradually returns to the baseline as the subjects 'escape' from the salt-retaining effect of the mineralocorticoid (Oates *et al.*, 1980).

By comparison with the effect of intravenous sodium chloride, Faucheux *et*

Figure 7.4: The Response of Urine and Plasma Dopamine to Added Dietary Sodium Chloride in Normal Volunteers

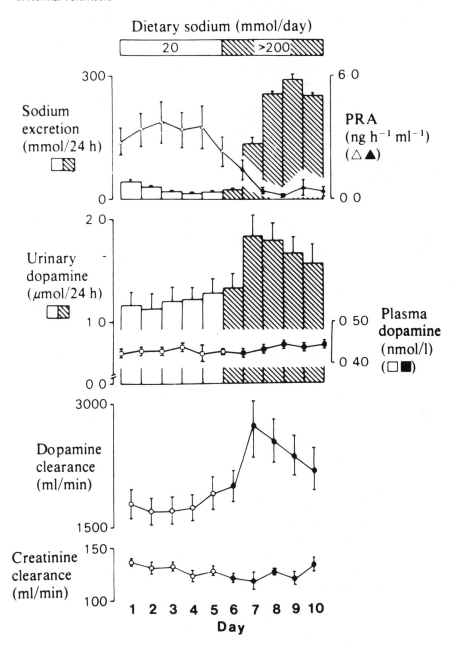

al. (1977) have shown that if albumin is given intravenously there is no change in urine dopamine output. This would suggest that the kidney can distinguish between crystalloid and colloid solutions, at least in regard to the renal production of dopamine. Kuchel *et al.* (1978a) have also demonstrated that the loop diuretic frusemide, when given intravenously, can increase the urinary output of dopamine significantly. Frusemide inhibits chloride transport in the ascending limb of the loop of Henle and this could result in an increase in chloride concentration at a distal sensing structure (perhaps the macula densa). As was pointed out earlier, chloride concentration in the tubule may be an important determinant of renal dopamine production. Whether other diuretics, such as the benzothiadiazines, or those of the distal tubular type, can affect urine dopamine output is at present unknown.

Frusemide can also increase renal blood flow (Birtch *et al.*, 1967) and it is tempting to speculate whether any part of this action could be due to intrarenal production of dopamine and indeed whether dopamine could then stimulate renal prostaglandin production. Experiments could be carried out in which animals (and man) are pretreated with sulpiride (or an alternative dopamine receptor antagonist) to establish whether the renal vascular response to frusemide can be attenuated or prevented.

Renal Dopamine and the Renin/Angiotensin System

Dopamine in intact animals or in the isolated perfused kidney preparation can increase renin release from the juxtaglomerular cells (Chokshi *et al.*, 1972). Generally, however, the dose levels and infusion rates employed for the catecholamine were far in excess of the physiological, and would be expected to activate both α_1 and β_1 adrenoceptors within the renal vasculature and on the surface of the juxtaglomerular cells, both being capable of stimulating renin release, either directly or indirectly (Wilcox *et al.*, 1974; Henry *et al.*, 1977).

Ball *et al.* (1981) investigated renin release in the conscious beagle dog with exteriorised carotid loop. The physiological range for plasma dopamine in the dog is of the order of 0.2–5.0 nmol litre^{-1}. When these workers infused 1.6 nmol min^{-1}kg^{-1} of dopamine, plasma levels rose to 13 nmol litre^{-1}, that is, at least twice the physiological level, but there was no effect on plasma renin concentration. A further ten-fold increase in infusion rate to 16 nmol min^{-1}kg^{-1} produced only a very small increase in plasma renin levels. These results suggest that it is unlikely that circulating dopamine can be an important controlling factor in renin release under normal conditions.

At an infusion rate of 160 nmol min^{-1}kg^{-1} there was an approximate doubling, both in plasma renin concentration and in plasma angiotensin II. The mechanism for this increase is debated. Imbs and Schwartz (1979) claim that haloperidol, a dopamine antagonist, blocks the effect, but others maintain that propranolol prevents the increase (Quesada *et al.*, 1979). The latter proposition is much more convincing, with the known β-adrenergic innervation of the juxtaglomerular cells and the known β-effect of dopamine at high concentrations.

In the light of this controversy, our recent work on two renal dopaminergic agonists is of interest. SKF 82526, an oral dopaminergic agent, is a renal vasodilator in animals and man (see below), and our results (Harvey *et al.*, 1984b) suggest that the renal vasodilatation produced by this compound, when given orally, produces an increase in plasma renin activity, reminiscent of that produced by other powerful renal vasodilators such as hydralazine and minoxidil (Freis *et al.*, 1953; Dormois *et al.*, 1975). In contrast gludopa (see above) inhibits the increase in plasma renin activity normally associated with natriuresis.

The answer may lie in the site of production of dopamine within the kidney and the route by which the catecholamine reaches the juxtaglomerular cells. It is likely that dopamine formed within the renal tubules will reach the receptors on the surface of the juxtaglomerular cells first (perhaps via the tubular lumen and the macula densa) and only later gain access to vascular receptors in the afferent and efferent arterioles of the glomeruli. As a result *physiological* release of dopamine within the kidney may inhibit renin release from the juxtaglomerular cells, whereas *pharmacological* activation of renal dopaminergic vasodilator systems may lead to renin release, as for example when oral SKF 82526 gains access to the renal blood vessels in the first instance.

Renal Dopamine in the Menstrual Cycle and Normal Pregnancy

During normal pregnancy in women there is a substantial increase in both renal blood flow and glomerular filtration rate (Sims and Krantz, 1958). The cause of these changes in the renal circulation remains obscure.

As an essential preliminary to studies on normal pregnancy, Perkins and co-workers studied 12 women over the course of a normal menstrual cycle and found no longitudinal change in urine dopamine output from menses, to midcycle, to premenstruation (Figure 7.5; Perkins *et al.*, 1981). Urine dopamine outputs tended to be 20–30 per cent lower than those of men of the same age, but when corrected for height and weight showed no significant difference. Surprisingly, when women were studied who were taking a combined oral contraceptive, there was a significant drop in urine dopamine output at midcycle, which recovered when the oral contraceptive agent was discontinued after the 21st day (Figure 7.6). The basis on which the oestrogen/progesterone combination suppresses renal dopamine production is unknown, but it is possible that this fall in renal dopamine production is one of the factors in the sodium and water retention seen commonly for the first few months when women take the combined oral contraceptive preparation.

Figure 7.5: Urine Free Dopamine Levels in Women Taking the Combined Oral Contraceptive Pill

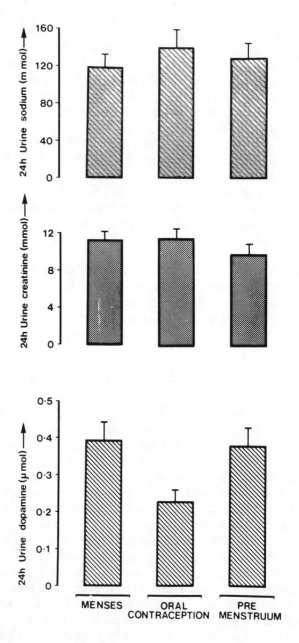

Figure 7.6: Urine Free Dopamine in Normal Pregnancy and Six Weeks *post partum*

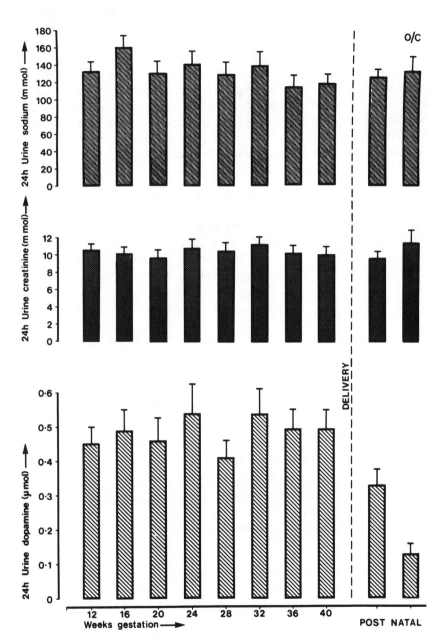

Reproduced by permission of *Clinical Science*

In a study of changes in urine dopamine in normal pregancy, 19 women attended the antenatal clinic monthly and gave 24 h urine samples for dopamine assay. Urine was again collected six weeks after parturition (Figure 7.6). There was an increase of approximately 30 per cent in urine dopamine in pregnancy and this was detectable from the 16th week onwards (Perkins *et al.*, 1981). After delivery some women received norethisterone as a contraceptive agent and in these individuals urine dopamine fell to lower levels than in women not receiving this treatment. It must be recognised that the studies during the menstrual cycle and normal pregnancy were not carried out under strict dietary control for sodium intake. However, no large variation was observed in the 24 h urine output for sodium, suggesting that wide divergence in sodium intakes did not take place.

Urine Dopamine in Experimental and Clinical Hypertensive States

At the moment the evidence in this area is disorganised and fragmentary. Nevertheless it must be considered in view of the recent development of compounds acting on the renal dopaminergic receptors (see next section) which may well be effective therapeutically in hypertensive and oedematous states in man.

(A) Studies in the Animal

Cope (1982) studied urinary dopamine following salt loading in two inbred strains of hypertensive rat, the New Zealand and the Okamoto (Japanese), both of which showed a prompt increase in urine dopamine on salt loading. It would be extremely interesting to repeat Cope's work on other strains of rat such as the Dahl 'S' and the Milan, where the fault is more clearly located to the kidney; and also in the Goldblatt Type I and II models for renal hypertension (see Chapter 8).

(B) Human Hypertensive Syndromes

When it became apparent that renal dopamine production could be mobilised by oral salt loading, this renal capacity was investigated in individuals with various states of clinical hypertension. These studies have concerned themselves with a number of different groups:

  (a) essential hypertension;
  (b) chronic renal failure with hypertension;
  (c) primary aldosteronism;
  (d) hypertensive disease of pregnancy.

(a) Essential Hypertension. There is a long-standing and wide-ranging debate on the relationship, if any, between dietary salt and essential hypertension (see Chapter 8). The fault in salt-sensitive individuals may well

lie in the kidney. We examined the dopamine response to salt loading in a small group of patients with essential hypertension when compared with normal volunteers under identical in-patient conditions.

By comparison with the normal volunteers, the patients with essential hypertension showed not a blunted dopamine response, as we had anticipated, but a paradoxical fall in urine dopamine output which was highly significant (Harvey *et al.*, 1984a). Moreover they tended to develop a more positive sodium balance and gain more weight than did the normal volunteers. Blood pressure rose little over the short period of salt loading (5 days).

This bizarre response may be a marker to the renal abnormality in essential hypertension, or it may be the fault itself. Certainly the abnormality cannot be attributed to chronic renal damage for two reasons:

(1) the mean plasma creatinine was within the normal range in the patients;
(2) in patients with chronic renal damage due to glomerulonephritis, the dopamine response to sodium loading is blunted, not inverted (see section (b) below).

(b) Chronic Renal Failure with Hypertension. Casson *et al.* (1983b) studied eight patients with chronic glomerulonephritis and five age-matched normal volunteers, under conditions of metabolic balance, when they were given additional oral sodium chloride. Urine dopamine excretion during a low-salt diet was much lower in the patients than in the controls and did not rise significantly in the patients on salt loading. Although plasma renin activity in the patients was suppressed on sodium loading, this change was not as prolonged (or as rapid) as that in the control subjects, in keeping with the proposal by other workers that plasma renin activity is inappropriately high in chronic renal disease (Warren and Ferris, 1970).

Casson (1984) also found in another series of patients with chronic renal failure that there was a critical relationship between urinary dopamine excretion and plasma creatinine. Below a plasma creatinine of 180 μmol litre^{-1} (approximately 2 mg 100 ml^{-1}) urine dopamine appears to be independent of GFR, whereas above 180 μmol litre^{-1} urine dopamine correlates positively with GFR. Similar observations had been made previously by Itskovitz and Gilberg (1981) who found that with increasing degrees of renal failure, urine free dopamine diminished, almost disappearing when plasma creatinine concentration was greater than 530 μmol litre^{-1} (6 mg 100 ml^{-1}).

It will be most interesting to establish whether, if endogenous dopamine production decreases to very low levels in the chronically damaged kidney, the dopamine receptors can be preserved to a degree, and indeed if they 'up' regulate. Can renal dopaminergic drugs like γ-glutamyl-L-dopa and SKF 82526 (see below) restore sodium handling to normal in these circumstances of chronic renal failure?

(c) Primary Aldosteronism. The acute studies on fludrocortisone administration described in an earlier section suggest that urine dopamine is depressed by short courses of mineralocorticoid. However, the situation is different when there is chronic overproduction of aldosterone and chronic expansion of the ECF as in Conn's syndrome (benign adenoma of the adrenal gland). Here Kuchel *et al.* (1978b) report that both free and conjugated dopamine levels in the urine are high and that after the surgical removal of the adenoma the excretion of free dopamine in the urine falls towards normal.

(d) Hypertensive Disease of Pregnancy. Studies on urine dopamine in hypertensive pregnancy have shown two patterns (Perkins *et al.*, 1982) in both cross-sectional and longitudinal studies. In those with significant proteinuria (> 0.5 g litre^{-1} of urine) urine dopamine increased to levels greater than in normotensive pregnancy, suggesting that in these women, the kidney was attempting to compensate for sodium retention and an expanded extracellular fluid volume. In contrast in the non-proteinuric hypertension of pregnancy, there seems to be a relative failure to generate dopamine. The post-delivery patterns of sodium excretion in the urine also confirm the existence of two types of hypertension in pregnancy, previously suggested by Chesley (1978). Pre-eclamptic toxaemia appears to be a disease *sui generis* with an immunological (or immunogenetic) basis, whereas gestational hypertension appears to be a form of essential hypertension brought on by the hormonal changes of pregnancy. In this respect the effects of the combined contraceptive pill or the progestogen-only contraceptive (norethisterone) on urine dopamine, described in an earlier section, will be recalled as perhaps presenting a paradigm for gestational hypertension.

Development of Compounds Acting Specifically on Renal Dopamine Receptors

The abnormalities of dopamine mobilisation that have been identified in essential hypertension and in chronic renal failure raise the possibility of correcting these abnormalities by the administration of dopaminergic drugs which act on the kidney and perhaps also on the mesenteric and peripheral arterioles. Three compounds are under consideration at the present time, and others will certainly emerge in due course:

(1) ibopamine;
(2) SKF 82526 (fenoldopam);
(3) γ-glutamyl-L-dopa.

(1) Ibopamine (Diisobutyryl-N-methyl-dopamine; Figure 7.7)

This esterified derivative of epinine was developed in Italy by the Simes

Figure 7.7: The Molecular Structure of Ibopamine (Diisobutyryl-N-methyl-dopamine)

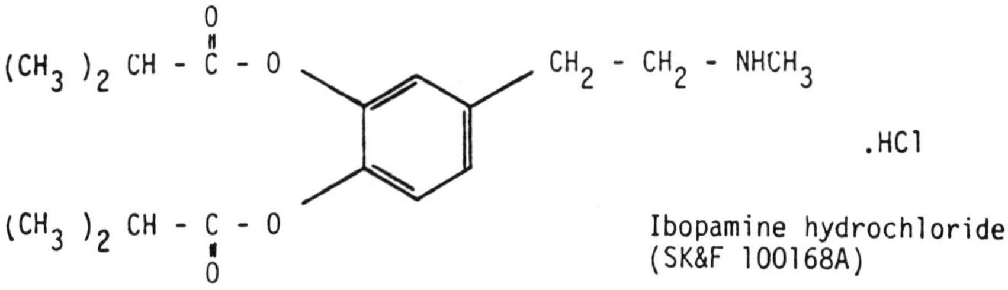

$$(CH_3)_2\ CH - \overset{\overset{O}{\|}}{C} - O \qquad\qquad CH_2 - CH_2 - NHCH_3$$

$$.HCl$$

$$(CH_3)_2\ CH - \underset{\underset{O}{\|}}{C} - O \qquad\qquad \text{Ibopamine hydrochloride}$$
$$(SK\&F\ 100168A)$$

company of Milan. In one study the drug was given in a dose of 50 mg twice a day for seven days to 12 patients; six with normal renal function and six with varying degrees of chronic renal impairment (Stefoni *et al.*, 1981). In both groups the compound gave a prompt increase in urinary excretion of water, sodium and potassium, and creatinine clearance also increased. The response of the patients with chronic renal failure to ibopamine was less marked than that in the volunteers with normal renal function. At this dose of ibopamine, heart rate and arterial blood pressure were unaffected. The authors concluded that ibopamine was of potential clinical value in chronic renal failure.

With such potentially important results our group decided to repeat the observations, confining ourselves in the first instance to placebo-controlled double-blind studies in normal volunteers, employing two single doses of ibopamine, 150 mg and 600 mg (Harvey *et al.*, 1984b). We have found no evidence of an effect on renal function of either 150 or 600 mg by mouth. Even with the 600 mg dose of ibopamine, the compound seemed to be remarkably devoid of pharmacological action, producing only minor changes in heart rate. These results with ibopamine are perhaps not surprising; it is likely that there will be substantial first-pass metabolism of ibopamine (in the liver and gut), to epinine, and then conjugation of epinine to its inactive sulphate and glucuronide. As epinine is much less active than dopamine on the renal circulation and also possesses considerable α-agonist effect, it is unlikely to form a sound basis for an effective renal dopaminergic drug.

(2) SKF 82526 (Fenoldopam)

This compound, developed recently as a specific dopamine agonist, is shown in Figure 7.8; it is a substituted benzazepine, and in animal studies it has been shown to be a selective dopamine DA_1 agonist which is devoid of central activity *in vivo* (Hahn *et al.*, 1982). Racemic fenoldopam is a powerful renal vasodilator in the dog (Stote *et al.*, 1983) and this effect could be blocked by bulbocapnine, a peripheral dopamine antagonist. The same authors also showed that the compound was six times more effective than dopamine on renal vascular resistance.

Figure 7.8: The Molecular Structure of Fenoldopam (SKF 82526)

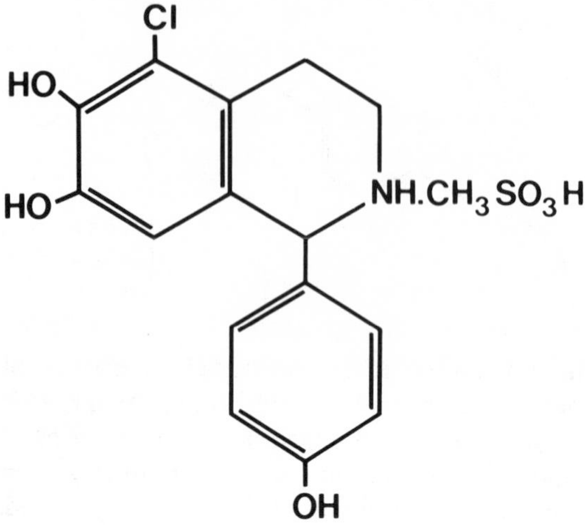

Fenoldopam

Although both the R and the S enantiomers of fenoldopam are powerful renal vasodilators, only the R enantiomer is hypotensive. In normal subjects, fenoldopam administered orally elicits increases in renal plasma flow (clearance of PAH) and sodium clearance at doses of 25, 50 and 100 mg. The renal vasodilatation results in a fall in filtration fraction but the acompanying natriuresis may be the result of direct tubular action of the dopamine agonist. Metoclopramide antagonised the renal effects of fenoldopam, and as this compound has DA_1 and DA_2 blocking properties, this suggested that action at the dopamine receptors was the basis of fenoldopam's activity.

Two recent studies with this compound have shown a hypotensive action in normal volunteers. Cregeen *et al.* (1984) administered 100 mg of fenoldopam four times daily for 14 days to normal subjects. Diastolic blood pressure fell by a mean of 4.4 mmHg by the 14th day. Heart rate and plasma catecholamines rose on the first day, probably reflecting reflex activation of noradrenaline release via the baroreceptors. By the 14th day these changes in heart rate had disappeared. Harvey *et al.* (1985) studied the effects of oral fenoldopam in a single dose of 100 mg on blood pressure, renal blood flow, glomerular filtration rate, plasma renin activity and urine sodium output in normal volunteers. They confirmed the hypotensive effect of the compound and also found a marked increase in renal blood flow, a modest increase in glomerular filtration rate and a small increase in urine sodium output. Plasma renin activity increased by two- to three-fold, probably reflecting a relative fall in arterial pressure in the afferent arterioles of the glomeruli, the result both of the fall in diastolic blood pressure and the intrarenal vasodilatation. These results are encouraging on the one hand but disappointing in other respects. The general theory of peripheral dopamine receptors in the arterioles of the peripheral circulation and in the renal vascular bed is supported by the hypotensive effect of fenoldopam. The disappointing feature of its spectrum of activity is the marked stimulation of renin release from the kidney. As has been pointed out in a previous section, γ-glutamyl-L-dopa, which probably mimics most closely the release of dopamine *physiologically* within the kidney, depresses plasma renin activity. The effect of fenoldopam is not physiological in that it is acting via the bloodstream and the vascular receptors, in contrast to dopamine mobilised within the tubules (by NaCl) which will act initially via tubular receptors. I would expect as a consequence that the hypotensive effect of fenoldopam would be limited eventually by increased production of angiotensin II, resulting in sodium retention and vasoconstriction. We also have preliminary results that suggest that fenoldopam may inhibit aldosterone production from the zona glomerulosa of the adrenal cortex, and this may extend the hypotensive effect of this substance.

Other compounds are also under investigation at the present time, for example FPL 60278, dopexamine, an agonist at peripheral dopamine DA_1-, DA_2- and β_2-adrenoceptors (Brown *et al.*, 1984). This compound can significantly reduce renal vascular resistance in the dog and the response is blocked by bulbocapnine (a known dopamine antagonist). No doubt the number of peripheral dopamine agonists and renal dopaminergic prodrugs will multiply rapidly in the next year or two. They may need to be combined with β-adrenoceptor antagonists (to combat reflex tachycardia) and/or angiotensin-converting enzyme inhibitors to produce an optimum hypotensive response in the clinical situation.

(3) γ-Glutamyl-L-Dopa

This compound has been discussed extensively in a previous section but it is mentioned again here to emphasise that it must represent at the present time the closest approach to physiological activation of the dopamine receptors from within the kidney; in particular in its ability to produce a natriuresis with concomitant inhibition of renin release. Preliminary studies are now taking place in our laboratory with intravenous infusion of this peptide in patients with stable chronic renal failure and essential hypertension. The therapeutic potential of gludopa may be limited by its lack of bioavailability as an oral drug, as a consequence of hydrolysis of the peptide in the gut wall (or liver) by γ-glutamyl transferase. One final point may be made concerning the hypotensive effect of dopamine agonists in essential hypertension. If there is a specific fault in dopamine mobilisation within the kidney in essential hypertension (see above), then the renal tubular and vascular receptors for the catecholamine may be 'up' regulated and the hypotensive effect of dopaminergic compounds may be potentiated in patients.

Unanswered Questions

There is little doubt that dopamine, produced intrarenally, is a natriuretic factor. However, in some respects, our understanding of the detailed renal physiological mechanisms that underpin our knowledge of this catecholamine need considerable strengthening:

(1) In which parts of the nephron is dopamine formed? Proximal tubule, distal tubule, other parts of the nephron?
(2) Where are the presumed tubular receptors for dopamine? Proximal tubule, distal tubule, other parts of the nephron? The recent work of Higashi and Bello-Reuss (1981) demonstrated a natriuretic effect of dopamine at 10^{-6} M concentration on the straight segments of rabbit proximal tubules.
(3) Does dopamine generated at the tubular level gain access to the juxtaglomerular cells to inhibit renin release? Is the pathway via the macula densa or via the bloodstream in a hitherto undescribed manner?
(4) How does dopamine produced intrarenally relate to kallikrein, the prostaglandins, and natriuretic peptides?
(5) In the control of dopamine mobilisation within the kidney, what are the effects of chloride, calcium, magnesium and acid-base status?
(6) Does dopamine have any part to play in the natriuresis of fasting and the sodium retention of refeeding? Preliminary evidence from our studies in may suggest that it may do so.

As far as the clinical studies are concerned, the major task that lies ahead is to establish the prevalence of faults in mobilisation of renal dopamine in patients with essential hypertension and their first-degree relatives. There is no doubt that effective peripheral dopaminergic agonists will be developed for the treatment of clinical situations in man. However, at the time of writing it would appear that for such compounds to imitate the physiological role of intrarenally generated dopamine will prove impossible, unless an oral equivalent to γ-L-glutamyl-L-dopa can be developed that will deliver a prodrug of L-dopa to the kidney.

It would appear that the intrarenal relationship between dopamine (a salt-eliminating substance) and renin (a salt-retaining hormone) must be crucial with regard to the overall regulation of sodium chloride in the body. A combined attack upon both homeostatic systems, with dopamine agonists and angiotensin I converting enzyme inhibitors, may therefore be effective in the treatment of oedematous and hypertensive states in man.

References

Albert, Z., Orlowski, M. and Szewczuk, A. (1961) 'Histochemical Demonstration of Gamma Glutamyl Transpeptidase', *Nature (Lond.)*, *191*, 767–8

Alexander, R.W., Gill, J.R., Jr, Yamabe, H., Lovenberg, W. and Keiser, H.R. (1974) 'Effect of Dietary Sodium and of Acute Saline Infusion on the Inter-relationship between Dopamine Excretion and Adrenergic Activity in Man', *J. Clin. Invest.*, *54*, 194–200

Akpaffiong, M.J. (1981) 'Studies on Renal Dopamine in the Rat', PhD Thesis, University of Bath

Anton, A.H. and Sayre, D.F. (1964) 'The Distribution of Dopamine and Dopa in Various Animals and a Method for their Determination in Diverse Biological Material', *J. Pharmacol. Exp. Ther.*, *145*, 326–36

Axelrod, J. (1973) 'The Fate of Noradrenaline in the Sympathetic Neurone', *Harvey Lectures*, *67*, 175–97

Baines, A.D. and Chan, W. (1980) 'Production of Urine-free Dopamine from DOPA: a Micropuncture Study', *Life Sci.*, *26*, 253–9

Ball, S.G. (1978) 'The Origin and Function of Urinary Dopamine', PhD thesis, University of Leeds

Ball, S.G. and Lee, M.R. (1977) 'The Effect of Carbidopa Administration on Urinary Sodium Excretion in Man. Is Dopamine an Intrarenal Natriuretic Hormone? *Brit. J. Clin. Pharmacol.*, *4*, 115–19

Ball, S.G., Oates, N.S. and Lee, M.R. (1978) 'Urinary Dopamine in Man and Rat: Effects of Inorganic Salts on Dopamine Excretion', *Clin. Sci. Mol. Med.*, *55*, 167–73

Ball, S.G., Tree, M., Morton, J.J., Inglis, G.C. and Fraser, R. (1981) 'Circulating Dopamine: its Effect on the Plasma Concentrations of Catecholamines, Renin, Angiotensin, Aldosterone and Vasopressin in the Conscious Dog', *Clin. Sci. Mol. Med.*, *61*, 417–22

Ball, S.G., Gunn, I.G. and Douglas, I.H.S. (1982) 'Renal Handling of Dopa; Dopamine; Norepinephrine and Epinephrine in the Dog', *Am. J. Physiol.*, *242*, section F, 56–62

Bell, C. and Lang W.J. (1973) 'Neural Dopaminergic Vasodilator Control in the Kidney', *Nature (Lond.)*, *246*, 27–9

Bell, C., Lang, W.J. and Laska, R. (1978) 'Dopamine-containing Vasomotor Nerves in the Dog Kidney', *J. Neurochem.*, *31*, 77–83

Birtch, A.G., Zakheim, R.M. and Jones, C.G. (1967) 'Redistribution of Renal Blood Flow Produced by Furosemide and Ethacrynic Acid', *Circ. Res.*, *21*, 869–79

Brotzu, G. (1970) 'Inhibition by Chlorpromazine of the Effects of Dopamine on the Dog Kidney', *J. Pharm. Pharmacol.*, *22*, 664–7

Brown, M.J. and Allison, D.J. (1981) 'Renal Conversion of Plasma DOPA to Urine Dopamine', *Brit. J. Clin. Pharmacol.*, *12*, 251–3

Brown, R.A., Farmer, J.B., Hall, J., Humphries, R.G., O'Connor, S.E. and Smith, G.W. (1984) 'FPL 60278. A Novel Agonist at Peripheral Dopamine Receptors and β_2-adrenoreceptors: Cardiovascular Effects in the Dog', Communication 10 to British Pharmacological Society, London Meeting, January 1984

Cadnapaphornchai, P., Taher, S.M. and McDonald, F.D. (1977) 'Mechanism of Dopamine-induced Diuresis in the Dog', *Am. J. Physiol.*, *232*, F524–8

Casson, I.F. (1984) 'Urine Dopamine in Acute and Chronic Renal Failure', MD Thesis, University of Leeds

Casson, I.F., Anderson, C.K., Cope, G.F. and Lee, M.R (1982) 'The Effect of Dietary Sodium Chloride and γ-Glutamyl Dopa on Tubular Necrosis Following Glycerol Administration in the Rat', *Brit. J. Exp. Pathol. Bacteriol.*, *63*, 426–31

Casson, I.F., Clayden, D.A., Cope, G.F. and Lee, M.R. (1983a) 'The Protective Effect of γ-Flutamyl L-Dopa on the Glycerol Treated Rat Model of Acute Renal Failure', *Clin. Sci. Mol. Med.*, *65*, 159–64

Casson, I.F., Lee, M.R., Brownjohn, A.M., Parsons, F.M., Davison, A.M., Will, E.J. and Clayden, A.D. (1983b) 'Failure of Renal Dopamine Response to Salt Loading in Chronic Renal Disease', *Brit. Med. J.*, *286*, 503–6

Chan, Y.L. (1976) 'Cellular Mechanisms of Renal Tubular Transport of L-Dopa and its Derivatives in the Rat: Microperfusion Studies', *J. Pharmacol. Exp. Ther.*, *199*, 17–24

Chapman, B.J., Horn, N.M., Munday, K.A. and Robertson, M.J. (1980) 'The Actions of

Dopamine and of Sulpiride on Regional Blood Flows in the Rat Kidney', *J. Physiol. (Lond.)*, *298*, 437–52

Chesley, L.C. (1978) *Hypertensive Disorders in Pregnancy*, Appleton-Century-Crofts, New York

Chokshi, D.S., Yeh, B.K. and Sambhi, P. (1972) 'Effects of Dopamine and Isoproterenol on Renin Secretion in the Dog', *Proc. Soc. Exp. Biol. Med.*, *140*, 54–7

Cope, G.C. (1982) 'Urine Free Dopamine Excretion and Salt Loading in Two Strains of Spontaneously Hypertensive Rat', MIBiol Dissertation, Manchester Polytechnic

Cregeen, R.J., Marr, G.M., Cassels, E. and Dalton, N. (1984) 'Acute and Chronic Cardiovascular Effects of Fenoldopam, a Novel Oral Dopamine Agonist in Healthy Subjects', *Proceedings of the International Society of Hypertension*, Interlaken Meeting

Crout, J.R. (1963) 'Sampling and Analysis of Catecholamines and Metabolites', *Anesthesiology*, *29*, 661–9

Cuche, J.L. Barbeau, A., Boucher, R. and Genest, J. (1972) 'Relationship between the Adrenergic Nervous System and Renin during Adaptation to Upright Posture. A Possible Role for 3,4-Dihydroxyphenethylamine (Dopamine)', *Clin. Sci. Mol. Med.*, *43*, 481–9

Da Prada, M. and Zurcher, G. (1976) 'Simultaneous Radioenzymatic Determination of Plasma and Tissue Adrenaline, Noradrenaline and Dopamine within the Femtomole Range', *Life Sci.*, *19*, 1161–74

Deis, R.P. and Alonso, N. (1970) 'Diuretic Effect of Dopamine in the Rat', *J. Endocrinol.*, *47*, 129–30

Dinerstein, R.J., Henderson, R.C., Goldberg, L.I. and Hoffman P.C. (1978) 'Evidence for Dopaminergic Innervation in the Kidney', *Fed. Proc.*, *37*, 713

Dinerstein, R.J., Vannice, J., Henderson, R.C., Roth, L.J., Goldberg, L.I. and Hoffmann, P.C. (1979) 'Histofluorescence Techniques Provide Evidence for Dopamine-containing Neuronal Elements in Canine Kidney', *Science*, *205*, 497–9

Dormois, J.C., Young, J.L. and Nies, A.S. (1975) 'Minoxidil in Severe Hypertension: Value when Conventional Drugs Have Failed', *Am. Heart. J.*, *90*, 360–8

Eble, J.N. (1964) 'A Proposed Mechanism for the Depressor Effect of Dopamine in the Anaesthetized Dog', *J. Pharmacol. Exp. Ther.*, *145*, 64–70

Faucheux, B., Buu, N.T. and Kuchel, O. (1977) 'Effects of Saline and Albumin on Plasma and Urinary Catecholamines in Dogs', *Am. J. Physiol.*, *232*, F123–7

Fox, M.,Thiers, S., Rosenberg, L. and Segal, S. (1964) 'Ionic Requirements for Amino Acid Transport in the Rat Kidney Cortex Slice. I Influence of Extracellular Ions', *Biochem. Biophys. Acta*, *79*, 167–76

Freis, E.D., Rose, J.C., Riggins, T.F., Finnerty, F.A., Jr, Kelley, R.T. and Partenop, E.A. (1953) 'The Haemodynamic Effects of Hypotensive Drugs in Man IV. 1-Hydrazino-phthalazine', *Circulation*, *8*, 199–204

Glenner, G.G., Folk, J.E. and McMillan, P.J. (1962) 'Histochemical Demonstration of a Gamma-glutamyl Transpeptidase-like Activity', *J. Histochem. Cytochem.*, *10*, 481–9

Goldberg, L.I. and Kohli, J.D. (1983) 'Peripheral Dopamine Receptors: a Classification Based on Potency Series and Specific Antagonism', *Trends Pharmacol. Sci.*, February, 64–6

Goldberg L.I., Sonneville, P.F. and McNay, J.L. (1968) 'An Investigation of the Structural Requirements for Dopamine Like Renal Vasodilation: Phenethylamines and Apomorphine', *J. Pharmacol. Exp. Ther.*, *163*, 188–97

Goldstein, M., Fuxe, K. and Hokfelt, T. (1972) 'Characterisation and Tissue Localisation of Catecholamine-synthesising Enzymes', *Pharmacol. Rev.*, *24*, 293–308

Hahn, R.A., Wardell, J.R., Jr, Sarau, H.M. and Ridley, P.T. (1982) 'Characterisation of the Peripheral and Central Effects of SKF 82526, a Novel Dopamine Receptor Agonist', *J. Pharmacol. Exp. Ther.*, *223*, 305–13

Harvey, J.N., Casson, I.F., Clayden, A.D., Cope, G.F., Perkins, C.M. and Lee, M.R. (1984a) 'A Paradoxical Fall in Urine Dopamine Output when Patients with Essential Hypertension are Given Added Dietary Salt', *Clin. Sci.*, *67*, 83–8

Harvey, J.N., Clayden, D., Brown, J. and Lee, M.R. (1984b) 'Lack of Effect of Ibopamine (Diisobutyryl-N-methyl dopamine) on Renal Function in Normal Subjects', *Brit. J. Clin. Pharmacol.*, *17*, 671–7

Harvey, J.N., Clayden, D., Worth, D.P. and Lee, M.R. (1985) 'The Effects of Fenoldopam on Blood Pressure and Renal Function in Normal Volunteers', *Brit. J. Clin. Pharmacol.*, *19*, 21–7

Henry, D.P., Aoi, W. and Weinberger, M.H. (1977) 'The Effects of Dopamine on Renin Release *in vitro*', *Endocrinology*, *101*, 279–83

Higashi, Y. and Bello-Reuss, E. (1981) 'Dopamine Decreases Fluid Reabsorption in Straight Portions of Rabbit Proximal Tubule', *Kidney Int.*, *19*, 244

Hornykiewicz, O. (1958) 'The Action of Dopamine on the Arterial Blood Pressure of the Guinea Pig', *Brit. J. Pharmacol.*, *13*, 91–4

Imbs, J. and Schwartz, J. (1979) 'Peripheral Dopaminergic Receptors', *Adv. Biosci.*, *20*, IX–XI

Itskovitz, H.D. and Gilberg, N. (1981) 'Renal Function and Patterns of Catecholamine Excretion', *Kidney Int.*, *19*, 168

Kebabian, J.W. and Calne, D.B. (1979) 'Multiple Receptors for Dopamine', *Nature (Lond.)*, *277*, 93–6

Kotake, C., Hoffmann, P.C., Goldberg, L.I. and Cannon, J.G. (1981) 'Comparison of the Effects of Dopamine and Beta-Adrenergic Agonists on Adenylate Cyclase of Renal Glomeruli and Striatum', *Mol. Pharmacol.*, *20*, 429–34

Kotchen, T.A., Galla, J.H. and Luke, R.G. (1976) 'Failure of $NaHCO_3$ and $KHCO_3$ to Inhibit Renin Release in the Rat', *Am. J. Physiol.*, *231*, 1050–6

Kuchel, O., Buu, N.T. and Unger, T. (1978a) 'Dopamine-Sodium Relationship, is Dopamine a Part of the Endogenous Natriuretic System?', *Contrib. Nephrol.*, *13*, 27–36

Kuchel, O., Buu, N.T. Unger, T. and Genest, T. (1978b) 'Free and Conjugated Catecholamines in Human Hypertension', *Clin. Sci. Mol. Med.*, *55*, Suppl. 4, 775–805

Lovenberg, W., Weissbach, H. and Udenfriend, S.(1962) 'Aromatic L-amino acid Decarboxylase', *J. Biol. Chem.*, *237*, 89–93

McDonald, R.H. Jr, Goldberg, L.I., McNay, J.L. and Tuttle, E.P. Jr, (1964) 'Effect of Dopamine in Man: Augmentation of Sodium Excretion, Glomerular Filtration Rate and Renal Plasma Flow', *J. Clin. Invest.*, *43*, 1116–24

McGiff, J.C. and Burns, C.R. (1967) 'Separation of Dopamine Natriuresis from Vasodilation: Evidence for Dopamine Receptors', *J. Lab. Clin. Med.*, *70*, 892

McNay, J.L., McDonald, R.H. Jr, and Goldberg, L.I. (1965) 'Direct Renal Vasodilation Produced by Dopamine in the Dog', *Circ. Res.* , *16*, 510–17

May, D.G. and Carter, M.K. (1970) 'Effect of Vasoactive Agents on Urine and Electrolyte Excretion in the Chicken', *Am. J. Physiol.*, *218*, 417–22

Morimoto, S. (1968) 'Pharmacological Studies of Dopamine 2. Effects of Dopamine on the Renal Functions in the Dog', *Fol. Pharmacol. Jap.*, *63*, 386–401

Nagatsu, T. (1973) *The Biochemistry of the Catecholamines*, University Park Press, Baltimore, pp. 50–60; 108–31

Oates, N.S. (1979) 'Studies on Renal Dopamine in Man and the Rat', PhD Thesis, University of Leeds, pp. 44–64

Oates, N.S., Ball, S.G., Perkins, C.M. and Lee, M.R. (1979) 'Plasma and Urine Dopamine in Man Given Sodium Chloride in the Diet', *Clin. Sci. Mol. Med.*, *56*, 261–4

Oates, N.S., Perkins, C.M. and Lee, M.R. (1980) 'The Effect of Mineralocorticoid Administration on Urine-free Dopamine in Man', *Clin. Sci. Mol. Med.*, *58*, 77–82

Orlowski, M. and Wilk, S. (1976) 'Metabolism of γ-Glutamyl Amino Acids and Peptides in Mouse Liver and Kidney *in vivo.*, *Eur. J. Biochem.*, *71*, 541–55

Orlowski, M. and Wilk, S. (1978) '*In vivo* Synthesis of Ophthalmic Acid in Liver and Kidney', *Biochem. J.*, *170*, 415–19

Perkins, C.M., Hancock, K.W., Cope, G.F. and Lee, M.R. (1981) 'Urine Free Dopamine in Normal Primigravid Pregnancy and Women Taking Oral Contraceptives',*Clin. Sci. Mol. Med.*, *61*, 423–8

Perkins, C.M., Hancock, K.W., Cope, G.F. and Lee, M.R. (1982) 'Urine Dopamine in Normal and Hypertensive Pregnancies', *Brit. J. Obstet. Gynaecol.*, *89*, 123–7

Quesada, T., Garcia Torres, L. Alba, F. and Garcia del Rio, C. (1979) 'The Effects of Dopamine on Renin Release in the Isolated Perfused Rat Kidney', *Experientia*, *35*, 1205

Rennick, B.R. (1968) 'Dopamine: Renal Tubular Transport in the Dog and Plasma Binding Studies', *Am. J. Physiol.*, *215*, 532–4

Rossum, J.M. van, (1966) 'The Significance of Dopamine Receptor Blockade for the Mechanism of Action of Neuroleptic Drugs', *Arch. Int. Pharmacodyn. Ther.*, *160*, 492–4

Sanner, E. (1963) 'Tubular Excretion of Dopamine (3-Hydroxytyramine) by the Chicken Kidney', *Acta Pharmacol. Toxicol.*, *20*, 375–84

Seely, J.F. and Dirks, J.H. (1967) 'The Effect of Vasomotor Agents on Proximal Tubular Sodium Reabsorption in the Dog', *Abstracts Ann. Meeting Amer. Soc. Nephrol.*, p. 60

Sims, E.A.H. and Krantz, K.E. (1958) 'Serial Studies of Renal Function throughout Pregnancy and the Puerperium in Normal Women', *J. Clin. Invest.*, *37*, 1764–74

Stefoni, S., Coli, L., Mosconi, G. and Prandini, R. (1981) 'Ibopamine (SB 7505) in Normal Subjects and in Chronic Renal Failure', *Brit. J. Clin. Pharmacol.*, *1*, 69–72

Stote, R.M., Dubb, J.W., Familiar, R.G., Erb, B.B. and Alexander, F. (1983) 'A New Oral Renal Vasodilator, Fenoldopam', *Clin. Pharmacol. Ther.*, *34*, 309–15

Ullrich, K.J., Rumrich, G. and Kloss, S. (1974) 'Sodium Dependence of the Amino Acid Transport in the Proximal Convolution of the Rat Kidney', *Pflügers Arch.*, *351*, 49–60

Unger, T., Buu, N.T. and Kuchel, O. (1980) 'Conjugated Dopamine: Peripheral Origin, Distribution and Response to Acute Stress in the Dog', *Can. J. Physiol. Pharmacol.*, *58*, 22–7

Warren, D.J. and Ferris, T.F. (1970) 'Renin Secretion in Renal Hypertension', *Lancet, i*, 159–62

Wilcox, C.S., Aminoff, M.J., Kurtz, A.B. and Slater, J.D.H. (1974) 'Comparison of the Renin Response to Dopamine and Noradrenaline in Normal Subjects and Patients with Autonomic Insufficiency', *Clin. Sci. Mol. Med.*, *46*, 481–8

Wilk, S., Mizoguchi, H. and Orlowski, M. (1978) 'γ-Glutamyl DOPA: a Kidney Specific Dopamine Precursor', *J. Pharmacol. Exp. Ther.*, *206*, 227–32

Worth, D., Brown, J., Cooke, J. Harvey, J. and Lee, M.R. (1984) 'The Effect of Intravenous γ-Glutamyl L-Dopa on Renal Function in Normal Volunteers', *Clin. Sci.*, *66*, 13P

Yeh, B.K., McNay, J.L. and Goldberg, L.I. (1969) 'Attenuation of Dopamine Renal and Mesenteric Vasodilation by Haloperidol: Evidence for a Specific Receptor', *J. Pharmacol. Exp. Ther.*, *168*, 303–9

8 HYPERTENSION AND THE KIDNEY

J.D. Swales

Introduction

Changes in renal function may be both a cause and a consequence of high blood pressure. In some situations the interrelationship between cause and effect may be more complex, so that renal abnormalities produced by elevated blood pressure may give rise to circulatory changes that maintain hypertension. In this review I shall deal exclusively with the kidneys as a potential cause of elevated blood pressure: renal consequences of hypertension will be discussed only to the extent that they are believed to influence blood-pressure control.

The second point central to any discussion of experimental and clinical hypertension is the heterogeneity of mechanisms involved, reflecting in turn the physiological systems by which blood pressure is controlled. Several different mechanisms may be responsible for the elevation of peripheral resistance which is the common feature of most types of hypertension (Folkow, 1982). This is reflected in the various clinical forms of secondary hypertension which may be due to overactivity of the sympathetic-adrenal system, adrenal cortex, or juxtaglomerular apparatus, or to impairment of sodium excretion by the kidney (Table 8.1). Experimental models in the laboratory animal parallel these clinical states (Table 8.2), although to what extent is still highly debatable (McGiff and Quilley, 1981).

In the majority of hypertensive patients, however, no obvious single cause for high blood pressure can be found. It is important to bear in mind that such patients are identified by drawing an arbitrary dividing line between normal and elevated blood pressures. Although this manoeuvre is clinically convenient in that it allows a high-risk group to be identified, there is no natural dividing line, in terms of blood-pressure distribution, to distinguish between the normotensive and the hypertensive (Pickering, 1968). Even in the event of a single factor giving rise to hypertension, it is improbable that such an abnormality is present *only* in those patients classified as hypertensive. Claims for a discrete abnormality in hypertensive populations should therefore be viewed with great suspicion. A more likely explanation for apparent differences between normotensive and hypertensive populations is that they have been artificially created by comparison of populations that differ biologically in other respects than blood pressure because of poor matching (see below). The unimodal nature of the blood-pressure distribution curve in unselected populations suggests that blood pressure is a multi-factorially determined characteristic. This will be manifest in considerable

Table 8.1: Forms of Clinical Hypertension

Sodium and fluid retention
   Bilateral nephrectomy
   Advanced bilateral renal disease (most)

Mineralocorticoid hypertension
   Primary aldosteronism
   Excessive synthesis of other mineralocorticoids

Renovascular
   Renal artery stenosis, bilateral/unilateral

Renal parenchymal
   Unilateral renal disease, e.g. chronic pyelonephritis

Renin-induced
   Renin-secreting tumour
      renal
      ectopic
   Chronic glomerulonephritis (occasionally)

Sympathetic nervous system lesions
   Bulbar lesions
   Raised intracranial pressure
   Spinal cord lesions
   ? Baroreceptor denervation

Increased circulating catecholamines
   Phaeochromocytoma

Coarctation of the aorta

Hypertension of pregnancy

Drug induced
   Contraceptive pill, steroid treatment
   Non-steroidal anti-inflammatory drugs, monoamine oxidase-inhibiting
   and tyramine-containing foods, liquorice

Essential hypertension

Table 8.2: Experimental Models of Hypertension (only models discussed are listed)

Renovascular
   Goldblatt 2-kidney 1-clip
   Goldblatt 1-kidney 1-clip
   Figure-of-eight ligature (Grollman hypertension) (1- or 2-kidney)
   Cellophane wrap (1- or 2-kidney) (Page hypertension)
   Coarctation

Mineralocorticoid
   DOC salt (deoxycorticosterone acetate injections, 1% saline to drink, usually
      combined with unilateral nephrectomy)

Genetic strains
   Spontaneously hypertensive rat (SHR)
   SHR stroke-prone strain
   Dahl salt-sensitive strain (DS)
   Milan hypertensive strain

---

overlap in measured variables where 'normotensive' and 'hypertensive' populations are compared, or in a relatively weak correlation between blood pressure and a measure of one of the several processes that contribute to blood-pressure control.

The kidney influences blood pressure through its two major functions as an excretory and as an endocrine organ. It is also possible that the kidney may play a role in blood-pressure control via renally originating sympathetic afferents.

The excretory functions of the kidneys may have important effects for blood pressure when they are responsible for the clearance of vasoactive materials. There is little available information on the role of renal clearance of endogenous vasoactive substances, but there is abundant evidence that impaired excretion of some antihypertensive drugs or their metabolites may have important consequences in patients with renal failure (Anderson *et al.*, 1976). Under physiological conditions, however, the excretion of sodium and water by the kidney is the aspect of renal excretory function that has attracted most attention in blood-pressure research.

Renal Control of Sodium and Fluid Balance

Fluid Volumes and Body Sodium in Hypertension

Bilateral nephrectomy is associated with elevated blood pressure in laboratory animals (Braun-Menendez and Von Euler, 1947; Grollman *et al.*, 1949) and man (Merrill *et al.*, 1961). There is a close relationship between sodium retention (as assessed by total exchangeable sodium) and blood pressure in such patients (Carlberger and Collste, 1968) and in patients with advanced renal disease where blood pressure is also usually correlated with the degree of sodium retention (Blumberg *et al.*, 1967). However, in some cases, severe hypertension persists despite fluid depletion: in these patients renin hypersecretion appears to be responsible (see below).

Despite the evidence that sodium retention plays a role in renoprival hypertension and in the hypertension associated with advanced renal disease, it seems that other factors are also important. Grollman *et al.* (1949) reported that hypertension in nephrectomised dogs could be prevented when a kidney was present, although its excretory function had been abolished by diverting the ureter into the vena cava; and Kolff *et al.* (1954) were able to demonstrate a vasodepressor action of transplanted kidneys, not mediated by sodium excretion. This work led to later attempts to characterise the renal medullary vasodepressor system (see below).

It is possible to demonstrate volume expansion in certain other forms of hypertension. Mineralocorticoid hypertension in the rat is produced by injection of deoxycorticosterone (DOC), usually combined with saline administration and unilateral nephrectomy. Exchangeable sodium is elevated in this model: however, when DOC is discontinued, blood pressure remains high despite a major fall in exchangeable sodium, indicating that other mechanisms are responsible for maintenance of high blood pressure at this stage (McAreavey *et al.*, 1985). The clinical counterpart of this is probably seen in hypertension associated with aldosterone-secreting tumours (adenoma) of the adrenal gland, where exchangeable sodium is elevated approximately in proportion to the degree of blood-pressure elevation: after removal of the adenoma there is a fall in blood pressure related to the fall in exchangeable sodium (Beretta-Piccoli *et al.*, 1983).

Hypertension produced by renal artery constriction in the absence of a contralateral kidney (Goldblatt 1-kidney 1-clip hypertension) is associated with a positive sodium balance (Swales *et al.*, 1972) and elevated exchangeable sodium (Tobian *et al.*, 1969). This is reflected in reduced renal renin content (Regoli *et al.*, 1962), reduced juxtaglomerular granulation (Heptinstall, 1965), and plasma renin levels which are normal or low despite the presence of renal ischaemia which would normally be expected to produce renin hypersecretion (Miksche *et al.*, 1970). Where a normal contralateral kidney is present, sodium retention cannot be demonstrated, and cumulative sodium-balance studies indicate sodium balance to be normal or negative (Swales *et al.*, 1972; Mohring *et al.*, 1975). The important determinant of sodium balance in such cases is probably the degree of blood-pressure elevation and the consequent perfusion pressure natriuresis (see below). Conversely, during the reversal of Goldblatt 2-kidney 1-clip hypertension (hypertension produced by restricting the blood supply to one kidney with the other intact) by removal of the renal artery clip or the ischaemic kidney, sodium retention occurs (Thurston *et al.*, 1980). The analogous clinical state in man is unilateral renal artery stenosis where a negative correlation can also be demonstrated between blood pressure and exchangeable sodium (McAreavey *et al.*, 1983). In both Goldblatt 2-kidney 1-clip hypertension in the rat and unilateral renal artery stenosis in man, quite profound sodium depletion may be observed when renovascular hypertension enters the malignant phase (Barraclough 1966; Mohring *et al.*, 1976b). The severity of renal sodium and water losses may have an adverse influence upon the natural history of malignant hypertension since there is evidence for improvement both in the rat and in man when sodium losses are replaced (Mohring *et al.*, 1976b; Thomas and Lee, 1976).

Reversal of Goldblatt 1-kidney 1-clip hypertension in the rat by removal of the renal artery clip is associated with a natriuresis: it seems unlikely, however, that negative sodium balance causes the fall in blood pressure, since replacement of sodium and water losses does not inhibit the fall (Neubig and Hoobler, 1975).

There is a short phase of positive sodium balance after application of the renal artery clip in the Goldblatt 2-kidney 1-clip model. Fundamental importance has been attributed to this phenomenon in the light of the autoregulatory theory of hypertension (Mohring *et al.*, 1975). It has not, however, been shown that this phase is an essential prerequisite for the later development of hypertension, rather than a non-specific consequence of renal artery constriction which may not play a direct role in blood pressure elevation.

Sodium retention and fluid volume expansion does not appear to be associated with hypertension in the Okamoto-Kyoto spontaneously hypertensive rat (SHR) (Trippodo *et al.*, 1978; Bianchi *et al.*, 1981; Toal and Leenen, 1983a). Exchangeable sodium is reduced in the Dahl salt-sensitive rat (Schackow and Dahl, 1966). The development of hypertension in the Milan hypertensive strain of rat (MHS) is associated with sodium retention as measured by cumulative sodium balance when compared with the normotensive strain: however, in established hypertension in this model exchangeable sodium is normal (Bianchi *et al.*, 1975).

It is not possible to study sodium balance during the development of essential hypertension in man. It is only feasible to measure fluid volumes or body elecrolytes in a group of hypertensive patients and compare the results with normotensive controls. This procedure is fraught with hazard since, unless extreme care is taken, hypertensive patients may differ from controls in such relevant factors as body weight, diet and age. This has clearly not been appreciated by several workers in this area. Nevertheless, most early reports detect no differences between exchangeable sodium and extracellular fluid volumes in hypertensive and normotensive subjects (for review see Swales, 1975a). More recent studies have described a slight reduction in exchangeable sodium and extracellular fluid in mildly hypertensive and young hypertensive subjects (Bing and Smith, 1981; Bauer and Brooks, 1982; Beretta-Piccoli *et al.*, 1982), suggesting that the earliest phases of hypertension are associated with a mild natriuresis produced by increased renal perfusion pressure, analogous with a negative sodium balance observed in Goldblatt 2-kidney 1-clip hypertension. One group described a positive correlation between body sodium and blood pressure in older subjects, which was interpreted as indicating secondary renal changes resulting in sodium retention (Beretta-Piccoli *et al.*, 1982).

In contrast to the minor changes observed in body sodium, plasma volume is reduced in most patients with essential hypertension (Tarazi *et al.*, 1968; Bing and Smith, 1981; Bauer and Brooks, 1982). Further, there is an association between the elevation of blood pressure and the degree of plasma volume contraction (Tarazi *et al.*, 1968). Where extracellular fluid and plasma volume have been measured simultaneously, there is a reduction in the ratio of plasma to interstitial fluid volume (Tarazi, 1976). The most likely explanation of this is increased venular tone resulting in enhanced transcapillary filtration of fluid from the vascular compartment. A minority of hypertensive patients, however, are apparently hyper- rather than hypovolaemic (Tarazi, 1976, 1983). Whether hypertension in these patients is caused by a different mechanism is, however, doubtful: this group is markedly more obese than the hypertensives and this calls into question the part played by the standard of reference used, since body composition in such subjects is clearly different from that in controls. The standard of reference (i.e. body weight or an expression of body mass) has a significant influence upon the demonstration of hypervolaemia in these subjects (Tarazi, 1976).

A proportion of patients with essential hypertension exhibits low basal plasma renin levels which respond subnormally to such stimuli as sodium restriction or diuretic therapy. Early workers suggested that renin suppression in 'low renin hypertension' is analogous to that observed in primary aldosteronism: fluid volume measurements were cited in favour of sodium retention. However, this evidence did not stand up to critical evaluation (Dunn and Tannen, 1974), and careful investigations have failed to reveal any evidence of volume expansion in 'low renin hypertension' (Schalekamp *et al.*, 1974). Renin secretion is influenced by several factors in addition to sodium balance (e.g. sympathetic nerve activity, renal arterial perfusion pressure, structural changes in the afferent arteriolar wall), which could account for the observed abnormalities in renin secretion (Swales, 1975b; Esler *et al.*, 1978).

Changes in Fluid Volume Distribution

Hypertension may involve changes in the partitioning of fluid between the different body compartments which is not reflected in overall changes in fluid volumes. Thus it has been claimed that there is a redistribution of fluid from the systemic to the pulmonary circulations in borderline hypertension (Safar *et al.*, 1974) and in renovascular but not essential hypertension (Tarazi, 1983). The conflicting results point to a considerable problem in making reliable measurements (Birkenhager and de Leeuw, 1984). Even accepting the possibility of cardiopulmonary diversion, there are physiological considerations which render the phenomenon of doubtful significance in the pathogenesis of hypertension. If it is the result of a selective increase in sympathetic efferent activity, cardiopulmonary diversion may be simply a manifestation of the primary abnormality and not necessarily a mediator of hypertension. Such diversion also occurs following sodium depletion (Ferrario *et al.*, 1981), a condition in which autonomic activity is also increased. Further, if diversion is a result of increased pulmonary vein compliance, pulmonary venous pressure will not be elevated and it is therefore difficult to see how cardiac output and consequently blood pressure can be influenced (Birkenhager and de Leeuw, 1984).

Others have postulated that the kidney influences fluid distribution in more subtle ways. Lucas and Floyer (1974) studied interstitial fluid and venous pressure during the development and reversal of Goldblatt 1-kidney hypertension in the rat, and concluded that renal-artery constriction resulted in a decrease in tissue compliance, perhaps as a result of secretion of a humoral factor. More recent studies of renal medullary vasodepressor substances with a possible effect upon venular resistance provided a possible explanation for some of these findings (see below). Mohring *et al.* (1976a) suggested that sodium and fluid move from the intra- to the extracellular compartments during the development of Goldblatt 2-kidney hypertension in female Sprague-Dawley rats: this was attributed to marked elevation of corticosterone in animals of this strain and sex. It was concluded that under some circumstances extracellular fluid volume expansion could occur even in the presence of external losses of sodium and fluid (Haack *et al.*, 1977). Although such a phenomenon may explain, as the authors propose, some of the anomalies in rat models, it is not consistent with the contracted blood volume that has now been repeatedly demonstrated in essential and renovascular hypertension in man, and it seems possible that changes in the volume of distribution of fluid space markers may have created an experimental artefact.

Summary of Fluid Volume Studies

Elevated blood pressure is associated with renal retention of sodium and fluid only in situations where sodium excretion is grossly altered by the specific manoeuvre or disease which gives rise to hypertension, e.g. bilateral nephrectomy, Goldblatt 1-kidney hypertension or mineralocorticoid hypertension. Where an apparently normal kidney is present, e.g. in Goldblatt 2-kidney hypertension, sodium retention is not observed, and if hypertension is severe enough, perfusion pressure natriuresis produces negative sodium balance. Established essential hypertension resembles the latter model in showing characteristics suggestive of a mechanism independent of sodium retention with plasma volume contraction which is related to the degree of blood-pressure elevation. The partition of fluid between plasma and interstitium is probably modified in favour of the latter by post-capillary venoconstriction. Sodium retention is not a feature of genetic hypertension in the rat except to a small extent in the stage of development of hypertension in the Milan hypertensive strain.

Induced Changes in Sodium Balance

In most patients, dialytic removal of sodium and water alleviates hypertension associated with advanced renal disease or bilateral nephrectomy (Vertes *et al.*, 1969; Wilkinson *et al.*, 1970; Brown *et al.*, 1971). Studies have also been carried out in which dietary sodium intake has been varied in healthy volunteers. In short-term studies (up to 4 weeks) blood pressure is markedly resistant to changes in sodium intake (10–410 mmol sodium per day: Kirkendall *et al.*, 1976; Burstyn *et al.*, 1980). More extreme degrees of salt loading with daily intakes up to 1500 mmol sodium cause only a very modest increase in blood pressure (Murray *et al.*, 1978). This resistance to the pressor effect of sodium cannot be attributed to renal excretion of the dietary load since increased total exchangeable sodium (Kirkendall *et al.*, 1976) and clinical evidence of fluid overload (Murray *et al.*, 1978) could be demonstrated in these experiments.

It is possible that blood-pressure responsiveness to changes in salt intake varies between different individuals. Skrabal *et al.* (1984) observed no overall change in blood pressure when dietary salt intake was varied from moderately low to high levels. However, they were able to define a group of 'salt-sensitive' normal subjects who showed significantly lower blood pressures on low compared with high salt intakes. This group was characterised by an increased incidence of hypertension in the family, enhanced pressor response to noradrenaline and lower plasma renin and aldosterone. Skrabal *et al.* argue that noradrenergic hypersensitivity causes increased proximal tubular sodium reabsorption and the resulting sodium retention is countered by elevated systemic arterial pressure and a consequent perfusion-pressure natriuresis. 'Salt-sensitive' hypertensive patients whose blood pressure rises when sodium intake is increased from low to high levels have also been described: these patients appeared to retain more sodium and had higher plasma noradrenaline levels than normal, although only when receiving a high-salt diet (Fujita *et al.*, 1980). Again, increased autonomic drive was implicated in the pathogenesis of 'salt-sensitive' hypertension. The hypothesis that a rise in blood pressure is a homeostatic adaptation by which sodium retention is opposed by perfusion pressure natriuresis will be discussed below. The concept of 'salt-sensitive' blood pressure does, however, deserve comment. First, no evidence has been produced from distribution studies in unselected populations that such salt-sensitive subjects are a separate subgroup: this does not of course negate the evidence but does make discrete mechanisms unlikely. Secondly, reproducibility of such salt sensitivity on different occasions has not been examined and it is by no means certain that the phenomenon is not one of blood-pressure variability. Thirdly, the fact that some individuals show a positive relationship between sodium intake and blood pressure does not necessarily implicate dietary sodium in the pathogenesis of hypertension in such individuals. If, for instance, the renin-aldosterone system is important in protecting blood pressure in the face of sodium depletion, individuals with an impaired renin response will show a fall in blood pressure with dietary salt restriction because they have lost one protective mechanism. The same line of reasoning explains the increased blood pressure response to diuretics of patients with 'low-renin' hypertension (Laragh, 1976). A marked fall in blood pressure during sodium depletion is not necessarily an indication that volume expansion is responsible for maintaining blood pressure.

The heterogeneity of renin response in essential hypertension may go some way towards explaining the disputed efficacy of low-salt diets in reducing blood pressure in patients with essential hypertension where evidence both for (Morgan *et al.*, 1978; MacGregor *et al.*, 1982) and against (Watt, 1983; Richards *et al.*, 1984) such an effect has been produced. It is noteworthy, however, that the change in blood pressure produced by salt restriction is indirectly correlated with the plasma-renin response so that a blood-pressure reduction only tended to be seen in those patients whose plasma renin failed to rise on a low-salt diet (Richards *et al.*, 1984).

Manipulation of sodium balance in animal models has yielded different responses depending upon the model studied. Anephric animals, like bilaterally nephrectomised man, show sodium-dependent hypertension (Leonards and Heisler, 1952; Houck, 1954), although Muirhead *et al.* (1953) were able to produce hypertension in anephric dogs in which sodium and water balance was carefully controlled. It is difficult to define normal sodium balance in nephrectomised animals, however, and it is undeniable that in the absence of kidneys sodium retention can produce hypertension: whether it is a necessary cause in this situation is less certain. As in man, the presence of normal kidney tissue seems to make animals' blood pressure resistant to the effect of changes in sodium balance. Thus, whereas dialytic removal of sodium lowered blood pressure in sodium-loaded bilaterally nephrectomised rats, the same procedure had no effect upon normal animals and indeed produced a slightly pressor response in Goldblatt 2-kidney 1-clip hypertension. In Goldblatt 1-kidney 1-clip hypertension, a moderate reduction in blood pressure was observed, although animals remained hypertensive (Swales and Tange, 1971). It is interesting (retrospectively) to observe that the blood pressure fall was only noted in situations where renin secretion was impaired or inhibited by the previous surgical procedure.

By contrast, sustained sodium depletion induced by dietary salt restriction neither prevents the development of hypertension nor reduces blood pressure in either the Goldblatt 2-kidney 1-clip or the Goldblatt 1-kidney 1-clip models in the rat (Thurston and Swales, 1976; Munoz-Ramirez *et al.*, 1980). In the latter study sham-operated control animals with one or two kidneys showed an increase in blood pressure with sodium depletion. An analogous finding was independently reported in unoperated Sprague-Dawley rats by Seymour *et al.* (1980) who further showed that unilateral nephrectomy combined with sodium depletion produced significant hypertension. Dietary sodium depletion also failed to modify the development of Goldblatt 1-kidney 1-clip hypertension in the dog (Stephens *et al.*, 1979), but salt restriction, or withdrawal of drinking water, does prevent development of DOC-salt hypertension both in the pig and the rat (Cohen *et al.*, 1980; Bing *et al.*, 1982).

Dietary salt loading exacerbates hypertension in the Okamoto-Kyoto SHR (Chrysant *et al.*, 1979). This effect is only seen several weeks after dietary salt supplementation has been started and is antedated by histologically demonstrable arterial wall thickening due to an increase in smooth-muscle mass, suggesting a direct effect of sodium loading upon the vasculature which is not a consequence of high blood pressure (Limas *et al.*, 1980). Hypertension in this model is much more resistant to salt depletion, and only the severest degrees of dietary salt restriction sufficient to retard the growth of the animals prevents or reduces blood-pressure elevation (Toal and Leenan, 1983b). The most widely studied model of salt-dependent hypertension is the Dahl salt-sensitive rat. Dahl bred two strains of rat. The salt-sensitive as opposed to salt-resistant rat develops hypertension on the high-salt diet and blood pressure remains elevated even after the diet is discontinued (Dahl *et al.*, 1962). The daily sodium intake required to produce hypertension in this model is extremely high (approximately 8 NaCl/100 g food). The corresponding intake in man exceeds the tolerable limits but would give rise to significant hypertension judging by the results of Murray *et al.* (1978) if these can be extrapolated to higher intakes. However, despite such extreme increases in salt intake, it was not possible to demonstrate an increase in exchangeable sodium (Schackow and Dahl, 1966). Although hypertension in the Dahl-sensitive strain is often assumed to be specific to NaCl, this is not the case: a later report by Dahl describes the strain as showing sensitivity to 'various noxious stimuli' (Dahl *et al.*, 1974).

In summary, changes in sodium balance are most effective in influencing blood pressure in renoprival hypertension: sodium restriction also prevents hypertension in one other volume-expanded model (DOC salt hypertension). In another volume-expanded model (Goldblatt 1-kidney 1-clip hypertension), severe acute sodium depletion has only a modest effect in limiting hypertension. In other forms of hypertension (except for the special case of the Dahl salt-sensitive rat) salt depletion is ineffective in preventing hypertension unless extreme. In some laboratory strains of rat, sodium depletion may raise blood pressure, an effect that is amplified by unilateral nephrectomy.

Renal Function in Hypertension

The experimental approach to renal function in patients with essential hypertension is constrained by the relative inaccessibility of the organ. Observations on animal models have therefore necessarily been extrapolated to man.

Renal Blood Flow and Glomerular Filtration Rate

Essential hypertension is characteristically associated wtih a normal glomerular filtration rate and a reduction in renal plasma flow so that filtration fraction is maintained or increased (Goldring *et al.*, 1941). Very severe or malignant hypertension, on the other hand, gives rise to significant renal failure by direct vascular damage. Renal blood flow declines and renal vascular resistance increases with ageing. However, even when compared with age-matched normotensive controls, patients with essential hypertension show a reduction in renal plasma flow which is directly related to the degree of blood pressure elevation (de Leeuw and Birkenhager, 1983a). (These differences can even be observed in patients receiving a controlled sodium intake.)

In contrast, in young subjects with a family history of hypertension (Bianchi *et al.*, 1979) and a minority of patients with essential hypertension (Hollenberg *et al.*, 1978), renal blood flow is increased: there is no clinical evidence that this phenomenon represents an early stage in the development of hypertension although such evidence is difficult to secure. Hollenberg and his co-workers claim that patients with increased renal blood flow constitute a discrete subgroup and suggest on this basis that hypertension may have a separate aetiology in such individuals (characteristically males with a family history of hypertension). However, the numbers fall well short of those required to demonstrate bimodality: in addition the population studied was not an unselected one and their suggestion must therefore be treated with caution. In the study reported by Bianchi and co-workers (1979, 1984) glomerular filtration rate as well as renal plasma flow was increased in the normotensive relatives of hypertensive patients. These findings are interpreted in the light of studies of the Milan hypertensive strain of rat. Renal blood flow (expressed as a percentage of cardiac output) and GFR (expressed per unit of kidney weight) were higher in the pre-hypertensive phase in this strain (Bianchi and Barlassina, 1983). They argue that these changes, together with increased renal tubular sodium transport, represent a fundamental genetically deter- mined cellular abnormality which gives rise to the later development of high blood pressure and glomerulosclerosis. Both Bianchi's and Hollenberg's groups therefore attach fundamental significance to changes in renal blood flow, although these changes are in opposite directions in the majority of the subjects studied by these two groups. The unresolved question is: how far do these changes result in abnormalities which cause hypertension, or how far do they simply reflect a subtle haemodynamic abnormality in the particular organ which has been most intensively studied, i.e. the kidney? Thus, Hollenberg's group emphasised the variability of renal blood-flow measurements in hypertensive patients (Hollenberg *et al.*, 1978). It is also noteworthy that mental stress depresses cortical blood flow in hypertensives to a greater extent than in normotensives (Hollenberg *et al.*, 1981). Relatives of hypertensive patients show an increased pressor response to stimuli such as mental stress, suggesting changes in vascular responsiveness which are not reflected, at an early stage, in high blood pressure but which may involve the kidney as part of the circulation (Falkner *et al.*, 1979).

A recent study has identified patients with essential hypertension, who failed to alter renal blood flow in response to changes in salt intake. This appeared to be due to the absence of normal changes in vascular responses to angiotensin II induced by changes in salt balance: the normal alteration in adrenal aldosterone release in response to angiotensin II (induced by changes in salt intake) was also absent (Hollenberg and Williams, 1983). It was suggested that a subgroup of hypertensives had been defined with an abnormality of angiotensin II receptor regulation. The role of this phenomenon in the pathogenesis of hypertension still has to be assessed.

In particular it remains to be established whether these patients form a discrete subgroup, whether the abnormality is characteristic and sustained in particular individuals, and whether it antedates rather than follows hypertension and its sequelae.

The development of changes in renal blood flow and GFR has been more carefully analysed in SHR. During the early stages of hypertension (3–4 months), there is no change in renal blood flow and GFR. Since perfusion pressure has been increased, vascular resistance has therefore 'reset', probably as a result of autoregulatory preglomerular vasoconstriction (Folkow *et al.*, 1977; Arendshorst and Beierwaltes, 1979), and hyperfiltration does not occur. Another study showed glomerular ultrafiltration forces almost identical at this stage despite raised renal perfusion pressure (Azar *et al.*, 1979). A small increase of renal vascular resistance at maximal vasodilatation suggests a modest structural component in this change (Folkow, 1982), but the vasoconstriction is most likely to be primarily the consequence of efferent sympathetic activity. Later an increase in postglomerular resistance and a further increase in total renal vascular resistance has been observed (Folkow, 1982); but by this stage GFR has fallen (probably as a result of loss of nephron mass due to nephrosclerosis).

Although luminal narrowing was reported in the afferent arterioles of the Dahl sensitive strain of rat (Jaffe *et al.*, 1970) this has not been confirmed by functional studies. Thus renal blood flow and GFR are normal in the early stages of hypertension in this strain (Ben-Ishay *et al.*, 1967). However, studies of single nephron function have revealed more subtle abnormalities. Preglomerular resistance was unchanged in comparison with salt-resistant control animals. As a result of elevated systemic pressure, the transcapillary hydraulic pressure was increased, with a single nephron GFR almost twice that of controls (Azar *et al.*, 1978). Although histological evidence for nephrosclerosis was minimal, these results indicated a substantial reduction in the number of functioning nephrons, with an adaptive increase in function in the remainder. It is difficult to decide how far a genetically determined decrease in nephron number, or how far hypertension-induced nephrosclerosis, accounted for this loss of functional nephrons. Nevertheless, the stage would seem set for a vicious circle in which hyperfiltration induced further nephron loss with further adaptive changes in the residual nephrons. Studies of overall renal blood flow in the isolated kidney of both Dahl sensitive rats and Okamoto-Kyoto SHR showed loss of autoregulatory function with increases of renal blood flow in response to increased perfusion pressure (Tobian *et al.*, 1975).

In both patients and animals a reduction of renal blood flow by renal artery stenosis gives rise to hypertension (Goldblatt *et al.*, 1934). In patients with such renovascular hypertension, renal blood flow remains reduced: blood flow to the opposite kidney is normal (Hollenberg *et al.*, 1978). Blood flow in the contralateral kidney of dogs with unilateral renal artery stenosis increases with the rise in systemic pressure, although elevation of blood flow is not proportional to the increase in weight so that the kidney is relatively hypoperfused (Zimmerman and Mommsen, 1981). Blood flow and GFR in the ischaemic kidney are initially reduced but then rise towards preoperative values (Deforrest *et al.*, 1978). The effect of renal artery stenosis upon renal blood flow reflects not only the alterations in luminal diameter at the site of the stenosis, and renal artery perfusion pressure, but also the resistance offered by the renal vasculature which is in series with the resistance produced by the stenosed renal artery. Selig *et al.* (1983) have shown that pressure distal to the stenosis recovers with progressive vasoconstriction. Since this effect can be blocked by converting enzyme inhibition, it is probably renin mediated. It is noteworthy that such blockade also produced a disastrous fall in GFR, probably indicating a critical effect of angiotensin II in maintaining efferent arteriolar tone. A similar fall in GFR has been reported in patients with renal artery stenosis to a single kidney or bilateral renal artery stenosis treated with converting enzyme inhibitors (Curtis *et al.*, 1983; Hricik *et al.*, 1983) and in the ischaemic kidney of patients with unilateral renal artery stenosis (Wenting *et al.*, 1984).

Sodium and Water Excretion

Systemic hypertension influences sodium and water excretion: conversely in some patients a primary change in sodium and water excretion causes high blood pressure. Increased renal perfusion pressure induces natriuresis and diuresis (Selkurt, 1951). Increased peritubular capillary hydrostatic pressure could be responsible for perfusion-pressure natriuresis. Thus natriuresis can be produced by exposure of these vessels to increased hydrostatic pressure by the combination of a vasodilator and elevated renal artery pressure (Earley and Friedler, 1966) and by partial occlusion of the renal vein (Lewy and Windhager, 1968).

Perfusion pressure natriuresis probably accounts for the increased sodium excretion by the untouched kidney which is observed in Goldblatt 2-kidney 1-clip hypertension (Lowitz *et al.*, 1968; Deforrest *et al.*, 1978) and which gives rise to negative sodium balance. It may also play a role in the accelerated natriuresis of hypertension.

Accelerated Natriuresis. Extracellular fluid volume expansion of hypertensive patients with saline (Farnsworth, 1946) or mannitol (Brodsky and Graubarth, 1953) results in a chloruresis and diuresis which is more rapid than in normal subjects. The same phenomenon can be reproduced in normal subjects although to a much lesser extent by the infusion of metaraminol (Vaamonde *et al.*, 1964). Some evidence supports the hypothesis that peritubular physical forces are responsible for the accelerated natriuresis of hypertension; natriuresis produced by mannitol in hypertensive patients was accompanied by elevated renal venous wedge pressures (Lowenstein *et al.*, 1970) and by raised renal interstitial pressure in acutely hypertensive dogs

(Raeder *et al.*, 1974). In the latter experiments two factors were postulated: (a) impaired autoregulation of renal blood flow after saline loading exposing peritubular capillaries to increased hydrostatic pressure; (b) a reduction in filtration fraction leading to a reduction in peritubular oncotic pressure. Other evidence is against a role for peritubular physical forces. Thus Willassen and Ofstad (1980) were unable to detect any rise in renal venous wedge pressures and calculated efferent arteriolar oncotic pressure showed a similar fall in normotensive and hypertensive subjects during saline loading. They suggest that the changes observed by Lowenstein *et al.* were the result of mannitol-induced diuresis. DiBona and Rios (1978) likewise found no evidence of changes in cortical peritubular and colloid osmotic pressure in SHR and control rats during volume expansion, and concluded that changes in the loop of Henle were responsible for the exaggerated diuresis and natriuresis. Normalisation of renal perfusion pressure by aortic constriction abolished the exaggerated response. It seems, therefore, that the exaggerated natriuresis is an acute response at the level of the loop of Henle. Although the sequence of events which occurs at this point is obscure in view of the acuteness with which it can be abolished, it seems unnecessary to postulate extrarenal mechanisms, and a local haemodynamic change seems most likely. At the same time, systemic hypertension is not an essential prerequisite since accelerated natriuresis is also observed in the normotensive relatives of hypertensive propositi (Wiggins *et al.*, 1978) and in the prehypertensive phase of genetic hypertension in the rat (Ben-Ishay *et al.*, 1973).

These observations and the controversy are also relevant to the control of sodium excretion in hypertension. In one study acute hypertension produced by baroreceptor denervation was associated with decreased proximal tubular sodium reabsorption (Koch *et al.*, 1968). However, indirect studies on hypertensive man (Buckalew *et al.*, 1969) and other micropuncture studies on chronically (Stumpe *et al.*, 1970) and acutely (Bank *et al.*, 1970) hypertensive rats suggest changes in sodium reabsorption in the loop of Henle. A similar effect has been observed at this level in the untouched kidney of rats with 2-kidney 1-clip hypertension (Lowitz *et al.*, 1968).

How far is elevated systemic pressure transmitted to the peritubular capillaries? Evidence against such transmission has been produced in SHR (DiBona and Rios 1978; Arendshorst and Beierwaltes, 1979). On the other hand, in NaCl-loaded Dahl salt-sensitive rats, high pressure appears to extend as far as the peritubular capillaries (Azar *et al.*, 1974), although this may be a particular feature of this strain.

Whatever the mechanism of pressure natriuresis, it is undoubtedly acute, consistent and profound. This led Borst and Borst (1963) to propose that perfusion pressure natriuresis was of fundamental importance in hypertension. They point out that 'escape' from sodium retention produced by DOC and liquorice is associated with elevation in systemic blood pressure and could therefore be due to high perfusion pressure natriuresis. This hypothesis has been elaborated by Guyton's group (Guyton *et al.*, 1972, 1974; Coleman *et al.*, 1975). Analysis of the relationship between renal perfusion pressure and sodium and water output was used to construct a perfusion pressure-natriuresis curve. This is extremely steep so that a small increase in renal perfusion pressure produces a several-fold increase in sodium excretion. Whenever blood pressure is elevated, without a shift in the pressure-natriuresis curve progressive sodium depletion would occur and inhibit the blood pressure rise. Because of this, renal excretion of sodium and water are considered to exert an overriding effect on blood pressure control. Although steady-state sodium excretion is modestly increased in some experimental models (e.g. Goldblatt 2-kidney 1-clip hypertension), this is much less than would be predicted on the basis of renal perfusion pressure. Construction of *in vivo* perfusion pressure natriuresis curves indicated a substantial shift to favour constant sodium excretion with increasing arterial pressure in Goldblatt 1-kidney 1-clip hypertensive rats and SHR (Norman *et al.*, 1978). Reducing the renal perfusion pressure of SHR and Dahl salt-sensitive rats to levels observed in normotensive controls produces subnormal excretion of sodium and water (Tobian *et al.*, 1975; Nagaoka *et al.*, 1981). In both studies, therefore, the kidneys' ability to excrete sodium and water is altered to maintain these at normal levels despite high renal perfusion pressures.

This hypothesis raises two interrelated questions: is a change in the natriuresis–perfusion pressure relationship a primary one in hypertension, and, secondly how is such a striking effect produced? Norman *et al.* (1978) define two components in their curves. A shift in both the slope and the position of the curve was observed in response to reduced renal mass so that an increase of renal perfusion pressure produced little further elevation of urinary output. This change in slope was also a feature of such sodium-retaining substances as angiotensin II and aldosterone. By contrast SHR showed a parallel shift to the right which is attributed to diffuse vasoconstriction. In other studies from the same group, small direct intrarenal infusions of angiotensin II produced sodium retention and hypertension in unilaterally nephrectomised dogs, whereas intravenous infusions which were calculated to raise plasma AII levels to the same extent had much less marked effects on sodium balance and blood pressure (Lohmeier and Cowley, 1979). A relatively modest elevation of angiotensin II levels in, for instance, renovascular hypertension could therefore have an important effect on the perfusion pressure/natriuresis relationship. The presence of renal cortical vasoconstriction in SHR, and in patients with essential hypertension, could be a consequence of increased renal sympathetic activity (Coote and Sato, 1977; Hollenberg *et al.*, 1978; Norman and Dzielak, 1982). Circulating catecholamines could also play a role in modifying the relationship between perfusion pressure and sodium excretion (Johnson and Barger, 1981). Later, increased vascular wall-to-lumen ratio in the afferent vessels as a result of hypertension-induced hypertrophy could play a role (Folkow, 1982). Other workers have suggested other mechanisms. For example, Brown *et al.* (1974) suggested that the increased filtration fraction described in essential hypertension could enhance renal tubular sodium reabsorption by an increase in efferent arteriolar oncotic pressure. Baer and Bianchi (1978) reported decreased glomerular hydraulic conductivity in Milan hypertensive rats, but later modified this in favour of elevated glomerular filtration rate with a genetically determined increased proximal tubular sodium reabsorption (Bianchi *et al.*, 1984). Tobian's group implicated reduced renal medullary PGE_2 (Tobian *et al.*, 1982) and reduced renal capillary flow in the reduced sodium excretion observed in isolated kidneys of Dahl salt-sensitive rats (Tobian *et al.*, 1978): the latter abnormality was also detected in SHR (Ganguli *et al.*, 1976). Restoration of medullary PGE_2 by increased dietary linoleic acid delayed the onset of hypertension in the Dahl salt-sensitive rats (Tobian *et al.*, 1982). The role of prostaglandins in sodium excretion is considered more fully in Chapter 5. In other situations, such as after partial nephrectomy or following the administration of mineralocorticoid, there are clearly factors present that may influence perfusion pressure natriuresis.

The demonstration of a shift in the perfusion pressure/natriuresis curve does not imply that it is the cause of hypertension. Two other important influences have to be borne in mind. First, the renal vessels participate in the general rise in total peripheral resistance which is observed in most forms of chronic hypertension. The effects of such a rise in renal vascular resistance upon blood pressure and flow in intrarenal vessels may result in different consequences from those produced by an acute rise in cardiac output (induced, for instance, by liquorice or mineralocorticoids). Secondly, even when an initial pressure natriuresis and diuresis occur, the resultant volume contraction will itself inhibit pressure natriuresis. This effect has been demonstrated in two situations. Thus although perfusion pressure natriuresis occurs during the development of Goldblatt 2-kidney 1-clip hypertension in the rat, the natriuresis is not as great as would be anticipated from the blood pressure levels attained (Figure 8.1). However, the animals are in negative sodium balance, and sodium depletion prevents the development of pressure natriuresis (despite the development of severe hypertension): the need to conserve volume therefore exerted an overriding effect upon pressure natriuresis (Swales, 1977). Omvik *et al.* (1980) constructed pressure–natriuresis curves in hypertensive patients during blood pressure lowering by sodium nitroprusside, and showed that the greater the degree of plasma volume contraction in the hypertensive patients, the lower the natriuretic response.

There are other reasons to reject the widely cited hypothesis that a shift in the pressure-natriuresis curve is the primary abnormality in hypertension. First, there is the evidence in some clinical and experimental models of hypertension for plasma volume contraction: the possibility of over-compensation by an excessive pressor response to volume loading would seem unlikely. Secondly, there is no evidence that the pressor response to fluid

Figure 8.1: Urinary Sodium Excretion in Goldblatt 2-Kidney 1-Clip Hypertension (2-k 1-c) in Relation to the Blood Pressure. The 'pressure-natriuresis curve' is much less steep than that observed in normal rats (data from Norman *et al.*, 1978). However, during the development of hypertension, animals showed a progressively negative cumulative sodium balance (columns below). When hypertension in this model was allowed to develop in rats on a sodium-restricted diet, cumulative sodium balance was more severely negative (dotted columns below) and no pressure natriuresis was seen (dotted line above). Thus, changes in sodium balance can override the normal pressure-natriuresis relationship. Both 24 h urinary Na output and cumulative Na balance are expressed in millimoles

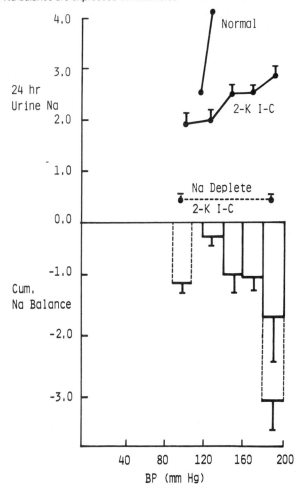

volume expansion is of overwhelming importance compared with the other mechanisms for regulating sodium and fluid excretion. Thus, dietary sodium loading in normal individuals produces at the very most an extremely modest pressor response despite volume expansion (Kirkendall *et al.*, 1976; Murray *et al.*, 1978). Unless other assumptions are made about the time span needed for the development of the pressor response to sodium loading, it seems that a shift of the pressure-natriuresis curve is a secondary rather than a primary change, although an important one in preventing or limiting sodium and fluid losses during the development of hypertension by other mechanisms.

There is other evidence that renal sodium handling may be abnormal in subjects genetically predisposed to essential hypertension. Relatives of hypertensive patients show enhanced renal retention of sodium in response to mental stress (Light *et al.*, 1983); likewise stress-induced sodium retention has been shown in young SHR (Lundin and Thoren, 1982). In both cases an increased sympathetic nervous system response could be incriminated. The catecholamine response to stress is increased in the normotensive relatives of hypertensive patients, and the change in catecholamines could produce increased sodium retention (Johnson and Barger, 1981). It is not therefore necessary to relate the probable later development of hypertension in the human subjects and the young SHR directly to sodium retention, since this could simply be evidence of enhanced sympathetic activity.

Two studies of the renal excretion of a sodium load by normotensive first-degree relatives of hypertensive patients have yielded opposite results. Wiggins *et al.* (1978) reported that these subjects had an accelerated natriuresis in comparison with control subjects, and there was a correlation between sodium excretion and blood pressure in control subjects which was not seen in the relatives of hypertensives. By contrast, Luft *et al.* (1982) reported a lesser natriuresis in first-degree relatives of hypertensive subjects, older subjects and blacks. This was interpreted as indicating a primary impairment of renal sodium excretion in subjects genetically predisposed to hypertension, analogous to that reported in the Dahl sensitive rat (Roos *et al.*, 1984). There are important differences in the protocol since the study reported by Luft *et al.* (1982) measured sodium excretion throughout a 24 h period of free activity. The subject was supine only for 4 h of saline infusion and the reduction in sodium excretion largely reflected nocturnal excretion. By contrast Wiggins *et al.* (1978) studied sodium excretion in seated subjects for 220 min only. It is therefore difficult to compare these two investigations directly. It does seem likely, however, that the reduction in sodium excretion observed by Luft *et al.* reflected more complex factors operating during free activity. Of these the sympathetic nervous system may again be a prime factor. In this context it is noteworthy that plasma renin activity was higher in the relatives of hypertensive subjects in the study of Luft but not in that reported by Wiggins *et al.* This would argue against extracellular fluid volume expansion in the relatives, but would favour increased sympathetic activity.

Renal Transplantation Studies. Transplantation of kidneys offers another approach to the role of renal excretory and non-excretory functions in hypertension. Renoprival hypertension in the dog (Muirhead *et al.*, 1956), DOC salt and figure-of-eight unilateral nephrectomy hypertension in the rat (see Gomez *et al.*, 1960, for explanation) are relieved by a functioning renal transplant. The effect on blood pressure in the rat model is associated with a fall in cardiac output (Rosas *et al.*, 1964). Restoration of blood pressure to normal occurs within minutes, and in the rat studies was too rapid to be mediated by sodium and water excretion. Measurement of external balances and radiosulphate space in the dog supports this interpretation (Muirhead *et al.*, 1956). Cross-transplantation between Dahl salt-sensitive and salt-resistant rats showed that hypertension 'followed the kidney' so that a kidney transplanted from a sensitive to a resistant strain raised the blood pressure and vice versa (Dahl *et al.*, 1974). When Dahl salt-sensitive and salt-resistant strains were linked in a parabiotic union, sensitivity was transferred, suggesting humoral transmission (Dahl *et al.*, 1969). Other reports document the transmission of hypertension from hypertensive to normotensive strains of the Milan rat (Bianchi *et al.*, 1974) and SHR (Kawabe *et al.*, 1979). In none of these later studies was the mechanism of transplantation-induced change in blood pressure further analysed, although a renomedullary antihypertensive function was postulated in one (Dahl *et al.*, 1974) and an effect on sodium excretion was postulated in another (Bianchi and Barlassina, 1983). Strong evidence for an endocrine function was produced by Muirhead *et al.* (1972a, 1977) with a demonstration of a blood pressure-lowering action of fragmented renal medullary transplants.

In summary, renal transplantation studies have repeatedly shown the action of a transplanted kidney in raising or lowering blood pressure depending upon the nature of the donor and recipient animals. The evidence suggests an endocrine rather than an excretory mechanism for this effect.

Mechanism of Salt-induced Hypertension

Under some circumstances (for instance after bilateral nephrectomy) sodium retention undoubtedly does cause high blood pressure. Early theories suggested that elevated peripheral resistance is an autoregulatory consequence of increased cardiac output produced by volume expansion (Guyton *et al.*, 1974). However, in both experimental hypertension and in hypertension produced by volume expansion, the initial change is often elevated peripheral resistance; there is no suggestion that an initial rise in cardiac output is mandatory (Fletcher *et al.*, 1976; Kim *et al.*, 1976; Ferrario and Page, 1978). Indeed, depending upon the state of sodium balance, the initial change in Goldblatt hypertension may be either in cardiac output or peripheral resistance (Stephens *et al.*, 1979). Further, in mineralocorticoid hypertension, when an early rise in cardiac output could be detected, the development of the subsequent elevation of peripheral resistance was extremely variable, suggesting that a simple cause-and-effect relationship did not obtain (Man in t'Veld *et al.*, 1984).

Other suggestions have been made to explain how sodium retention may cause hypertension. The most widely discussed has been the hypothesis put forward originally by Blaustein (1977). According to this a sodium-calcium exchange process in vascular smooth muscle is affected by elevation of intracellular sodium, resulting in the accumulation of intracellular calcium which enhances smooth-muscle contractility. Intracellular sodium could be elevated as a result of an increase in total body sodium. There is evidence of this in the mesenteric arterial wall when hypertension is produced by extreme dietary sodium loading (Madden *et al.*, 1979). However, it is further argued that intracellular sodium may also be increased as a result of reduced ouabain-sensitive sodium pumping inhibited by a circulating ouabain-like substance. This hypothesis was developed with a further postulate that this inhibitor is identical with 'natriuretic hormone' produced as a result of impaired renal sodium excretion (de Wardener and MacGregor, 1982). In favour of this view, leucocytes from essential hypertensive patients show reduced ouabain-sensitive sodium pumping (Edmondson *et al.*, 1975): further, this defect can be induced in normal leucocytes by incubation in plasma from hypertensive patients (Poston *et al.*, 1981) and material which inhibited a membrane-bound $(Na^+ + K^+)$ ATPase was found in the plasma of hypertensive patients (Hamlyn *et al.*, 1982). Another group described a factor that inhibited ouabain-sensitive rubidium uptake by rat arterial tissue (Haddy and Pamnani, 1983; Huot *et al.*, 1983) and was present in the plasma of volume-expanded animals (with experimental hypertension) and in low-renin hypertension in man.

Blaustein's hypothesis and de Wardener and MacGregor's development of it require primary renal retention of sodium if they are to be applied to essential hypertension in man and to other forms of hypertension. However, in most forms of hypertension, volume expansion cannot be demonstrated. In a later modification, de Wardener and MacGregor (1982) argue in favour of cardiopulmonary volume diversion as a primary event. This has been discussed previously. The interpretation of events at a cellular level is also open to criticism. Although a cardiac calcium-sodium exchange channel has been well documented, it is debatable whether such a process operates at the vascular smooth-muscle level under physiological conditions (Van Breeman *et al.*, 1979; Aaronson and Van Breeman, 1981; Mulvaney *et al.*, 1982). In nucleated cells of both man and rat (Bradlaugh *et al.*, 1984; Swales *et al.*, 1984) sodium pump inhibition is a feature of sodium depletion rather than sodium loading. In the Dahl salt-sensitive rat used as a model for the de Wardener–MacGregor hypothesis, vascular ouabain-sensitive sodium pumping is increased (Overbeck *et al.*, 1981). Increased rather than decreased sodium and potassium turnover by arterial tissue has been a characteristic feature of the majority of models of hypertension examined: the most likely explanation of this is that increased permeability to sodium leads to a compensatory increase in sodium pumping (Bohr, 1981). Though this could be due to a dissociation of a putative inhibitor from its binding site as these studies were carried out *in vitro*, such loose binding is not a feature of inhibition of the sodium pump observed in the leucocytes from hypertensive subjects. Whereas Dahl's experiments implicated a humoral factor in the pathogenesis of hypertension in his sensitive strain, later studies, using perfusion of isolated kidneys by plasma from Dahl-sensitive and resistant rats indicated that the former had sodium-retaining rather than natriuretic properties relative to the latter (Tobian *et al.*, 1979). It seems unlikely, therefore, that 'natriuretic-hormone'-induced inhibition of the sodium pump is responsible for Dahl hypertension in the rat or essential hypertension in man.

It should also be borne in mind that several disturbances of sodium transport have been demonstrated in erythrocytes from patients with essential hypertension. Such changes include a reduction in sodium-potassium co-transport (Garay and Meyer, 1979), and an increase in lithium-sodium counter-transport (Canessa *et al.*, 1980). These findings have been confirmed in some populations but not in others, and it is likely that ethnic factors are of considerable importance. It is also likely that some of the abnormalities in essential hypertension are due to poor matching for age, sex, diet, the effect of previous treatment, body composition and ethnic factors (Swales, 1983). The importance of such factors has not been adequately considered in many reports in this area. Of particular importance may be elevated catecholamine levels, which can be produced as a result of the stress of venepuncture, and which may induce substantial sodium-pump inhibition in the human leucocyte (Riozzi *et al.*, 1984). Where ion-transport disturbances in hypertension are not an experimental artefact, it seems probable that, in view of their multiple nature, they are manifestations of an intrinsic disturbance of cell-membrane physicochemical structure, perhaps in some circumstances induced or influenced by circulating catecholamines (Swales, 1983). The connection with blood pressure may be through disturbances of membrane calcium handling rather than indirectly through impairment of renal sodium excretory function (Kwan *et al.*, 1979; Postnov and Orlov, 1984).

Bohr (1981) has put forward an intriguing interpretation of the significance of changes in membrane electrolyte transport. The haemodynamic abnormality during the development of high blood pressure is not either consistently one of vascular resistance or cardiac output. This suggests an abnormality of central neurogenic control of blood pressure. The critical membrane disturbance, Bohr suggests, is one involving the vasomotor neurones of the hypothalamus and brainstem, and consequent changes in sympathetic efferent activity. The inaccessibility of these sites to ion-transport measurement renders this hypothesis speculative, but progress in this field may render it ultimately testable.

Summary and Conclusions

Retention of sodium as a result of bilateral nephrectomy or advanced renal failure produces hypertension by a mechanism which is still uncertain. Theories postulating an autoregulatory response to increased cardiac output or alteration of calcium-sodium exchange in vascular smooth muscle are not consistent with much of the experimental evidence. In the most common forms of clinical and experimental hypertension, there is no convincing evidence for a primary disturbance of sodium excretion although secondary changes probably prevent a disastrous perfusion pressure natriuresis in response to elevated blood pressure. There is no persuasive evidence that abnormalities of ion transport by blood cells and vascular smooth muscle in hypertension are a consequence of changes in renal function.

Renin-Angiotensin System in Hypertension

Although renin induces high blood pressure through production of angiotensin II, renin secretion is sensitive to several factors which may be altered as a result of hypertension, e.g. extracellular fluid volume, renal arterial perfusion pressure and sympathetic nervous system activity. Plasma renin may therefore be either high or low when compared with values in a normotensive subject or animal, but still in the strict sense of the term 'normal' in relation to the multifactorial determinants of plasma renin. Renin hypersecretion by the kidney appears to be responsible for hypertension in two fairly rare clinical situations: these are renin-secreting tumours and dialysis-resistant hypertension in patients with advanced renal disease.

Renin-secreting Tumours

Benign tumours of the juxtaglomerular cells (haemangiopericytomata) may secrete large amounts of renin. Hypersecretion of renin has also been reported in other non-renal malignant tumours, e.g. pulmonary carcinomata and pancreatic adenocarcinomata (MacKay *et al.*, 1983a). Renal tumours may also cause renin hypersecretion by local compression and ischaemia, and this is probably more common than tumour synthesis of renin.

Hypertension in patients with renin-secreting tumours is associated with very high plasma renin and angiotensin II levels, together with secondary hyperaldosteronism which may produce severe hypokalaemia. When measured plasma levels of angiotensin II are compared with blood-pressure levels obtained at the same time, the degree of hypertension is much greater than observed when angiotensin II is elevated to similar plasma levels by short-term infusions (Brown *et al.*, 1979; MacKay *et al.*, 1983a). From this it appears that long-standing exposure to high plasma renin levels amplifies the immediate pressor response. This may therefore represent the clinical counterpart of the 'slow' pressor response to angiotensin II (see below).

Hypertension in Advanced Renal Failure

Hypertension in the majority of patients on intermittent dialysis for advanced renal disease is sodium-dependent. However, a minority of patients with advanced renal failure develop a severe form of hypertension which is not relieved by reducing body sodium, although it can be controlled by bilateral nephrectomy. Kolff *et al.* (1964) suggested that secretion of pressor material by damaged kidneys was responsible. Hyperreninaemia seems the most likely explanation in most situations (Wilkinson *et al.*, 1970; Weidmann *et al.*, 1976). High plasma renin levels could be a consequence of attempts to control blood pressure by sodium and fluid withdrawal. However, Weidmann and Maxwell (1975) noted that bilateral nephrectomy reduced blood pressure in 92 patients with elevated renin, and failed to reduce it in only five. Even in this minority of cases it is possible that compliance with dietary sodium control was not adequate. Further evidence incriminating the renin-angiotensin system was produced when it was shown that blood pressure fell substantially with infusion of saralasin (MacGregor and Dawes, 1976). It therefore seems that the normal control of renin secretion is disturbed in some patients with severe renal disease, and that this results in renin hypersecretion and hypertension.

Renovascular and Renal Parenchymal Disease

Hypertension may occur in combination with unilateral or bilateral renal disease. The renin-angiotensin system probably plays at least a partial role in some cases, although the extent of this role is still controversial.

Two major difficulties occur in analysing the role of renin in renal hypertension in man. First, atheromatous renal artery stenosis is frequently found at necropsy in patients who are normotensive (Heptinstall, 1974), and since essential hypertension is a common disorder, the association between the two must often be coincidental. The second problem is that it is rarely possible to follow the natural history of human hypertension from its outset to the phase of sustained high blood pressure levels which may occur many years later. As there are important differences in the pathophysiology of early and late experimental renovascular hypertension, studies of clinical reno-vascular hypertension may only throw light on the latter stage of the illness, and may not provide a great deal of information about the earlier stages of hypertension. These difficulties can be overcome by means of animal studies of experimental hypertension, but there are species differences in the relative importance of the processes that control blood pressure and therefore it is at times difficult to extrapolate from experimental hypertension to man.

There is a transient rise in plasma renin immediately after the induction of renal artery stenosis: this reflects the normal physiological response to a fall in perfusion pressure. The short-lived elevation of plasma renin in this situation is probably responsible for the postoperative rise in blood pressure that occurs since this transient hypertension can be prevented by converting enzyme inhibition (Miller *et al.*, 1975). After a latent period of variable duration, blood pressure gradually rises again over a period of days or weeks. This phase is sometimes classified as acute but is probably preferably called early to avoid confusion with the postoperative phase of hypertension. Early-phase hypertension is usually associated with elevated plasma renin in the Goldblatt 2-kidney 1-clip model so long as hypertension is severe: renin elevation is much more variable where hypertension is modest (Miksche *et al.*, 1970; Mohring *et al.*, 1975; Morton and Wallace, 1983). After blood-pressure elevation has been present for a period of time, plasma renin levels begin to decline in experimental Goldblatt 2-kidney hypertension. There is marked species variation in duration of the early hyperreninaemic phase. Renin is elevated for up to 3 weeks in the dog (Watkins *et al.*, 1976), is elevated to a modest degree only in the rabbit (Lohmeier and Davis, 1976), and in the rat it is elevated for several weeks or months (Miksche *et al.*, 1970; Morton and Wallace, 1983). After hypertension of more than 4 months' duration ('chronic'), plasma renin is usually (although not always) normal (Russell *et al.*, 1983). Changes in plasma renin are reflected by changes in the depressor response to angiotensin II blockade with saralasin. During the early phase of hypertension, when plasma renin is usually elevated, blood pressure shows an immediate fall in response to infusions of saralasin, whereas after 3 or 4 months' hypertension no depressor response is observed (Bing *et al.*, 1981a).

Patients with renal artery stenosis only come under observation when hypertension is established. It is therefore not possible to say whether all such patients pass through a phase of elevated plasma renin or not. There is no agreement on the proportion of patients who have surgically correctable renovascular hypertension in the presence of elevated plasma renin. According to some groups, elevated plasma renin is found in the majority of such patients (Bath *et al.*, 1968; Vaughan *et al.*, 1974), whereas, according to others, plasma renin is elevated in only a minority (MacKay *et al.*, 1983b). However, there is no doubt that in a proportion of patients with renal artery stenosis, corrective renal artery surgery restores blood pressure to normal, despite plasma renin levels that fall within the normal range preoperatively. Conversely, in some patients, corrective surgery restores a high plasma renin to normal, although blood pressure remains elevated (Maskill *et al.*, 1980).

There are three possibilities to explain these changes.

(1) Other factors independent of the renin-angiotensin system could maintain blood pressure and such factors could become progressively more important with the passage of time.
(2) Renin hypersecretion might act as an essential trigger activating other processes which are then responsible for blood pressure maintenance.
(3) The renin-angiotensin system could still be responsible for blood pressure maintenance, even in chronic experimental hypertension, despite normal plasma renin levels and in the absence of a significant blood pressure response to acute renin-angiotensin system blockade.

One possible blood pressure maintenance system that could be triggered by an initial renin-induced hypertension is vascular hypertrophy.

Vascular Hypertrophy. Increased perfusion pressure leads to structural changes in precapillary resistance vessels. The initial change is smooth-muscle hypertrophy (within 1 to 2 weeks), followed by an increase in collagen and other interstitial material (Ooshima *et al.*, 1974). Precapillary vessel hypertrophy has important consequences for hypertension. Vasoconstriction is initiated from the adventitial side of the muscle layer where the neuroeffector junctions lie, and there is subsequent activation of the inner layers by myogenic spread of excitation. Thus the wall mass is pushed inwards on contraction to narrow the luminal diameter. As a consequence, thickening of the wall, which increases wall-to-lumen ratio, amplifies the increase in resistance produced by vasoconstrictor stimuli (Folkow *et al.*, 1973; Folkow, 1982). There are two features of hypertension-induced vessel hypertrophy. Resistance to flow is higher, even at maximal vasodilation, and pressor dose-response curves are steeper since, for any given degree of vascular smooth muscle shortening induced by agents such as noradrenaline, a greater increase in resistance to flow is produced. Vascular hypertrophy therefore produces a generalised (non-specific) hypersensitivity to pressor agents such as nor-adrenaline and angiotensin II (Folkow *et al.*, 1973).

Vascular hypertrophy could therefore act as a blood pressure maintaining system triggered by angiotensin II induced hypertension. This would explain some observations reported by Freis *et al.* (1972). When SHR are treated with antihypertensive medication during the period in which arterial pressure would normally be expected to increase, the pressure remains substantially lower even when the medication is discontinued, suggesting that a vicious circle is normally established by which hypertension induces changes which then maintain hypertension. There are, however, good reasons to believe that a combination of renin hypersecretion and vascular hypertrophy does not provide the complete explanation for blood pressure maintenance in reno-vascular hypertension. Thus regression of smooth muscle hypertrophy occurs where blood pressure is restored to normal over a 2- or 3-week period (Lundgren *et al.*, 1974). When hypertension is long-standing, the process is slower and incomplete (Lundgren and Weiss, 1979). However, when experimental renovascular hypertension is corrected by removal of a constricting clip or by unilateral nephrectomy of the ischaemic kidney, peripheral resistance decreases to normal values within 24 h even after hypertension has been present for many months (Russell *et al.*, 1983). It therefore seems that, whatever role vascular hypertrophy plays, it can readily be overcome when renovascular hypertension is corrected. This is not of course to argue that vascular hypertrophy is unimportant in the steady-state control of blood pressure in renovascular hypertension.

'Slow' Pressor Response to Angiotensin II. It has long been known that when low doses of angiotensin II, which are not sufficient to cause an acute rise in blood pressure, are infused into patients (or animals), there is a gradual rise in

blood pressure over a period of days (Dickinson and Lawrence, 1963). It seems likely that a similar phenomenon is responsible for blood pressure levels that are disproportionately high relative to concurrent plasma angiotensin II, in patients with renin-secreting tumours (MacKay *et al.*, 1983a). There is still no certainty, however, as to the mechanism for this. Several hypotheses have been advanced.

(1)   Sodium retention. The slow pressor response to angiotensin II in dogs can be prevented by dietary salt restriction (Muirhead *et al.*, 1975) and exacerbated by dietary salt loading (Cowley and DeClue, 1976). More detailed studies of the relationship between angiotensin and sodium excretion have been carried out (DeClue *et al.*, 1978). Normal dogs showed a trivial pressor response to prolonged isotonic sodium chloride infusions. However, when low doses of angiotensin II were infused as well, a marked pressor response occurred. This was reversed by frusemide, and when frusemide was discontinued, hypertension returned, although the urinary output of sodium was the same in hypertensive angiotensin/saline-infused animals as in the normotensive saline-infused animals. It was therefore concluded that angiotensin resulted in a shift of the pressure-natriuresis curve, leading to inhibition of the normal natriuretic response to elevated pressure. In a later study, low doses of angiotensin II were infused directly into the renal artery. This produced a reduction in urinary sodium excretion and a much greater pressor response than would have been expected on the basis of calculated peripheral plasma angiotensin II levels (Lohmeier and Cowley, 1979). An alternative possibility which would explain the antinatriuretic action of subpressor doses of angiotensin II is stimulation of aldosterone by angiotensin II, but this is unlikely as the slow pressor response to angiotensin II is not prevented by adrenalectomy and cannot be reproduced by chronic aldosterone infusion into normal or nephrectomised dogs (Lohmeier *et al.*, 1978). In other studies the slow pressor response was not blocked by spironolactone, nor associated with elevation of plasma aldosterone (DeClue *et al.*, 1978).

Brown *et al.* (1981) have argued against involvement of renal excretion of sodium in the development of the slow pressor response in rats. During the development of hypertension, there was no evidence of sodium retention; neither was there a significant natriuresis during reversal of hypertension after discontinuation of the angiotensin infusion (Brown *et al.*, 1981). It could, however, be argued that angiotensin II was preventing the anticipated negative sodium balance which would normally have accompanied elevated pressure, and on current evidence the direct renal action of angiotensin II on sodium excretion appears to be an important factor in the slow pressor response to angiotensin II.

(2)   Other workers have postulated an interaction between angiotensin II and the sympathetic nervous system. Thus angiotensin II infused directly into

vertebral arteries produces a pressor response by an action on vaso-motor neurones in the area postrema of the medulla oblongata and the subfornical region of the third ventricle (Buckley and Jandhyala, 1977). Dickinson (1981) has argued for a primary disturbance in these centres as a cause of essential hypertension, and some characteristics of early essential hypertension (e.g. increased heart rate and cardiac output, and decreased plasma volume) are consistent with a slight increase in sympathetic activity. There is, however, no evidence to implicate angiotensin II in the mechanism postulated by this persuasive hypothesis, and there is no direct evidence that this centrally mediated cardiovascular effect of angiotensin II has the necessary slow characteristics.

Angiotensin II also potentiates the vasoconstrictor action of sympathetic nerve stimulation (Malik and Nasjletti, 1976; Zimmerman, 1981), so acutely subpressor doses of angiotensin II could produce a slow pressor effect through increased sympthetic nervous activity. There is no direct evidence in support of such a hypothesis but the blood pressure fall produced by converting enzyme inhibition is associated with a decrease in baroreceptor-mediated sympathetic reflexes (Clough *et al.*, 1982).

(3) Pressor sensitivity to angiotensin II at the peripheral vascular level could be enhanced. Since the slow pressor effect is seen with angiotensin II and not with noradrenaline, specific receptor-mediated hypersensitivity would have to be involved. Direct measurement of angiotensin receptors suggests, however, that down- rather than up-regulation of receptors occurs as a result of increased agonist concentration (see below), and this explanation therefore seems an unlikely one.

Does the slow pressor response to angiotensin II play a role in renovascular hypertension? Theoretically the slow pressor response to angiotensin II provides a mechanism which would account for the renin-angiotensin system maintaining elevated blood pressure despite the presence of near-normal circulating plasma renin and angiotensin II levels (Brown *et al.*, 1979; MacKay *et al.*, 1983a). This is not an easy hypothesis to test. However, one study does favour such a role for the renin-angiotensin system. When hypertension in the Goldblatt 2-kidney 1-clip model in the rat is reversed by removal of the constricting clip or by nephrectomy, the fall in blood pressure occurs over the next 6 to 12 h. The characteristics of this slow fall of blood pressure can be mimicked precisely by discontinuing a prolonged infusion of angiotensin II into normal rats. Discontinuation of a noradrenaline infusion on the other hand produces an immediate fall in blood pressure, which is quite dissimilar in characteristics (Kumar *et al.*, 1984). A similarly slow blood pressure fall should also be produced by angiotensin blockade. Riegger *et al.* (1977) reported that the fall in blood pressure observed in Goldblatt 2-kidney 1-clip hypertensive rats infused with saralasin was progressive over a 12 h period, and not related to basal angiotensin II levels. However, this observation has not been confirmed (se e.g. Bing *et al.*, 1981a) and the maximal fall in blood pressure with saralasin occurs within 30 min, even in chronically hypertensive rats. This pattern of response is different from that observed as a result of declipping or removal of the ischaemic kidney.

Increased Responsiveness to Angiotensin II. 'Normal' levels of angiotensin II could give rise to hypertension if vascular contractile responsiveness were increased. Non-specific hyperresponsiveness to vasoconstrictor agents (such as angiotensin and noradrenaline) as a result of vascular hypertrophy occurs when hypertension has been present for prolonged periods (Folkow *et al.*, 1973; Folkow, 1982). In addition, local humoral and biochemical factors may produce non-specific hypersensitivity through changes in chemomechanical coupling within the vascular smooth muscle. Such non-specific hypersensitivity to both angiotensin II and noradrenaline has been shown in isolated tissue beds before vascular hypertrophy has developed in renovascular hypertension (Collis and Alps, 1975), DOC hypertension in the rat (Beilin *et al.*, 1970) and the pig (Berecek *et al.*, 1980), SHR (Lais and Brody, 1978) and in Goldblatt 1-kidney hypertension in the rabbit (Ichikawa *et al.*, 1978). In other studies it has been possible to demonstrate increased responsiveness to the renin-angiotensin system after blood pressure has been restored to normal by removal of the clip in Goldblatt 2-kidney hypertension (Skulan *et al.*, 1974; Ten Berg and de Jong, 1980). Michelakis *et al.* (1975) reported that plasma from hypertensive patients enhances the pressor response of bilaterally nephrectomised rats to both noradrenaline and angiotensin II. Although it was suggested that this material acted by modulation of angiotensin receptor affinity, it seems more likely, in view of its lack of specificity, that it acts at a point distal to the receptor site.

The non-specific hyperresponsiveness demonstrated in these studies suggests that changes in chemomechanical coupling within the vascular smooth muscle cell, perhaps involving alterations in cytosolic calcium, may increase the contractile response to pressor agents such as noradrenaline and angiotensin II. In the case of DOC hypertension, a direct effect on ouabain-resistant sodium movements is a possibility (Bohr, 1981). In the other forms of hypertension the nature of the sensitising process remains obscure.

It is still uncertain whether specific hyperresponsiveness to angiotensin II (as distinct from the slow pressor response to acutely subpressor doses of angiotensin II discussed above) occurs. If so, this would suggest changes at the receptor level. Collis and Vanhoutte (1978) reported increased responsiveness to angiotensin II but not to electrical nerve stimulation or exogenous noradrenaline in the isolated kidney of rats with renovascular hypertension. Measurements of mesenteric artery angiotensin II receptors suggest that important changes in number can occur. Thus exposure of the vascular bed to high circulating concentrations of angiotensin II results in down-regulation of receptors (Gunther *et al.*, 1980a, b; Aguilera and Catt, 1981). This effect probably accounts in part for the increased response to angiotensin II produced by salt loading and the decreased response produced by salt depletion. However, it is difficult to distinguish between the consequences of such down-regulation of receptors and increased occupancy of available receptors by endogenous angiotensin II, since both of these would result in decreased sensitivity to exogenous angiotensin II. Such decreased overall pressor responsiveness, which can be reversed by converting enzyme inhibition, can be demonstrated in the early phase of Goldblatt 2-kidney hypertension and appears to outweigh the consequences of any morphological change which would have the opposite effects on vascular sensitivity (Marks *et al.*, 1982). Pressor dose-response studies in both experimental and mineralo-corticoid and renovascular hypertension in the rat indicate that changes in endogenous renin and angiotensin II play a major role in the alterations in responsiveness to angiotensin II (Bing *et al.*, 1982).

One other piece of evidence argues against vascular hyperresponsiveness to angiotensin II as a mechanism responsible for renovascular hypertension. There is a close relationship between the fall in blood pressure produced by angiotensin II blockade with saralasin, and initial plasma renin and angiotensin II measurements (MacDonald *et al.*, 1975; Streeten *et al.*, 1975; Bing *et al.*, 1981a). This applies to infusions of up to 36 h with saralasin. Studies using prolonged ACE inhibition in Goldblatt hypertension have yielded rather different results with a progressive fall in blood pressure (Bengis and Coleman, 1979); even the immediate pressor response to converting enzyme inhibition is not closely correlated with plasma renin in this model (Bing *et al.*, 1981a). It is possible, however, that this represents additional vasodepressor effects of converting enzyme inhibition, rather than renin-angiotensin blockade.

Renin-Angiotensin Blockade in Renovascular Hypertension. As noted previously, high renin models of renovascular hypertension show a depressor response to renin-angiotensin blockade. Sustained angiotensin converting enzyme (ACE) inhibition with teprotide prevented development of hyper-tension in the dog Goldblatt 1-kidney 1-clip model (Miller *et al.*, 1975). Deforrest *et al.* (1982) reported similar observations in Goldblatt 2-kidney 1-clip hypertension in the rat. Although such studies are consistent with the concept of a role for the renin-angiotensin system, they certainly do not prove such a role, since the mechanism of blood pressure reduction in such studies may well differ from the mechanism of blood pressure elevation in the first place.

Evidence against the Renin-Angiotensin System as a Sole Mediator of Renovascular Hypertension. Goldblatt 2-kidney 1-clip hypertension can be reversed by removal of the constricting clip under renin-angiotensin blockade either with captopril or with saralasin (Russell *et al.*, 1982a). The characteristics of the blood-pressure fall are not modified, despite the fact that the renin-angiotensin system has been blocked both before, during and after the surgical procedure. It seems likely, therefore, that other vasodepressor systems participate in the blood pressure fall at least during the 24 h after surgery. In another study it was possible to show that plasma angiotensin II was significantly correlated with arterial pressure in Goldblatt 2-kidney 1-clip hypertensive rats. However, the time relations of the rise in plasma angiotensin II and blood pressure were rather different (Morton and Wallace, 1983). Thus, two weeks after clipping the renal artery of the rat, plasma renin and angiotensin II had fallen from transiently high postoperative values to mean values no different from those observed in controls, although blood pressure remained high. Only from the fourth week after operation did mean values for plasma renin and angiotensin II again rise, although to a variable extent.

Vascular Renin. Renin and other components of the renin-angiotensin system accumulating within the resistance vessel wall could result in the local generation of angiotensin II. Thus, blood pressure could be maintained by the renin-angiotensin system independently of circulating angiotensin II. Renin-like activity can be detected in the aortic wall and in the wall of the large arteries (Swales, 1979), and immunofluorescent studies have demonstrated renin within the media of smaller-resistance vessels (Swales *et al.*, 1983).

Blood pressure changes induced by rapid fluctuations in plasma renin, which can be produced, for instance, by renin injections or by bilateral nephrectomy, correlate much better with changes in arterial-wall renin-like activity than with plasma renin (Swales, 1979; Loudon *et al.*, 1983). If such locally generated angiotensin II is a final determinant of blood pressure, this would explain the need to obtain very high plasma levels of saralasin (several orders of magnitude greater than those of concurrent plasma angiotensin II) to produce a maximal depressor response compared with the low dosage needed to block exogenous angiotensin II (Swales, 1979). In some studies, however, it has not been possible to detect a divergence between plasma and aortic-wall renin-like activity except in non-steady-state conditions (Loudon *et al.*, 1983): this would suggest that local accumulation of renin could not explain the renovascular hypertension in the presence of normal angiotensin II levels. However, others have demonstrated a divergence between plasma and aortic-wall renin in SHR (Barrett *et al.*, 1978; Asaad and Antonaccio, 1982). In another study an angiotensin I forming enzyme was described with kinetic characterisics that suggested that it was distinct from plasma renin (Rosenthal *et al.*, 1984). Such work supports the concept of locally synthesised renin, independent of plasma renin. At the same time it has to be borne in mind that other tissue proteases may have a renin-like activity, generating angiotensin from substrate *in vitro* (but perhaps not active in this respect *in vivo*). Fordis *et al.* (1983) demonstrated renin within the blood vessel wall which was derived from plasma, and which disappeared following bilateral nephrectomy: other renin-like activity appeared to be due to non-specific tissue proteases. This does not mean, of course, that small amounts of renin could not be synthesised locally at critical sites and produce a vasoconstrictor effect without detectable changes in the overall renin content of the vessel. Dzau *et al.* (1984) found that renin messenger RNA was present in several tissues, including submandibular gland, testis, kidney, small intestine, spleen, brain, liver and colon, suggesting that the renin gene was expressed in a wide variety of tissues, although with unknown functional consequences. On present evidence, it seems unlikely that blood pressure is maintained in steady-state conditions by high levels of vascular wall renin in the presence of a normal or low plasma renin. The close correlation between the depressor response to renin-angiotensin blockade and plasma renin would support such a view.

It would, nevertheless, be surprising if the renin-angiotensin system did not play any role in renovascular hypertension and particularly in hypertension associated with high plasma renin, although it is likely that other systems are involved, including the sympathetic nervous system (modulating sodium excretion), vascular hypertrophy, and the renal vasodepressor system (see below).

Renin-Angiotensin System in other Models of Hypertension

Plasma renin concentration and activity are elevated in a minority of patients with essential hypertension (high-renin essential hypertension). Hyper-reninaemia in such patients appears to be a secondary change and not causal. In some cases hyperreninaemia is associated with malignant hypertension and may reflect fibrinoid necrosis in the juxtaglomerular apparatus. Another possibility is pressure natriuresis in patients with severe hypertension (Barraclough, 1966). Patients with less severe degrees of essential hypertension associated with high renin levels have been found to have increased plasma noradrenaline levels and increased responsiveness of plasma noradrenaline to postural stimulation (Esler *et al.*, 1977, 1978). It seems reasonable to implicate the sympathetic nervous system in such cases.

In experimental coarctation of the aorta in rats, the pattern of change in plasma renin is analogous with that in Goldblatt 2-kidney 1-clip hypertension, i.e. an initial elevation of renin followed by a return to normal values (Yagi *et al.*, 1968). Both normal and elevated plasma renin levels have been reported in patients with coarctation, and the renin response to stimuli such as diuretics may be increased (Ribeiro and Krakoff, 1976). A fall in blood pressure during saralasin infusion occurs in some patients (Ribeiro and Krakoff, 1976; De Leeuw and Birkenhager, 1983b). In general, however, plasma renin levels are probably not of the same magnitude as those observed in, for example, hypertension associated with renal artery stenosis, but just as in that condition, renin may be more important in the early than in the chronic stages of hypertension. One report documents a significant fall in blood pressure (in five patients with hypertension due to Cushing's syndrome) produced by saralasin (Dalakos *et al.*, 1978). However, this was only demonstrated after salt depletion and it seems likely that the elevated levels of angiotensin II are not alone sufficient to account for hypertension. Renin levels are also somewhat elevated in the hypertension sometimes associated with hyperparathyroidism (Brinton *et al.*, 1975). Again, however, it seems unlikely that renin levels are sufficiently elevated to produce hypertension.

Humoral Antihypertensive Role of the Kidney

The renal transplantation studies reviewed above indicate that a normal kidney exerts a blood-pressure-lowering action in several models with experimental hypertension, and this action did not appear to be mediated by sodium excretion. Muirhead and co-workers (1960) implicated the renal medulla in the non-excretory antihypertensive function of the kidney. Renoprival hypertension in dogs was alleviated by the presence of the kidney even when a ureterocaval anastamosis was present. When the ureter was ligated, however, the kidney failed to reduce blood pressure. In the former case the renal medulla was intact whereas in the latter papillary necrosis was detected. Muirhead's group (Muirhead *et al.*, 1972a, 1977; Muirhead, 1980) carried out autotransplants from fragmented renal medulla in 1-clip, 1-kidney Goldblatt hypertension in rats and rabbits and in renoprival hypertension in dogs. In each case it was possible to demonstrate prevention or reversal of hypertension. Histological examination of the transplants showed proliferation of renomedullary interstitial cells with lipid-containing granules.

Renomedullary interstitial cells can be grown as a monolayer culture, and cultured cells lower blood pressure in Goldblatt 1- and 2-kidney hypertension, DOC-salt hypertension, and angiotensin-salt hypertension (Muirhead *et al.*, 1972a; Muirhead, 1980). The beneficial effect of renomedullary transplants has been confirmed by other groups (Manthorpe, 1973, 1975; Susic *et al.*, 1976). One study demonstrated that the fall in blood pressure observed in 1-kidney 1-clip hypertension in rats was associated with a fall in cardiac output (Susic *et al.*, 1978); a similar haemodynamic change has been detected with transplantation of a normal kidney into rats with renovascular hypertension (Rosas *et al.*, 1964). Interstitial-cell granularity is reduced in DOC salt, Goldblatt 1- and 2-kidney hypertension and partial nephrectomy, and in SHR (Ishii and Tobian, 1969; Muehrcke *et al.*, 1969; Bohman, 1980). However granularity was closely correlated with the medullary sodium gradient in kidneys from rats with Goldblatt 2-kidney 1-clip hypertension (Ishii and Tobian, 1969), and in another study reduction in granularity only occurred after the onset of hypertension: the possibility was raised that these changes are secondary to alterations in renal medullary blood flow (Muehrcke *et al.*, 1969). A later study showed a better correlation between operative trauma and interstitial cell granulation than between blood pressure and interstitial cell granulation in Goldblatt 2-kidney hypertension (Latta *et al.*, 1975). Interstitial granular cell counts may not be a sensitive or precise measure of interstitial-cell lipid secretory function, and it has been claimed that measurement of volume density of interstitial-cell granules is preferable (Muirhead, 1983).

Renal Medullectomy. The renal medulla can be removed surgically and the resultant hypertension in sodium-loaded rats is alleviated by medullary transplants (Susic and Kentera, 1980). A readily available and reproducible model of renomedullary hypertension is produced by selective ablation of the renal papilla by the compound 2-bromoethylamine hydrobromide. This produces hypertension in normal rats (Bing *et al.*, 1983) and is reported as exacerbating Goldblatt 2-kidney 1-clip hypertension (Heptinstall *et al.*, 1975). Hypertension in this chemically medullectomised model is attributable neither to sodium retention nor to renin hypersecretion (Bing *et al.*, 1983; Taverner *et al.*, 1985). Treatment with 2-bromoethylamine hydrobromide inhibits the antihypertensive action of renomedullary tissue transplants into rats with renovascular hypertension (Susic *et al.*, 1983). Chemical renal-medullectomy of rats with Goldblatt 2-kidney 1-clip hypertension, unlike pharmacological pretreatment with renin-angiotensin blockade or indomethacin, partially inhibits the fall in blood pressure observed when the renal artery clip is removed (Bing *et al.*, 1981b). Chemical renal medullectomy therefore offers an interesting demonstration of the circulatory importance of an intact renal medulla.

Renomedullary Interstitial Cell Secretion. Three groups of compounds which may have a circulatory action are secreted by the renal medulla.

(a) A glucocorticoid-stimulated peptide which is a cyclo-oxygenase inhibitor has been isolated from the medium when renomedullary interstitial cells are cultured (Russo-Marie *et al.*, 1980). This compound may have important consequences in controlling the local action of prostaglandins, which are important in regulating sodium and water excretion (Dunn and Hood, 1977); see also Chapter 5.

(b) Renomedullary cells in culture secrete large amounts of PGE_2 and lesser amounts of $PGF_{2\alpha}$ (Muirhead *et al.*, 1972b; Muirhead, 1983). Secretion is stimulated by angiotensin II, bradykinin and arginine vasopressin (Zusman and Keiser, 1977). Although PGE_2 and to a lesser extent $PGF_{2\alpha}$ can be detected in the renal venous effluent of anaesthetised dogs after the acute induction of ischaemia (McGiff *et al.*, 1970), it is unlikely that the vasodepressor action of the renal medulla is exerted through prostaglandin release. Indomethacin treatment has little effect upon total vascular resistance or blood pressure in the rat (Gerber and Nies, 1979). Further, indomethacin pretreatment does not alter the quantity of vasodepressor material in renal venous effluent after release of renal ischaemia in rat 1-kidney 1-clip hypertension (Muirhead *et al.*, 1982), neither does it inhibit the fall in blood pressure produced by unclipping in Goldblatt 2-kidney 1-clip hypertension (Russell *et al.*, 1982b), whereas chemical renal-medullectomy does have such an inhibitory effect (Bing *et al.*, 1981b).

(c) Two groups of antihypertensive non-prostanoid lipids have been isolated from the renal medulla and from renal venous effluent (Muirhead, 1980, 1983; Muirhead *et al.*, 1982). The antihypertensive polar renomedullary lipid (APRL) consists of a group of 1-0 alkyl ethers of phosphatidyl choline, with the predominant compounds having side-chain lengths C16: 0 (67%), C16: 1 (16%) and C18: 1 (11%). It produces both an acute blood-pressure-lowering effect within 2-3 s and a slow depressor effect lasting 30-60 h. A greater vasodepressor effect is observed in SHR. In lower doses the effect is mediated by vasodilatation, whereas in higher doses cardiac output is reduced as well (Prewitt *et al.*, 1980; Muirhead, 1983). Direct application to the rat cremaster muscle revealed a dilator effect on both arterioles and venules: the constrictor response to noradrenaline (but not other agonists) was blocked, suggesting that APRL has an α-adrenergic antagonist action (Smith *et al.*, 1981). Reflex tachycardia occurs in association with the fall in blood pressure induced by APRL (Muirhead *et al.*, 1983).

Antihypertensive neutral renomedullary lipid (ANRL) also has both acute and prolonged depressor effects, although there is a latent period of 2-3 min before any action is seen and the blood pressure fall is more gradual. However, this compound lowers both heart rate and directly measured sympathetic nerve traffic (Muirhead *et al.*, 1983), suggesting a direct effect with inhibition of baroreceptor-mediated circulatory reflexes.

Role of Renomedullary Lipids in Reversal of Hypertension. Chemically renal-medullectomised rats show partial inhibition of the fall in blood pressure produced by removal of the renal artery clip in the Goldblatt 2-kidney 1-clip model (Bing *et al.*, 1981b). This suggests a role for the renal medulla in reversal of renovascular hypertension. Muirhead *et al.* (1982) examined this possibility by studying the venous effluent from the unclipped kidney in 1-kidney 1-clip Goldblatt-hypertensive rats. As blood pressure fell, an ANRL-like lipid (measured by bioassay after extraction) was detectable in the effluent, and the renomedullary interstitial cells degranulated. Gothberg *et al.* (1982a) perfused isolated clipped kidneys from rats with Goldblatt 2-kidney 1-clip hypertension with blood from the circulation of conscious normotensive rats. Removal of the constricting clip produced a profound fall in blood pressure due to a reduction in cardiac output, with no tachycardia. It was concluded that a humoral agent was released which had a direct inhibitory effect on sympathetic activity. Later work demonstrated direct suppression of tonic sympathetic nerve activity (Gothberg *et al.*, 1982b). There is therefore strong supporting evidence for ANRL as a mediator of the blood pressure fall following surgical correction of Goldblatt hypertension. As Gothberg *et al.* (1982a) point out, there is one major anomaly in these findings. Whereas the fall in blood pressure is mediated by a fall in cardiac output in these studies and the previously reviewed studies of renal transplantation, the fall in blood pressure with declipping of the renal artery in Goldblatt hypertension is associated with a fall in total peripheral resistance, although in both cases no tachycardia was seen (Hallback-Nordlander *et al.*, 1979; Russell *et al.*, 1983). Whether this reflects measurement at different periods, or whether it reflects differences in hypertensive as opposed to normotensive animals as Gothberg *et al.* suggest, is uncertain, but the evidence from these divergent studies indicates that renomedullary lipids have a central inhibitory action resulting in blood pressure fall.

Other Vasoactive Renal Secretions

Several other putative renal humoral secretions have an action upon blood pressure. These include nephrotensin (Grollman and Krishnamurty, 1973), corticotensin (Risler and Fasciolo, 1974), renopressin (Skeggs *et al.*, 1977) and tonin (Boucher *et al.*, 1978). Only the last named has been satisfactorily characterised biochemically. In addition, Michelakis *et al.* (1975) have described a circulating factor in patients with essential hypertension and experimental hypertension which potentiates the pressor response to agents such as angiotensin II. So far no satisfactory role has been established for any of these substances in either experimental (Huang *et al.*, 1978) or clinical hypertension.

Sympathetic Nervous System and the Kidneys in Hypertension

There is good evidence for increased sympathetic nerve activity in SHR (Folkow, 1976). Direct measurement of renal nerve activity shows a correlation with blood pressure in SHR cross-breeds (Judy *et al.*, 1976). These phenomena have been implicated in the pathogenesis of hypertension in SHR with the hypothesis that enhanced cardiovascular reactivity and transient blood-pressure changes induce structural hypertrophy of the resistance vessels (Folkow, 1982).

Winternitz and Oparil (1982) attributed a specific role to the renal nerves; renal denervation delayed the onset and slowed the rise in blood pressure in SHR, and the blood-pressure-lowering action of renal denervation was associated with natriuresis whereas escape produced by reinnervation was associated with sodium retention. Renal denervation in the early stages (3 weeks) of DOC-salt hypertension also produced a natriuresis and attenuation of the blood-pressure rise: at 10 weeks no effect was seen (Katholi *et al.*, 1983). The beneficial effect on blood pressure at 3 weeks was associated with an inhibition of the normal elevation in wall-to-lumen ratio in the renal precapillary arterioles produced by DOC and salt. These authors therefore suggest that denervation acts by shifting the pressure-natriuresis curve, as a result of the intrarenal haemodynamic changes produced. There is some direct support for the view that sympathetic nerve activity is increased in DOC-salt hypertension, based upon measurements of splanchnic nerve activity (Iriuchijima *et al.*, 1975) and demonstration of elevated plasma noradrenaline levels (Reid *et al.*, 1975; Dargie *et al.*, 1977b). Renal denervation also attenuated Goldblatt 1- and 2-kidney 1-clip hypertension in the rat; the effect was not associated with natriuresis, but was associated with a fall in plasma noradrenaline (Katholi *et al.*, 1982a, b). These findings were interpreted as indicating that renal afferent nerve activity was important in regulating efferent sympathetic activity to the cardiovascular system (and hence peripheral resistance) through central connections. Although other workers have confirmed the elevation of plasma noradrenaline in Goldblatt 1-kidney 1-clip hypertension, this finding is debatable in the 2-kidney model, where there is otherwise no evidence of increased sympathetic activity when either central or peripheral catecholamines are measured (Dargie *et al.*, 1977a). It should also be noted that in these studies changes in afferent activity were assumed rather than demonstrated. It is difficult to see how afferent nerves would mediate the blood pressure-lowering action of a transplanted kidney, and also difficult to exclude the possibility that interruption of renal efferent activity activates a renal vasodepressor or inhibits the renal pressor system.

If confirmed, it is possible that these findings may have relevance to essential hypertension in man, where there is some evidence for increased sympathetic nerve activity (Dickinson, 1981), based on studies of circulating noradrenaline levels which have yielded results with a trend favouring increased levels in hypertensive patients (Goldstein, 1981). One major warning has been made by Folkow's group in this context (Folkow *et al.*, 1983). Both positive and negative evidence on the possible role of the sympathetic nervous system based upon alterations in plasma noradrenaline should be regarded with caution since resistance-vessel innervation makes overall a relatively small contribution to total noradrenaline production.

Recent work has suggested a region of the brain which appears to be critical for the development of several models of hypertension (Brody *et al.*, 1983). The AV3V region is situated in the periventricular tissue surrounding the anterior part of the third ventricle. This area appears to play a role in fluid-balance regulation as well as blood pressure. Lesions here inhibit the pressor response to angiotensin II and hypertonic sodium chloride, and protect rats against Goldblatt 1- and 2-kidney hypertension, DOC-salt hypertension and hypertension in Dahl sensitive rats. Lesions do not influence the development of hypertension in SHR. The mechanisms by which this lesion has such widespread effects are unknown, although it has been suggested that vasopressin or the sodium-pump inhibitory 'natriuretic hormone' may play a role (Brody *et al.*, 1983; Haddy, 1984; see also Chapter 6).

The Kidney in Hypertension: Is an Integrated Approach Possible?

Changes in renal function can elevate blood pressure by several mechanisms. Experimental and clinical models exist in which the prime cause is clear, i.e. hypersecretion of renin in patients with renin-secreting tumours, sodium retention in bilaterally nephrectomised patients and animals, and inhibition of renomedullary vasodepressor lipid secretion after chemical medullectomy. In other situations such as renovascular hypertension or mineralocorticoid hypertension, it is possible with less certainty to implicate renal mechanisms although these are by no means simple or straightforward. Two unanswered questions exist. How do the known pressor systems produce hypertension, and how do they interrelate? To the present reviewer, although Guyton's analysis of the physiology of hypertension has been of enormous value, his concept of the overriding importance of the renal excretion of sodium and water has been misleading and has led to attempts to force experimental data on hypertension into a conceptual straightjacket in which changes in sodium excretion are central. Undoubtedly an unmodified perfusion pressure natriuresis would negate any other pressor mechanism, but it seems clear that such modification of the perfusion-pressure natriuresis relationship is universal in hypertension and a readily accomplished secondary change rather than a primary one in most cases. As this review has shown, in some cases (such as the renin-angiotensin system) the pressor processes are well characterised whereas other systems (such as the renomedullary vasodepressor system) are not well defined at present. Bohr (1981) has commented that blood pressure, rather than vascular resistance or cardiac output, appears to be the regulated variable, and this makes it unlikely that a primary abnormality in the peripheral blood vessels or in cardiac function alone can be incriminated in hypertension. This naturally leads to the conclusion that whatever the primary abnormalities may be, integration occurs at the level of the brain vasomotor neurones, and these may play a role in regulating blood pressure in the hypertension of sustained hyperreninaemia and volume expansion. Work over the next decade will, it is hoped, be directed at determining how abnormalities in several different homeostatic processes produce the final result of elevated blood pressure.

References

Aaronson, P. and Van Breeman, C. (1981) 'Effects of Sodium Gradient Manipulation upon Cellular Calcium, 45Ca Fluxes and Cellular Sodium in the Guinea Pig *Taeni coli*', *J. Physiol. (Lond.)*, *319*, 443–61

Aguilera, G. and Catt, K. (1981) 'Regulation of Vascular Angiotensin II Receptors in the Rat during Altered Sodium Intake', *Circ. Res.*, *49*, 751–8

Anderson, R.J., Gambertoglio, J.G. and Schrier, R.W. (1976) 'Fate of Drugs in Renal Failure', in B.M. Brenner and F.C. Rector (eds), *The Kidney*, W.B. Saunders, Philadelphia, pp.1911–48

Arendshorst, W.J. and Beierwaltes, W.H. (1979) 'Renal and Nephron Hemodynamics in

Spontaneously Hypertensive Rats', *Am. J. Physiol.*, *236*, F246–51

Asaad, M.M. and Antonaccio, M.J. (1982) 'Vascular Wall Renin in Spontaneously Hypertensive Rats. Potential Relevance to Hypertension Maintenance and Antihypertensive Effect of Captopril', *Hypertension*, 4, 487–93

Azar, S., Tobian, L. and Johnson, M.A. (1974) 'Glomerular, Efferent Arteriolar, Peritubular Capillary, and Tubular Pressures in Hypertension', *Am. J. Physiol.*, 227, 1045–50

Azar, S., Johnson, M.A., Iwai, J., Bruno, L. and Tobian, L. (1978) 'Single Nephron Dynamics in 'Post-salt' Rats with Chronic Hypertension', *J. Lab. Clin. Med.*, *91*, 156–66

Azar, S., Johnson, M.A., Scheinman, J., Bruno, L. and Tobian, L. (1979) 'Regulation of Glomerular Capillary Pressure and Filtration Rate in Young Kyoto Hypertensive Rats', *Clin. Sci.*, *56*, 203–9

Baer, P.G. and Bianchi, G. (1978) 'Renal Micropuncture Study of Normotensive and Milan Hypertensive Rats Before and After Development of Hypertension', *Kidney Int.*, *13*, 452–66

Bank, N., Aymedjian, H.S., Barsal, V.K. and Goldman, D.M. (1970) 'Effect of Acute Hypertension in Sodium Transport by the Distal Nephron', *Am. J. Physiol.*, *219*, 275–80

Barraclough, M.A. (1966) 'Sodium and Water Depletion with Acute Malignant Hypertension', *Am. J. Med.* 40, 265–72

Barrett, J.D., Eggena, P. and Sambhi, M.P. (1978) 'Partial Characterization of Aortic Renin in the Spontaneously Hypertensive Rat and its Interrelationship with Plasma Renin, Blood Pressure and Sodium Balance', *Clin. Sci. Mol. Med.*, 55, 261–70

Bath, N.M., Gunnells, J.C. and Robinson,R.R. (1968) 'Plasma Renin Activity in Renovascular Hypertension', *Am. J. Med.*, *45*, 381–90

Bauer, J.H. and Brooks, C.S. (1982) 'Body-fluid Composition in Normal and Hypertensive Man', *Clin. Sci.*, *62*, 43–9

Beilin, L.J., Wade, N.D., Honour, A.J. and Cole, T.J. (1970) 'Vascular Hyper-activity with Sodium Loading with Deoxycorticosterone-induced Hypertension in the Rat', *Clin. Sci.*, *39*, 793–810

Bengis, R.G. and Coleman, T.G. (1979) 'Antihypertensive Effect of Prolonged Blockade of Angiotensin Formation in Benign and Malignant One- and Two-kidney Goldblatt Hypertensive Rats', *Clin. Sci.*, 57, 53–62

Ben-Ishay, D., Knudson, K.D. and Dahl, L.K. (1967) 'Renal Function Studies in the Early Stage of Salt Hypertension in Rats', *Proc. Soc. Exp. Biol. Med.*, *125*, 515–18

Ben-Ishay, D., Knudsen, K.D. and Dahl, L.K. (1973) 'Exaggerated Response to Isotonic Saline Loading in Genetically Hypertension-prone Rats', *J. Lab. Clin. Med.*, *82*, 597–604

Berecek, K.H., Stocker, M. and Gross F. (1980) 'Changes in Renal Vascular Reactivity at Various Stages of Deoxycorticosterone Hypertension in Rats', *Circ. Res.*, *46*, 619–24

Beretta-Piccoli, C., Davies, D.L., Boddy, K., Brown, J.J., Cumming, A.M.M., East, B.W., Fraser, R., Lever, A.F, Padfield, P.L., Semple, P.F., Robertson, J.I.S., Weidmann, P. and Williams, E.D. (1982) 'Relation of Arterial Pressure with Body Sodium, Body Potassium and Plasma Potassium in Essential Hypertension', *Clin. Sci.*, *63*, 257–70

Beretta-Piccoli, C. Davies, D.L., Brown, J.J., Ferriss, B. Fraser, R., Lasuridis, A., Lever, A.F., Morton, J.J., Robertson, J.I.S., Semple, P.F. and Watts, R. (1983) 'Relation of Blood Pressure with Body and Plasma Electrolytes in Conn's Syndrome', *J. Hypertension*, *1*, 197–205

Bianchi, G. and Barlassina, C. (1983) 'Renal Function in Essential Hypertension', in *Hypertension*, 2nd edn, J. Genest, O. Kuchel, P. Hamet and M. Cantin (eds), McGraw-Hill, New York, pp. 54–73

Bianchi, G., Fox, U., Di Francesco, G.F., Giovanetti, A.M. and Pagetti, D. (1974) 'Blood Pressure Changes Produced by Kidney Cross-transplantation between Spontaneously Hypertensive Rats and Normotensive Rats', *Clin. Sci. Mol. Med.*, 47, 435–48

Bianchi, G., Baer, P.G., Fox, U., Duzzi, L., Pagetti, D. and Giovannetti, A.M. (1975) 'Changes in Renin, Water Balance and Sodium Balance during Development of High Blood Pressure in Genetically Hypertensive Rats', *Circ. Res.*, Suppl. I., 36–7, I153–61

Bianchi, G., Gatti, M. Ferrari, P., Picotti, G.B., Colombo, G. Velis, O., Cusi, D., Lupi, G.P., Barlassina, C., Bracchi, G., Gori, D. and Mazzei, D. (1979) 'A Renal Abnormality as a Possible Cause of "Essential" Hypertension', *Lancet*, *i*, 174–7

Bianchi, M., Bellini, G., Hessan, H., Kim, K.E., Swartz, C. and Fernandes, M. (1981) 'Body

Fluid Volumes in the Spontaneously Hypertensive Rat', *Clin. Sci.*, *61*, 685–91

Bianchi, G., Ferrari, P., Casi, D., Guidi, E., Pati, C., Vezzoli, G., Tripodi, M.G. and Niutta, E. (1984) 'Genetic Hypertension and the Kidney', *J. Cardiovasc. Pharmacol.*, *6*, S162–70

Bing, R.F. and Smith, A.J. (1981) 'Plasma and Interstitial Volumes in Essential Hypertension: Relationship to Blood Pressure', *Clin. Sci.*, *61*, 287–93

Bing, R.F., Russell, G.I., Swales, J.D. and Thurston, H. (1981a) 'Effect of 12-hour Infusions of Saralasin or Captopril on Blood Pressure in Hypertensive Conscious Rats', *J. Lab. Clin. Med.*, *98*, 302–10

Bing, R.F., Russell, G.I., Swales, J.D., Thurston, H. and Fetcher, A. (1981b) 'Chemical Medullectomy: Effect upon Reversal of Two-kidney One-clip Hypertension in the Rat', *Clin. Sci.*, *61*, 335s–8s

Bing, R.F., Russell, G.I., Swales, J.D. and Thurston, H. (1982) 'Effect of Sodium, Deoxycorticosterone and Duration of Hypertension on Pressor Responses in Rats', *J. Physiol.*, *333*, 383–91

Bing, R.F., Russell, G.I., Thurston, H., Swales, J.D., Godfrey, N., Lazarus, Y. and Jackson, J. (1983) 'Chemical Renal Medullectomy: Effect upon Urinary Prostaglandin E2 and Plasma Renin in Response to Variations in Sodium Intake and in Relation to Blood Pressure', *Hypertension*, *5*, 951–7

Birkenhager, W.H. and de Leeuw, P.W. (1984) 'Cardiac Aspects of Essential Hypertension', *J. Hypertension*, *2*, 121–5

Blaustein, M.P. (1977) 'Sodium Ions, Calcium Ions, Blood Pressure Regulation, and Hypertension: a Reassessment and a Hypothesis', *Am. J. Physiol.*, *232*, C165–73

Blumberg, A. Hegstrom, R.M., Nelp, W.B. and Scribner, B.H. (1967) 'Extracellular Volume in Patients with Chronic Renal Disease Treated for Hypertension by Sodium Restriction', *Lancet*, *ii*, 69–73

Bohman, S.O. (1980) 'The Ultrastructure of the Renal Medulla and the Interstitial Cells', in A.K. Mandal and S.O. Bohman (eds), *The Renal Papilla and Hypertension*, Plenum, New York, pp.7–33

Bohr, D.F. (1981) 'What Makes the Pressure Group? A Hypothesis', *Hypertension*, *3*, Suppl. II, II–160 to II–165

Borst J.G.G. and Borst, D.G.A. (1963) 'Hypertension Explained by Starling's Theory of Circulating Homeostasis', *Lancet*, *i*, 677–82

Boucher, R., Garcia, R., Demassieux, S., Gutkowska, J. and Genest, J. (1978) 'Tonin-Angiotensin II System', *Clin. Sci. Mol. Med.*, *55*, Suppl. 4, 183s–6s

Bradlaugh, R., Heagerty, A.M., Bing, R.F., Swales, J.D. and Thurston, H. (1984) 'Rat Thymocyte Sodium Transport', *Hypertension*, *6*, 454–9

Braun-Menendez, E. and von Euler, U.S. (1947) 'Hypertension after Bilateral Nephrectomy in the Rat', *Nature (Lond.)*, *160*, 905

Brinton, G.S., Jubiz, W. and Lagerquist, L.D. (1975) 'Hypertension in Primary Hyperparathyroidism: the Role of the Renin-Angiotensin System', *J. Clin. Endocrinol. Metabol.*, *41*, 1025–9

Brodsky, W.A. and Graubarth, H.N. (1953) 'Excretion of Water and Electrolytes in Patients with Essential Hypertension', *J. Lab. Clin. Med.*, *41*, 43–55

Brody, M.J., Baron, K.W., Berecek, K.H., Faber, J.E. and Lappe, R.W. (1983) 'Neurogenic Mechanisms of Experimental Hypertension', in J. Genest, O. Kuchel, P. Hamet and M. Cantin (eds), *Hypertension*, 2nd edn, McGraw-Hill, New York, pp. 117–40

Brown, J.J., Dusterdieck, G., Fraser, R., Lever, A.F., Robertson, J.I.S., Tree, M. and Weir, R.J. (1971) 'Hypertension and Chronic Renal Failure', *Brit. Med. Bull.*, *27*, 128–35

Brown J.J., Lever, A.F., Robertson, J.I.S. and Schalekamp, M.A. (1974) 'Renal Abnormality of Essential Hypertension', *Lancet*, *ii*, 320–3

Brown, J.J., Casals-Stenzel, J., Cumming, A.M.M., Davies, D.L., Fraser, R., Lever, A.F., Morton, J.J., Semple, P.F., Tree, M. and Robertson, J.I.S. (1979) 'Angiotensin II, Aldosterone and Arterial Pressure: a Quantitative Approach', *Hypertension*, *1*, 159–79

Brown, J.J., Casals-Stenzel, J., Gofford, S., Lever, A.F. and Morton, J.J. (1981) 'Comparison of Fast and Slow Pressor Effects of Angiotensin II in the Conscious Rat', *Am. J. Physiol.*, *241*, H381–8

Buckalew, V.M., Puschett, J.E., Kintzel, and Goldberg, M. (1969) 'Mechanisms of Exaggerated Natriuresis in Hypertensive Man: Impaired Sodium Transport in the Loop of Henle', *J. Clin.*

Invest., *48*, 1007–16

Buckley, J.P. and Jandhyala, B.S. (1977) 'Central Cardiovascular Effects of Angiotensin', *Life Sciences*, *20*, 1485–94

Burstyn, E., Hornall, D. and Watchorn, C. (1980) 'Sodium and Potassium Intake and Blood Pressure', *Brit. Med. J.*, *281*, 537–9

Canessa, M., Adragna, N. Solomon, H.S., Connolly, T.M. and Tosteson, D.C. (1980) 'Increased Sodium-Lithium Countertransport in Red Cells of Patients with Essential Hypertension', *New Engl. J. Med.*, *302*, 772–6

Carlberger, G. and Collste, L.G. (1968) 'Hypertension and Sodium Restriction in Bilaterally Nephrectomized Man', *Scand. J. Urol. Nephrol.*, *2*, 151–6

Chrysant, S.G., Walsh, G.M., Kem, D.C. and Frohlich, E.D. (1979) 'Hemodynamic and Metabolic Evidence of Salt Sensitivity in Spontaneously Hypertensive Rats', *Kidney Int.*, *15*, 33–7

Clough, D.P.,Collis, M.G., Conway, J., Hatton, R. and Keddie, J.R. (1982) 'Interaction of Angiotensin-converting Enzyme Inhibitors with the Function of the Sympathetic Nervous System', *Am. J. Cardiol.*, *49*, 1410–14

Cohen, D.M. Grekin, R.J., Mitchell J., Rice W.H. and Bohr, D.F. (1980) 'Hemodynamic, Endocrine and Electrolyte Changes during Sodium Restriction in DOCA Hypertensive Pigs', *Hypertension*, *2*, 490–6

Coleman, T.G., Manning, R.D., Norman, A. and de Clue, J. (1975) 'The Role of the Kidney in Spontaneous Hypertension', *Am. J. Med.*, *89*, 94–8

Collis, M.G. and Alps, B.J. (1975) 'Vascular Reactivity to Noradrenaline, Potassium Chloride, and Angiotensin II in the Rat Perfused Mesenteric Vasculature Preparation, during the Development of Renal Hypertension', *Cardiovasc. Res.*, *9*, 118–26

Collis, M.G. and Vanhoutte, P.M. (1978) 'Increased Renal Vascular Reactivity to Angiotensin II but not to Nerve Stimulation or Exogenous Norepinephrine in Renal Hypertensive Rats', *Circ. Res.*, *43*, 544–52

Coote, J.H. and Sato, Y. (1977) 'Reflex Regulation of Sympathetic Activity in the Spontaneously Hypertensive Rat', *Circ. Res.*, *40*, 571–7

Cowley, A.W. and De Clue, J.W. (1976) 'Quantification of Baroreceptor Influence of Arterial Pressure Changes Seen in Primary Angiotensin-induced Hypertension in Dogs', *Circ. Res.*, *39*, 779–87

Curtis, J.J., Luke, R.G., Whelchel, J.D., Diethelm, A.G., Jones, P. and Duston, H.P. (1983) 'Inhibition of Angiotensin-converting Enzyme in Renal Transplant Recipients with Hypertension', *New Engl. J. Med.*, *308*, 377–81

Dahl, L.K., Heine, M. and Tassinari, L (1962) 'Effects of Chronic Excess Salt Ingestion: Evidence that Genetic Factors Play an Important Role in Susceptibility to Experimental Hypertension', *J. Exp. Med.*, *115*, 1173–90

Dahl, L.K., Heine, M. and Thompson, K. (1974) 'Genetic Influence of the Kidneys on Blood Pressure. Evidence from Chronic Renal Homografts in Rats with Opposite Predispositions to Hypertension'. *Circ. Res.*, *34*, 94–101

Dahl, L.K., Knudsen, K.D. and Iwai, J. (1969) 'Humoral Transmission of Hypertension. Evidence from Parabiosis', *Circ. Res.* (Suppl. 24), 21–33

Dalakos, T.G., Elias, A.N., Anerson, G.H., Streeten, D.H.P. and Schroeder, E.T. (1978) 'Evidence for an Angiotensinogenic Mechanism of the Hypertension of Cushing's Syndrome', *J. Clin. Endocrinol. Metab.*, *46*, 114–18

Dargie, H.J., Franklin, S.S. and Reid, J.L. (1977a) 'Central and Peripheral Noradrenaline in the Two-kidney Model of Renovascular Hypertension in the Rat', *Brit. J. Pharmacol.*, *61*, 213–15

Dargie, H.J., Franklin, S.S. and Reid, J.L. (1977b) 'Plasma Noradrenaline Concentrations in Experimental Renovascular Hypertension in the Rat', *Clin. Sci. Mol. Med.*, *52*, 477–83

DeClue, J.W., Guyton, A.C., Cowley, A.W., Coleman, T.G., Norman, R.A. and McCaa, R.E. (1978) 'Subpressor Angiotensin Infusion, Renal Sodium Handling, and Salt Induced Hypertension in the Dog', *Circ. Res.*, *43*, 503–12

Deforrest, J.M., Davis, J.O., Freeman, R.H., Watkins, B.E. and Stephens, G.A. (1978) 'Separate Renal Function Studies in Conscious Dogs with Renovascular Hypertension', *Am. J. Physiol*, *235*, F310–16

Deforrest, J.M., Knappenberger, R.C., Antonaccio, M.J., Ferrone, R.A. and Creekmore, J.S.

(1982) 'Angiotensin II is a Necessary Component for the Development of Hypertension in the Two-kidney, One-clip Rat', *Am. J. Cardiol.*, *49*, 1515–17

De Leeuw, P.W. and Birkenhager, W.H. (1983a) 'The Renal Circulation in Essential Hypertension', *J. Hypertension*, *1*, 321–31

De Leeuw, P.W. and Birkenhager, W.H. (1983) 'Coarctation of the Aorta', in J.I.S. Robertson (ed.), *Handbook of Hypertension*, vol. 2, Elsevier, Amsterdam, pp. 1–17

de Wardener, H.W. and MacGregor, G.A. (1982) 'The Natriuretic Hormone and Essential Hypertension', *Lancet*, *i*, 1450–4

DiBona, G.F. and Rios, L.L. (1978) 'Mechanism of Exaggerated Diuresis in Spontaneously Hypertensive Rats', *Am. J. Physiol.*, *235*, F409–16

Dickinson, C.J. (1981) 'Neurogenic Hypertension Revisited', *Clin. Sci.*, *60*, 471–7

Dickinson, C.J. and Lawrence, F.R. (1963) 'A Slowly Developing Pressor Response to Small Concentrations of Angiotensin', *Lancet*, *i*, 1354–6

Dunn, M.J. and Hood, V.L. (1977) 'Prostaglandins and the Kidney', *Am. J. Physiol.*, *233*, F169–84

Dunn, M.J. and Tannen, R.L. (1974) 'Low Renin Hypertension', *Kidney Int.*, *5*, 317–25

Dzau, V.J., Ellison, K., McGowan, D., Gross, K.W. and Ouellette, A. (1984) 'Hybridization Studies with a Renin cDNA Probe: Evidence for Widespread Expression of Renin in the Mouse', *J. Hypertension*, *2*, Suppl. 3, 235–7

Earley, L.E. and Friedler, R.M. (1965) 'Changes in Renal Blood Flow and Possibly the Intrarenal Distribution of Blood during the Natriuresis Accompanying Saline Loading in the Dog', *J. Clin. Invest.*, *44*, 929–41

Earley, L.E. and Friedler, R.M. (1966) 'The Effects of Combined Renal Vasodilation and Pressor Agents on Renal Hemodynamics and the Tubular Reabsorption of Sodium', *J. Clin. Invest.*, *45*, 542–51

Edmondson, R.P.S., Thomas, R.D., Hilton, P.J., Patrick, J. and Jones, N.F. (1975) 'Abnormal Leucocyte Composition and Sodium Transport in Essential Hypertension', *Lancet*, *i*, 1003–5

Esler, M., Julius, S. Zweifler, A., Randall, O., Harburg, E., Gardiner, H. and de Quattro, V. (1977) 'Mild High-renin Essential Hypertension', *N. Engl. J. Med.*, *296*, 405–11

Esler, M., Zweifler, A., Randall, O., Julius, S. and de Quattro, V. (1978) 'The Determinants of Plasma-renin Activity in Essential Hypertension', *Ann. Int. Med.*, *88*, 746–52

Falkner, B., Onesti, G., Angelakos, E.T., Fernandes, M. and Langman, C. (1979) 'Cardiovascular Response to Mental Stress in Normal Adolescents with Hypertensive Parents: Hemodynamics and Mental Stress in Adolescents', *Hypertension*, *1*, 23–30

Farnsworth, E.B. (1946) 'Renal Reabsorption of Chloride and Phosphate in Normal Subjects and in Patients with Essential Arterial Hypertension', *J. Clin. Invest.*, *25*, 897–905

Ferrario, C.M. and Page, I.H. (1978) 'Brief Reviews: Current Views Concerning Cardiac Output in the Genesis of Experimental Hypertension', *Circ. Res.*, *43*, 821–31

Ferrario, C.M., Takishita, S., Lynn, M.P., Szilagyi, J.E. and Brosnihan, K.B. (1981) 'Effect of Dietary Sodium Depletion on Central and Peripheral Nervous System Mechanisms Regulating Arterial Pressure in the Dog', in F.M. Abboud, H.A. Fozzard, J.P. Gilmore and D.J. Reiss (eds), *Disturbances in Neurogenic Control of the Circulation*, American Physiological Society, Washington DC, pp.119–31

Fletcher, P.J., Korner, P.I., Angus, J.A. and Oliver, J.R. (1976) 'Changes in Cardiac Output and Total Peripheral Resistance during Development of Renal Hypertension in the Rabbit', *Circ. Res.*, *39*, 633–9

Folkow, B. (1976) 'The Neurogenic Component in Spontaneously Hypertensive Rats (SHR): a Survey', in S. Julius and M.D. Esler (eds), *The Nervous System in Arterial Hypertension*, Charles C. Thomas, Springfield, Illinois, pp. 3–16

Folkow, B. (1982) 'Physiological Aspects of Primary Hypertension', *Physiol. Rev.*, *62*, 347–504

Folkow, B., Hallback, M., Lundgren, Y., Sivertsson, R. and Weiss, L. (1973) 'Importance of Adaptive Changes in Vascular Design for Establishment of Primary Hypertension Studied in Man and in Spontaneously Hypertensive Rats', *Circ. Res.*, *32*, Suppl. 1, 2–16

Folkow, B., Gothberg, G. Lundin, S. and Ricksten, S.E. (1977) 'Structural "Resetting" of the Renal Vascular Bed in Spontaneously Hypertensive Rats', *Acta Physiol. Scand.*, *100*, 270–2

Folkow, B., DiBona, G. Hjemdahl, P., Toren, P.H. and Wallin, B.G. (1983) 'Measurement of

Plasma Norepinephrine Concentrations in Human Primary Hypertension. A Word of Caution on their Applicability for Assessing Neurogenic Contributions', *Hypertension*, 5, 399–402

Fordis, C.M., Megorden, J.S., Ropchak, T.G. and Keiser, H.R. (1983) 'Absence of Renin-like Activity in Rat Aorta and Microvessels', *Hypertension*, 5, 635–41

Freis, E.D., Ragan, D., Pillsbury, H. and Mathews, M. (1972) 'Alteration of the Course of Hypertension in the Spontaneously Hypertensive Rat', *Circ. Res.*, 31, 1–7

Fujita, T., Henry, W.L., Bartter, F.C. and Lake, C.R. (1980) 'Factors Influencing Blood Pressure in Salt-sensitive Patients with Hypertension', *Am. J. Med.*, 69, 334–44

Ganguli, M., Tobian, L. and Dahl, L. (1976) 'Low Renal Papillary Plasma Flow in Both Dahl and Kyoto Rats with Spontaneous Hypertension', *Circ. Res.* 39, 337–41

Garay R.P. and Meyer, P. (1979) 'A New Test Showing Abnormal Net Na^+ and K^+ Fluxes in Erythrocytes of Essential Hypertensive Patients', *Lancet*, i, 349–53

Gerber, J.G. and Nies, A.S. (1979) 'The Hemodynamic Effects of Prostaglandins in the Rat', *Circ. Res.* 44, 406–10

Goldblatt, H., Lynch, J., Hanzal, R.F. and Summerville, W.W. (1934) 'Studies on Experimental Hypertension. 1. The Production of Persistent Elevation of Systolic Blood Pressure by Means of Renal Ischemia', *J. Exp. Med.*, 59, 347–79

Goldring, W. Chasis, H.A. and Smith, H.W. (1941) 'Effective Renal Blood Flow in Subjects with Essential Hypertension', *J. Clin. Invest.*, 20, 637–53

Goldstein, D.S. (1981) 'Plasma Norepinephrine in Essential Hypertension. A Study of the Studies', *Hypertension*, 3, 48–52

Gomez, A.H., Hoobler, S.W. and Blaquier, P. (1960) 'Effect of Addition and Removal of a Kidney Transplant in Renal and Adrenocortical Hypertensive Rats', *Circ. Res.*, 8, 464–72

Gothberg, G., Lundin, S., Folkow, B. and Thoren, P. (1982a) 'Suppression of Tonic Sympathetic Nerve Activity by Depressor Agents Released from the Declipped Kidney', *Acta Physiol. Scand.*, 116, 93–5

Gothberg, G., Lundin, S. and Folkow, B. (1982b) 'Acute Vasodepressor Effect in Normotensive Rats Following Extracorporeal Perfusion of the Declipped Kidney of Two-kidney, One-clip Hypertensive Rats', *Hypertension*, 4, II–101 to II–105

Grim, C.E., Luft, F.C., Miller, J.Z., Brown, P.L., Gannon, M.A. and Weinberger, M.H. (1979) 'Effects of Sodium Loading and Depletion in Normotensive First-degree Relatives of Essential Hypertensives', *J. Lab. Clin. Med.*, 94, 764–71

Grollman, A. and Krishnamurty, V.S.R. (1973) 'Differentiation of Nephrotensin from Angiotensin I and II', *Proc. Soc. Exp. Biol. Med.*, 143, 85–8

Grollman, A., Muirhead, E.E. and Vanatta, J. (1949) 'Role of the Kidney in Pathogenesis of Hypertension as Determined by a Study of the Effects of Bilateral Nephrectomy and Other Experimental Procedures on the Blood Pressure of the Dog', *Am. J. Physiol.*, 157, 21–30

Gunther, S., Gimbrone, M.A. and Alexander, R.W. (1980a) 'Regulation by Angiotensin II of its Receptors in Resistance Blood Vessels', *Nature (Lond.)*, 287, 230–2

Gunther, S., Gimbrone, M.A. and Alexander, R.W. (1980b) 'Identification and Characterization of the High Affinity Vascular Angiotensin II Receptor in Rat Mesenteric Artery', *Circ. Res.*, 47, 278–86

Guyton, A.C., Coleman, T.G., Cowley, A.W., Scheel, K.W., Manning, R.D. and Norman, R.A. (1972) 'Arterial Pressure: Overriding Dominance of the Kidneys in Long-term Regulation Aid in Hypertension', *Am. J. Med.*, 52, 584–94

Guyton, A.C., Coleman, T.G., Cowle, A.W., Scheel, K.W., Manning, R.D. and Norman, R.A. (1974) 'Arterial Pressure Regulation', in J.H. Laragh (eds), *Hypertension Manual*, Yorke Medical Books, New York, pp. 111–34

Haack, D., Mohring, J., Mohring, M. Petri, M. and Hackenthal, E. (1977) 'Comparative Study on Development of Corticosterone and DOCA Hypertension in Rats', *Am. J. Physiol.*, 233, F403–11

Haddy, F.J. (1984) 'The Role of a Humoral Na^+ K^+-ATPase Inhibitor in Regulating Precapillary Vessel Tone', *J. Cardiovasc. Pharmacol.*, 6, S439–56

Haddy, F.J. and Pamnani, M.B. (1983) 'The Role of a Humoral Sodium-Potassium Pump Inhibitor in Low-renin Hypertension', *Fed. Proc.*, 42, 2673–80

Hallback-Nordlander, M., Noresson, E. and Lundgren, Y. (1979) 'Haemodynamic Alteration after Reversal of Renal Hypertension in Rats', *Clin. Sci.*, 57, 15s–17s

Hamlyn, J.M., Ringel, R., Schaeffer, J., Levinson, P.D., Hamilton,B.P., Avinoum Kowarski, A. and Blaustein, M.P. (1982) 'Circulating Inhibitor of (Na^+-K^+) ATPase Associated with Essential Hypertension', *Nature (Lond.)*, *300*, 650–2

Heptinstall, R.H. (1965) 'The Role of the Juxtaglomerular Apparatus in Experimental Hypertension in the Rat', *Lab. Invest.*, *14*, 2150–9

Heptinstall, R.H. (1974) *Pathology of the Kidney*, 2nd Edn, Little Brown and Company, Boston, pp. 173–4

Heptinstall, R.H., Salyer, D.C. and Salyer, W.R. (1975) 'Experimental Hypertension: the Effects of Chemical Ablation of the Renal Papilla on the Blood Pressure with and without Silver Clip Hypertension', *Am.J. Pathol.*, *78*, 297–308

Hollenberg, N.K. and Williams, G.H. (1983) 'Volume Control and Altered Renal and Adrenal Responsiveness to Angiotensin in Essential Hypertension: Implications for Treatment with Converting Enzyme Inhibition', *J. Hypertension*, *1*, Suppl. 1, 119–28

Hollenberg, N.K., Borucki, L.J. and Adams, D.F. (1978) 'The Renal Vasculature in Early Essential Hypertension: Evidence for a Pathogenetic Role', *Medicine*, *57*, 167–78

Hollenberg, N.K. Williams, G.H. and Adams, D.F. (1981) 'Essential Hypertension: Abnormal Renal Vascular and Endocrine Responses to a Mild Physiological Stimulus', *Hypertension*, *3*, 11–17

Houck, C.R. (1954) 'Effect of Hydration and Dehydration on Hypertension in the Chronic Bilaterally Nephrectomised Dog', *Am. J. Physiol.*, *176*, 183–9

Hricik, D.E., Browning, P.J., Kopelman, R., Goorno, W.E. Madias, N.E. and Dzau, V.J. (1983) 'Captopril-induced Functional Renal Insufficiency in Patients with Bilateral Renal-artery Stenosis in a Solitary Kidney', *N. Engl. J. Med.*, *308*, 373–6

Huang, C.T., Cardona, R. and Michelakis, A.M. (1978) 'Existence of a New Vasoactive Factor in Experimental Hypertensive', *Am. J. Physiol.*, *234*, E25–31

Huot, S.J., Pamnani, M.B., Clough, D.L., Buggy, J., Bryant, H.J., Harder, D.R. and Haddy, F.J. (1983) 'Sodium-Potassium Pump Activity in Reduced Renal-mass Hypertension', *Hypertension*, *5* (Suppl. 1), I-94 to I-100

Ichikawa, S., Johnson, J.A., Fowler, W.L., Payne, C.G., Kurz, K. and Keitzer, W.F. (1978) 'Pressor Responses to Norepinephrine in Rabbits with 3-day and 30-day Renal Artery Stenosis', *Circ. Res.*, *43*, 437–46

Iriuchijima, J., Mizogami, S. and Sokabe, H. (1975) 'Sympathetic Nervous Activity in Renal and DOC Hypertensive Rats', *Jap. Heart J.*, *16*, 236–43

Ishii, M. and Tobian, L. (1969) 'Interstitial Cell Granules in Renal Papilla and the Solute Composition of Renal Tissue in Rats with Goldblatt Hypertension', *J. Lab. Clin. Med.*, *74*, 47–52

Jaffe, D., Sutherland, L.E., Barker, D. and Dahl, L.K. (1970) 'Effects of Chronic Excess Salt Ingestion: Morphological Findings in Kidneys of Rats with Different Genetic Susceptibilities to Hypertension', *Arch. Pathol.*, *90*, 1–16

Johnson, M.D. and Barger, A.C. (1981) 'Circulating Catecholamines in Control of Renal Electrolyte and Water Excretion', *Am. J. Physiol.*, *240*, F192–9

Judy, W.V., Watanabe, A.M., Henry, D.P., Besch, H.R., Murphy, W.R. and Hockel, G.M. (1976) 'Sympathetic Nerve Activity. Role in Regulation of Blood Pressure in Spontaneously Hypertensive Rats', *Circ. Res.*, *38*, Suppl. II, II–21 to II–129

Katholi, R.E., Whitlow, P.L., Winternitz, S.R. and Oparil, S. (1982a) 'Importance of the Renal Nerves in Established Two-kidney, One-clip Goldblatt Hypertension', *Hypertension*, *4*, II–166 to II–174

Katholi, R.E., Winternitz, S.R. and Oparil, S. (1982b) 'Decrease in Peripheral Sympathetic Nervous System Activity Following Renal Denervation or Unclipping in the One-kidney One-Clip Goldblatt Hypertensive Rat', *J. Clin. Invest.*, *69* 55–62

Katholi, R.E., Naftilan, A.J., Bishop, S.P. and Oparil, S. (1983) 'Role of the Renal Nerves in the Maintenance of DOCA-Salt Hypertension in the Rat. Influence on the Renal Vasculature and Sodium Excretion', *Hypertension*, *5*, 427–35

Kawabe, K., Watanebe, T.X., Shiono, K. and Sokabe, H. (1979) 'Influence of Blood Pressure on Renal Isografts between Spontaneously Hypertensive and Normotensive Rats Utilizing the F1 Hybrids', *Jap. Heart J.*, *20*, 886–94

Kim, K.E., Onesti, G., Del Guercio, E.T. Greco, J., Fernandes, M. and Swartz, C. (1976) 'The Haemodynamic Response to Salt and Water Loading in Patients with End-stage Renal

Disease and Anephric Man', *Clin. Sci. Mol. Med.*, *51*, Suppl. 3, 223S–5s

Kirkendall, W.M., Cannor, W.E., Arboud, F., Rastogi, S.P., Anderson, T.A. and Fry, M. (1976) 'The Effect of Dietary Sodium Chloride on Blood Pressure, Body Fluids, Electrolytes, Renal Function, and Serum Lipids of Normotensive Man', *J. Lab. Clin. Med.*, *87*, 418–34

Koch, K.M., Aynedjian, H.S. and Bank, N. (1968) 'Effect of Acute Hypertension on Sodium Reabsorption by the Proximal Tubule', *J. Clin. Invest.*, *47*, 1696–1709

Kolff, W.J. and Page, I.H. (1954) 'Blood Pressure Reducing Function of the Kidneys: Reduction of Renoprival Hypertension by Kidney Perfusion', *Am. J. Physiol.*, *178*, 75–81

Kolff, W.J., Page, I.H. and Corcoran, A.C. (1954) 'Pathogenesis of Renoprival Cardiovascular Disease in Dogs', *Am. J. Physiol.*, *178*, 237–45

Kolff, W.J., Nakamoto, S., Poutasse, E.F., Straffon, R.A. and Figueroa, J.E. (1964) 'Effect of Bilateral Nephrectomy and Kidney Transplantation on Hypertension in Man', *Circ. Res.*, *30*, Suppl. II, 23–8

Kumar, S., Bing, R.F., Swales, J.D. and Thurston, H. (1984) 'Delayed Reversal of Goldblatt Hypertension by Angiotensin II Infusion in the Rat', *Am. J. Physiol.*, *15*, H811–17

Kwan, C.Y., Belbeck, L. and Daniel, E.E. (1979) 'Abnormal Biochemistry of Vascular Smooth Muscle Plasma Membrane as an Important Factor in the Initiation and Maintenance of Hypertension in Rats', *Blood Vessel*, *16*, 259–68

Lais, L.T. and Brody, M.J. (1978) 'Vasoconstrictor Hyperresponsiveness: an Early Pathogenic Mechanism in the Spontaneously Hypertensive Rat', *Eur. J. Pharmacol.*, *47*, 177–89

Laragh, J.H. (1976) 'Modern System for Treating High Blood Pressure Based on Renin Profiling and Vasoconstriction-Volume Analysis: a Primary Role for Beta-blocking Drugs Such as Propranolol', *Am. J. Med.*, *61*, 797–810

Latta, H., White, F.N., Osvaldo, L. and Johnston, W.H. (1975) 'Unilateral Renovascular Hypertension in Rats. Measurements of Medullary Granules, Juxtaglomerular Granularity and Cellularity, and Areas of Adrenal Zones', *Lab. Invest.*, *33*, 379–90

Leonards, J.R. and Heisler, C.R. (1952) 'Blood Pressure of Bilaterally Nephrectomised Dogs', *Fed. Proc.*, *11*, 247

Lewy, J.E. and Windhager, E.E (1968) 'Peritubular Control of Proximal Fluid Reabsorption in the Rat Kidney', *Am. J. Physiol.*, *214*, 943–54

Light, K.C., Koepke, J.P., Obrist, P.A. and Willis, P.W. (1983) 'Psychological Stress Induces Sodium and Fluid Retention in Men at High Risk for Hypertension', *Science*, *223*, 429–31

Limas, C., Westrum, B., Limas, C.J. and Cohn, J.N. (1980) 'Effect of Salt on the Vascular Lesions of Spontaneously Hypertensive Rats', *Hypertension*, *2*, 477–89

Lohmeier, T.E. and Cowley, A.W. (1979) 'Hypertensive and Renal Effects of Chronic Low Level Intrarenal Angiotensin Infusion in the Dog', *Circ. Res.*, *44*, 154–60

Lohmeier, T.E. and Davis, J.O. (1976) 'Renin-Angiotensin-Aldosterone System in Experimental Renal Hypertension in the Rabbit', *Am. J. Physiol.*, *230*, 311–18

Lohmeier, T.E, Cowley, A.W. DeClue, J.W. and Guyton, A.C. (1978) 'Failure of Chronic Aldosterone Infusion to Increase Arterial Pressure in Dogs with Angiotensin-induced Hypertension', *Circ. Res.*, *43*, 381–9

Loudon, M., Bing, R.F., Thurston, H. and Swales, J.D. (1983) 'Arterial Wall Uptake of Renal Renin and Blood Pressure Control', *Hypertension*, *5*, 629–34

Lowenstein, J., Berenbaum, E.R., Chasis, H. and Baldwin, D.S. (1970) 'Intrarenal Pressure and Exaggerated Natriuresis in Essential Hypertension', *Clin. Sci.*, *38*, 359–74

Lowitz, H.D., Stumpe, K.O. and Ochwadt, B. (1968) 'Natrium und Wasserresorption in den weirschredenen Abschnitten des Nephrons beim experimentellen renalen Hochduck der Ratte', *Pflügers Arch.*, *304*, 322–35

Lucas, J. and Floyer, M.A. (1974) 'Changes in Body Fluid Distribution and Interstitial Tissue Compliance during the Development and Reversal of Experimental Renal Hypertension in the Rat', *Clin. Sci. Mol. Med.*, *47*, 1–11

Luft, F.C., Weinberger, M.H. and Grim, C.E. (1982) 'Sodium Sensitivity and Resistance in Normotensive Humans', *Am. J. Med.*, *72*, 726–36

Lundgren, Y. and Weiss, L. (1979) 'Cardiovascular Design after Reversal of Longstanding Renal Hypertension', *Clin. Sci.*, *57*, Suppl. 5, 19s–21s

Lundgren, Y., Hallback, M., Weiss, L. and Folkow, B. (1974) 'Rate and Extent of Adaptive Cardiovascular Changes in Rats during Experimental Renal Hypertension', *Acta Physiol. Scand.*, *91*, 103–15

Lundin, S. and Thoren, P. (1982) 'Renal Function and Sympathetic Activity during Mental Stress in Normotensive and Spontaneously Hypertensive Rats', *Acta Physiol. Scand.*, *115*, 115–24

McAreavey, D., Brown, J.J., Cumming, A.M.M., Davies, D.L., Fraser, R., Lever, A.F., Mackay, A., Morton, J.J. and Robertson, J.I.S. (1983) 'Inverse Relation of Exchangeable Sodium and Blood Pressure in Hypertensive Patients with Renal Artery Stenosis', *J. Hypertension*, *1*, 297–302

McAreavey, D., Brown, J.J., Murray, G.D. and Robertson, J.I.S. (1985) 'Exchangeable Sodium in DOC-salt and Post-DOC-salt Hypertension in Rats', *J. Hypertension*, *3*, 275–9

MacDonald, G.J., Boyd, G.W. and Peart, W.S. (1975) 'Effect of the Angiotensin II Blocker 1-Sar-8-ala-angiotensin II on Rat Renal Artery Clip Hypertension in the Rat', *Circ. Res.*, *37*, 640–6

MacGregor, G.A. and Dawes, P.M. (1976) 'Angiotensin II Blockade in Hypertensive Dialysis Patients', in G.S. Stokes and K.D.G. Edwards (eds) *Drugs Affecting the Renin-Angiotensin-Aldosterone System, Progr. Biochem. Pharmacol.*, *12*, 190–9

MacGregor, G.A., Markandu, N., Best, F., Elder, D., Cam, J. and Squires, M. (1982) 'Double-blind Randomised Crossover Trial of Moderate Sodium Restriction in Essential Hypertension', *Lancet, i*, 351–4

McGiff, J.C. and Quilley, C.P. (1981) 'The Rat with Spontaneous Genetic Hypertension is not a Suitable Model of Human Essential Hypertension', *Circ. Res.*, *48*, 455–63

McGiff, J.C., Crowshaw, K., Terragno, N.A. Lonigro, A.J., Strand, J.C., Williamson, M.A., Lee, J.B. and Ng, K.K.F. (1970) 'Prostaglandin-like Substances Appearing in Canine Renal Venous Blood during Renal Ischaemia', *Circ. Res.*, *27*, 765–82

MacKay, A., Brown, J.J., Lever, A.F., Morton, J.J. and Robertson, J.I.S. (1983a) 'Unilateral Renal Disease in Hypertension', in J.I.S. Robertson (eds.), *Handbook of Hypertension*, Vol. 2, Elsevier, Amsterdam, pp. 33–79

MacKay, A. Boyle, P., Brown, J.J., Cumming, A.M.M., Forrest, H., Graham, A.G., Lever, A.F., Robertson, J.I.S. and Semple, P.F. (1983b) 'The Decision on Surgery in Renal Artery Stenosis', *Q. J. Med.*, *52*, 363–81

Madden, J.A., Smith, G.A. and Llaurado, J.G. (1979) 'Sodium Distribution in Mesenteric Arterial Wall of Rats with Hypertension Induced by Drinking Saline', *Clin. Sci.*, *56*, 471–8

Malik, K.U. and Nasjletti, A. (1976) 'Facilitation of Adrenergic Transmission by Locally Generated Angiotensin II in Rat Mesenteric Arteries', *Circ. Res.*, *38*, 26–30

Man in t'Veld, A.J., Wenting, G.J. and Schalekamp, M.A.D.H. (1984) 'Distribution of Extracellular Fluid over the Intra and Extravascular Space in Hypertensive Patients', *J. Cardiovasc. Pharmacol.*, *6*, S143–50

Manthorpe, T. (1973) 'The Effect on Renal Hypertension of Subcutaneous Isotransplantation of Renal Medulla from Normal or Hypertensive Rats', *Acta Pathol. Microbiol. Scand. A*, *81*, 725–33

Manthorpe, T. (1975) 'Antihypertensive and Hypertensive Effects of the Kidney', *Acta. Pathol. Microbiol. Scand. A*, *83*, 395–405

Marks, E.S., Bing, R.F., Thurston, H., Russell, G.I., and Swales, J.D. (1982) 'Responsiveness to Pressor Agents in Experimental Renovascular and Steroid Hypertension', *Hypertension*, *4*, 238–44

Maskill, M., Bing, R.F., Thurston, H., Bell, P.R.F. and Swales, J.D. (1980) 'Surgical Correction of Renovascular Hypertension. Dissociation between Post-operative Changes in Plasma Renin and Blood Pressure', *Q. J. Med.*, *49*, 179–90

Merrill, J.P. Giordano, C. and Heetderks, D.R. (1961) 'The Role of Kidney in Human Hypertension', *Am. J. Med.*, *31*, 931–40

Michelakis, A.M., Mizukoshi, H., Huang, C., Murakami, K. and Inagami, T. (1975) 'Further Studies on the Existence of a Sensitising Factor to Pressor Agents in Hypertension', *J. Clin. Endocrinol. Metab.*, *41*, 90–6

Miksche, L.W., Miksche, U. and Gross, F. (1970) 'Effect of Sodium Restriction on Renal Hypertension and on Renin Activity in the Rat', *Circ. Res.*, *27*, 973–84

Miller, E.D., Samuels, A.I., Haber, E. and Barger, A.C. (1975) 'Inhibition of Angiotensin Conversion and Prevention of Renal Hypertension', *Am. J. Physiol.*, *228*, 448–53

Mohring, J., Mohring, B., Naumann, H.J., Philippi, A., Homsy, E., Orth, H., Daud, G.,

Kazda, S. and Gross, F. (1975) 'Salt and Water Balance and Renin Activity in Renal Hypertension of Rats', *Am. J. Physiol*, *228*, 1847–55

Mohring, J., Mohring, B., Petri, M., Saur, W., Haack, D. and Hackenthal, E. (1976a) 'Sodium and Water Balance, ECFV and BV and Hormones in the Pathogenesis of Renal Hypertension in Rats', *Proc. 6th Congress of Nephrology*, Florence, Basel, Karger, pp. 255–65

Mohring, J., Petri, M., Szokol, M., Haack, D. and Mohring, B. (1976b) 'Effects of Saline Drinking on Malignant Course of Renal Hypertension in Rats', *Am. J. Physiol.*, *230*, 849–57

Morgan, T., Gillies, A., Morgan, G., Adam, W., Wilson, M. and Carney, S. (1978) 'Hypertension treated by Salt Restriction', *Lancet*, *i*, 227–33

Morton, J.J. and Wallace, E.C.H. (1983) 'The Importance of the Renin-Angiotensin System in the Development and Maintenance of Hypertension in the Two-Kidney One-clip Hypertensive Rat', *Clin. Sci.*, *64*, 359–70

Muehrcke, R.C., Mandal, A.K., Epstein, M. and Volini, F.I. (1969) 'Cytoplasmic Granularity of the Renal Medullary Interstitial Cells in Experimental Hypertension', *J. Lab. Clin. Med.*, *73*, 299–308

Muirhead, E.E. (1980) 'Antihypertensive Functions of the Kidney', Arthur C. Corcoran Memorial Lecture, *Hypertension*, *2*, 444–64

Muirhead, E.E. (1983) 'The Renomedullary Antihypertensive System and its Putative Hormone(s)', J. Genest, O. Kuchel, P. Hamet and M. Cantin (eds), *Hypertension*, 2nd edn, McGraw-Hill, New York, pp. 394–407

Muirhead, E.E., Jones, F. and Graham, P. (1953) 'Hypertension in Bilaterally Nephrectomized Dogs in the Absence of Exogenous Sodium Excess', *Arch. Pathol.*, *56*, 286–92

Muirhead, E., Stirman, J., Lesch, W. and Jones, F. (1956) 'Reduction of Post-nephrectomy Hypertension by Renal Homotransplant', *Surg. Gynecol. Obstet.*, *103*, 673–86

Muirhead, E.E., Jones, F., and Stirman, J.A. (1960) 'Hypertensive Cardiovascular Disease of Dog: Relation of Sodium and Dietary Protein to Ureterocaval Anastomosis and Ureteral Ligation', *Arch. J. Pathol.*, *70*, 108–16

Muirhead, E.E., Brooks, B., Pitcock, J.A. and Stephenson, P. (1972a) 'Renomedullary Antihypertensive Function in Accelerated (Malignant) Hypertension', *J. Clin. Invest.*, *51*, 181–90

Muirhead, E.E., Germain, G., Leach, B.E., Pitcock, J.A., Stephenson, P., Brooks, B., Brosius, W.L., Daniels, E.G. and Hinman, J.W. (1972b) 'Production of Renomedullary Prostaglandins by Renomedullary Interstitial Cells Grown in Tissue Culture', *Circ. Res.*, *31*, (Suppl. 2) 161–72

Muirhead, E.E., Leach, B.E., Davis, J.O., Armstrong, F.B. Jr, Pitcock, J.A. and Brosius, W.L. Jr (1975) 'Pathophysiology of Angiotensin-Salt Hypertension', *J. Lab. Clin. Med.*, *85*, 734–45

Muirhead, E.E., Rightsel, W.A., Leach, B.E., Byers, L.W., Pitcock, J.A. and Brooks, B. (1977) 'Reversal of Hypertension by Transplants and Lipid Extracts of Cultured Renomedullary Intestinal Cells', *Lab. Invest.*, *36*, 162–72

Muirhead, E.E., Byers, L.W., Desiderio, D.M., Pitcock, J.A., Brooks, B., Brown, P.S. and Brosius, W.L. (1982) 'Derivation of Antihypertensive Neutral Renomedullary Lipid from Renal Venous Effluent', *J. Lab. Clin. Med.*, *99*, 64–75

Muirhead, E.E., Folkow, B., Byers, L.W., Desiderio, D.M., Thoren, P., Gothberg, G., Dow, A.W. and Brooks, B. (1983) 'Cardiovascular Effects of Antihypertensive Polar and Neutral Renomedullary Lipids', *Hypertension*, *5*, 1112–18

Mulvaney, M.J., Nilsson, H., Flettman, J.A. and Korsgaard, N. (1982) 'Potentiating and Depressive Effects of Ouabain and Potassium-free Solutions in Rat Mesenteric Resistance Vessels', *Circ. Res.*, *51*, 514–24

Munoz-Ramirez, H., Chatelain, R.E., Bumpus, F.M. and Khairallah, P.A. (1980) 'Development of Two-kidney Goldblatt Hypertension in Rats under Dietary Sodium Restriction', *Am. J. Physiol.*, *238*, G889–94

Murray, R.H., Luft, F.C. Bloch, R. and Weyman, E. (1978) 'Blood Pressure Response to Extremes of Sodium Intake in Normal Man', *Proc. Soc, Exp. Biol. Med.*, *159*, 432–6

Nagaoka, A., Kakinhana, M., Suno, M. and Hamajo, K. (1981) 'Renal Hemodynamics and Sodium Excretion in Stroke-prone Spontaneously Hypertensive Rats', *Am. J. Physiol.*, *241*, F244–9

Neubig, R.R. and Hoobler, S.W. (1975) 'Reversal of Chronic Renal Hypertension: Role of Salt and Water Excretion', *Proc. Soc. Exp. Biol. Med.*, *150*, 254–6

Norman, R.A. and Dzielak, D.J. (1982) 'Role of Renal Nerves in Onset and Maintenance of Spontaneous Hypertension', *Am. J. Physiol.*, *243*, H284–8

Norman, R.A., Enobakhare, J.A., DeClue, J.W., Douglas, B.H. and Guyton, A.C. (1978) 'Arterial Pressure-Urinary Output Relationship in Hypertensive Rats', *Am. J. Physiol.*, *234*, R98–103

Omvik, P., Tarazi, R.C. and Bravo, E.L. (1980) 'Regulation of Sodium Balance in Hypertension', *Hypertension*, *2*, 515–23

Ooshima, A., Fuller, G.C., Cardinale, S., Spector, S. and Uderfriend, S. (1974) 'Increased Collagen Synthesis in Blood Vessels of Hypertensive Rats and its Reversal by Anti-hypertensive Agents', *Proc. Natl. Acad. Sci. USA*, *71*, 3019–23

Overbeck, H.W., Du, D.D. and Rapp, J.P. (1981) 'Sodium Pump Activity in Arteries of Dahl Salt-sensitive Rats', *Hypertension*, *3*, 306–12

Pickering, G.W. (1968) *High Blood Pressure*, Churchill-Livingstone, Edinburgh

Postnov, Y.V. and Orlov, S.N. (1984) 'Cell Membrane Alteration as a Source of Primary Hypertension', *J. Hypertension*, *2*, 1–6

Poston, L, Sewell, R.B., Wilkinson, S.P., Richardson, P.J. Williams, R., Clarkson, E.M., MacGregor, G.A. and de Wardener, H.E. (1981) 'Evidence for a Circulating Sodium Transport Inhibitor in Essential Hypertension', *Brit. Med. J.* , *282*, 847–9

Prewitt, R.L., Leach, B.E., Byers, L.W., Brooks, B., Lands, W.E.M. and Muirhead, E.E. (1980) 'Antihypertensive Polar Renomedullary Lipid, a Semi-synthetic Vasodilator', *Hypertension*, *1*, 299–308

Raeder, M., Omvok, P.Jr and Kiil, F. (1974) 'Effect of Acute Hypertension on the Natriuretic Response to Saline Loading', *Am. J. Physiol.*, *226*, 989–95

Regoli, D. Brunner, H., Peters, G., and Gross, F. (1962) 'Changes in Renin Content in Kidneys of Renal Hypertensive Rats', *Proc. Soc. Exp. Biol. (NY)*, *109*, 142–5

Reid, J.L., Zivin, J.A. and Kopin, I.J. (1975) 'Central and Peripheral Adrenergic Mechanisms in the Development of Deoxycorticosterone-Saline Hypertension in Rats', *Circ. Res*, *37*, 569–79

Ribeiro, A.B. and Krakoff, L.R. (1976) 'Angiotensin Blockade in Coarctation of the Aorta', *N. Engl. J. Med.*, *295*, 148–50

Richards, A.M., Espiner, E.A., Maslowski, A.H., Nicholls, M.G., Ikram, H., Hamilton, E.J. and Wells, J.E. (1984) 'Blood Pressure Response to Moderate Sodium Restriction and to Potassium Supplementation in Mild Essential Hypertension', *Lancet*, *i*, 757–61

Riegger, A.J.G., Millar, J.A., Lever, A.F., Morton, J.J. and Slack, B. (1977) 'Correction of Renal Hypertension in the Rat by Prolonged Infusion of Angiotensin Inhibitors', *Lancet*, *ii*, 1317–19

Riozzi, A., Heagerty A.M., Bing, R.F., Thurston, H and Swales, J.D. (1984) 'Noradrenaline: a Circulating Inhibitor of Sodium Transport', *Brit. Med. J.*, *289*, 1025–7

Risler, N.R. and Fasciolo, J.C. (1974) 'Vascular Effects of Corticotensin Peaks Separated by Gel Filtration', *Acta Physiol. Lat. Am.*, *24*, 503–8

Roos, J.C., Kirchner, K.A., Abernethy, J.D. and Langford, H.G. (1984) 'Differential Effect of Salt Loading on Sodium and Lithium Excretion in Dahl Salt-resistant and Sensitive Rats', *Hypertension*, *6*, 420–4

Rosas, R., Gomez, A., Montague, D., Gross, M. and Hoobler, S.W. (1964) 'Hemodynamic Effects of Renal Transplants in Hypertensive and Control Rats', *Proc. Soc. Exp. Biol. Med.*, *115*, 4–8

Rosenthal, J.H., Pfeifle, B., Michailov, M.L., Pschorr, J., Jacob, I.C.M. and Dahlheim, H. (1984) 'Investigation of Components of the Renin-Angiotensin System in Rat Vascular Tissue', *Hypertension*, *6*, 383–90

Russell, G.I., Bing, R.F., Thurston, H. and Swales, J.D. (1982a) 'Surgical Reversal of Two-kidney, One-clip Hypertension during Inhibition of the Renin-Angiotensin System', *Hypertension*, *4*, 69–76

Russell, G.I., Bing, R.F., Swales, J.D. and Thurston, H. (1982b) 'Indomethacin or Aprotinin Infusion: Effect on Reversal of Chronic Two-kidney, One-clip Hypertension in the Conscious Rat', *Clin. Sci.*, *62*, 361–6

Russell, G.I., Bing, R.F., Swales, J.D. and Thurston, H. (1983) 'Hemodynamic Changes Induced by Reversal of Early and Late Renovascular Hypertension', *Am. J. Physiol.*,

245, H734–40

Russo-Marie, F., Seillan, C. and Duval, D. (1980) 'Effect of Dexamethasone on Cyclooxygenase Activity in Reno-medullary Cells in Culture', *Agents Action*, *10*, 516–19

Safar, M.E., Weiss, Y.A., London, G.M., Frackowiak, R.F. and Milliez, P.L. (1974) 'Cardiopulmonary Volume in Borderline Hypertension', *Clin. Sci. Mol. Med.*, *47*, 153–64

Schackow, E. and Dahl, L.K. (1966) 'Effects of Chronic Excess Salt Retention in Salt-Hypertension', *Proc. Soc. Exp. Biol. Med.*, *122*, 952–7

Schalekamp, M.A., Lebel, M., Beevers, D.G., Fraser, R., Kolsters, G. and Birkenhager, W.H. (1974) 'Body-fluid Volume in Low-renin Hypertension', *Lancet*, *ii*, 310–11

Selig, S.E., Anderson, W.P., Korner, P.I. and Casley, D.J. (1983) 'The Role of Angiotensin II in the Development of Hypertension and in the Maintenance of Glomerular Filtration Rate during 48 Hours of Renal Artery Stenosis in Conscious Dogs', *J. Hypertension*, *1*, 153–8

Selkurt, E.E. (1951) 'Effect of Pulse Pressure and Mean Arterial Pressure Modification on Renal Hemodynamics and Electrolyte and Water Excretion', *Circulation*, *4*, 541–51

Seymour, A.A., Davis, J.O., Freeman, R.H., Deforrest, J.M., Rowe, B.P., Stephens, G.A. and Williams, G.M. (1980) 'Hypertension Produced by Sodium Depletion and Unilateral Nephrectomy: a New Experimental Model', *Hypertension*, *2*, 125–9

Skeggs, L.T., Kahn, J.R., Levine, M. Dorer, F.E. and Lentz, K.E. (1977) 'Chronic One-kidney Hypertension in Rabbits. III. Renopressin, a New Hypertensive Substance', *Circ. Res.*, *40*, 143–9

Skrabal, F., Hamberger, L. and Ledochowski, M. (1984) 'Inherited Salt Sensitivity in Normotensive Humans as a Course of Essential Hypertension: a New Concept', *J. Cardiovasc. Pharmacol.*, *6*, Suppl. 1, S215–S23

Skulan, T.W., Brousseau, A.C. and Leonard, K.A. (1974) 'Accelerated Induction of Two-kidney Hypertension in Rats and Renin-Angiotensin Sensitivity', *Circ. Res.*, 734–41

Smith, K.A., Prewitt, R.L., Byers, L.W. and Muirhead, E.E. (1981) 'Analogs of Phosphatidylcholine: α-Adrenergic Antagonists from the Renal Medulla', *Hypertension*, *3*, 460–70

Stephens, G.A., Davis, J.O., Freeman, R.H., DeForrest, J.M. and Early, D.M. (1979) 'Hemodynamic, Fluid and Electrolyte changes in Sodium-depleted, One kidney, Renal Hypertensive Dogs', *Circ. Res.*, *44*, 316–21

Streeten, D.H.P., Anderson, G.H., Freiberg, J.M. and Dalakos, T.G. (1975) 'Use of an Angiotensin II Antagonist (Saralasin) in the Recognition of "Angiotensinogenic" Hypertension', *N. Engl. J. Med.*, *292*, 657–62

Stumpe, K.O., Lowitz, H.D. and Ochwadt, B. (1970) 'Fluid Reabsorption in Henle's Loop and Urinary Excretion of Sodium and Water in Normal Rats and Rats with Chronic Hypertension', *J. Clin. Invest.*, *49*, 1200–12

Susic, D. and Kentera, D. (1980) 'Role of the Renal Medulla in the Resistance of Rats to Salt Hypertension', *Pflügers Arch.*, *384*, 283–5

Susic, D., Sparks, J.C. and Machado, E.A. (1976) 'Salt-induced Hypertension in Rats with Hereditary Hydronephrosis: the Effect of Renomedullary Transplantation', *J. Lab. Clin. Med.*, *87*, 232–9

Susic, D., Sparks, J.C., Machado, E.A. and Kentera, D. (1978) 'The Mechanism of Renomedullary Antihypertensive Action: Haemodynamic Studies in Hydronephrotic Rats with One-kidney Renal-clip Hypertension', *Clin. Sci. Mol. Med.*, *54*, 361–7

Susic, D., Mujovic, S. and Kentera, D (1983) 'The Effect of Chemical Damage to the Renal Medulla on its Antihypertensive Function', *Bas. Res. Cardiol.*, *78*, 8–18

Swales, J.D. (1975a) *Sodium Metabolism in Disease*, Lloyd-Luke, London, pp. 183–4

Swales, J.D. (1975b) 'Low Renin Hypertension: Nephrosclerosis?', *Lancet*, *i*, 75–7

Swales, J.D. (1977) 'On the Inappropriate in Hypertension Research', *Lancet*, *ii*, 702–4

Swales, J.D. (1979) 'Arterial Wall or Plasma Renin in Hypertension', *Clin. Sci.*, *56*, 293–8

Swales, J.D. (1983) 'Abnormal Ion Transport by Cell Membranes in Hypertension. *Handbook of Hypertension*, vol. 1, J.I.S. Robertson (ed.), Elsevier, Amsterdam, pp. 239–66

Swales, J.D. and Tange, J.D. (1971) 'The Influence of Acute Sodium Depletion on Experimental, Hypertension in the Rat', *J. Clin. Med.*, *78*, 369–79

Swales, J.D., Thurston, H., Queiroz, F.P. and Medina, A. (1972) 'Sodium Balance during the Development of Experimental Hypertension', *J. Lab. Clin. Med.*, *80*, 539–47

Swales, J.D., Abramovici, A., Beck, F., Bing, R.F., Loudon, M. and Thurston, H. (1983) 'Arterial Wall Renin', *J. Hypertension*, Suppl. 1, 17–22

Swales, J.D., Bing, R.F., Bradlaugh, R., El-Ashry, A., Godfry, N., Heagerty, A.M. and Thurston, H. (1984) 'Cell Membrane Handling of Sodium, Sodium Balance and Blood Pressure', *J. Cardiovasc. Pharmacol.*, 6, S42–48

Tarazi, R.C. (1976) 'Hemodynamic Role of Extracellular Fluid in Hypertension', *Circ. Res.*, 38, Suppl. II, 73–83

Tarazi, R.C. (1983) 'Haemodynamics, Salt and Water', in J. Genest, O. Kuchel, P. Hamet and M. Cantin (eds), *Hypertension*, McGraw-Hill, New York, pp. 15–42

Tarazi, R.C., Frohlich, E.D. and Dustan, H.P. (1968) 'Plasma Volume in Men with Essential Hypertension', *N. Engl. J. Med.*, 278, 762–5

Taverner, D., Fletcher, A., Russell, G.I., Bing, R.F., Jackson, J., Swales, J.D. and Thurston, H. (1983) 'Chemical Renal Medullectomy: Effect on Blood Pressure in Normal Rats', *J. Hypertension*, 1, (Suppl. 2), 43–5

Taverner, D., Bing, R.F., Swales, J.D. and Thurston, H. (1985) 'Fluid Volumes and Hemodynamics in Hypertension Produced by Chemical Renal Medullectomy', *Am. J. Physiol.*, 249, H415–20

Ten Berg, R. and De Jong, W. (1980) 'Mechanism of Enhanced Blood Pressure Rise after Reclipping Following Removal of a Renal Artery Clip in Rats', *Hypertension*, 2, 4–13

Thomas, R.D. and Lee, M.R. (1976) 'Sodium Repletion and Beta-adrenergic Blockade in Treatment of Salt Depletion with Accelerated Hypertension', *Brit. Med. J.*, 2, 1425–26

Thurston, H. and Swales, J.D. (1976) 'Influence of Sodium Restriction upon Two Models of Renal Hypertension', *Clin. Sci. Mol. Med.*, 51, 275–9

Thurston, H. Bing, R.F. and Swales, J.D. (1980) 'Reversal Two-kidney One-clip Renovascular Hypertension in the Rat', *Hypertension*, 2, 256–65

Toal, C.B. and Leenen, F.H.H. (1983a) 'Body Fluid Volumes during Development of Hypertension in the Spontaneously Hypertensive Rat', *J. Hypertension*, 4, 345–50

Toal, C.B. and Leenen, F.H.H. (1983b) 'Dietary Sodium Restriction and Development of Hypertension in Spontaneously Hypertensive Rats', *Am. J. Physiol.*, 245, H1081–6

Tobian, L., Coffee, K. and McCrea, P. (1969) 'Contrasting Exchangeable Sodium in Rats with Different Types of Goldblatt Hypertension', *Am. J. Physiol.*, 217, 458–60

Tobian, L., Lange, J. and Azar, S. (1978) 'Reduction of Natriuretic Capacity and Renin Release in Isolated, Blood-perfused Kidneys of Dahl Hypertension-prone Rats', *Circ. Res.*, 43, Suppl. I, 192–8

Tobian, L. Johnson, M.A., Lange, J. and Macgraw, S. (1975) 'Effect of Varying Perfusion Pressures on the Output of Sodium and Renin and the Vascular Resistance in Kidneys of Rats with 'Post-salt' Hypertension and Kyoto Spontaneous Hypertension', *Circ. Res.*, 36–37, Suppl I, 162–70

Tobian, L., Lange, J., Iwai, J., Hiller, K., Johnson, M.A. and Goossens, P. (1979) 'Prevention with Thiazide of NaCl-induced Hypertension in Dahl's Rats. Evidence for a Na-retaining Humoral Agent in 'S' Rats', *Hypertension*, 316–23

Tobian, L., Ganguli, M., Johnson, M.A. and Iwai, J. (1982) 'Influence of Renal Prostaglandins and Dietary Linoleate on Hypertension in Dahl Salt Rats', *Hypertension*, 4, II 149–53

Trippodo, N.C., Walsh, G.H. and Frohlich, E.D. (1978) 'Fluid Volumes during Onset of Spontaneous Hypertension in Rats', *Am. J. Physiol.*, 235, H52–5

Vaamonde, C.A., Sporn, I.N., Lamestremere, R.G., Belsky, J.L. and Papper, S. (1964) 'Augmented Natriuretic Response to Acute Sodium Infusion after Blood Pressure Elevation with Metaraminol in Normotensive Subjects', *J. Clin. Invest.*, 43, 496–502

Van Breeman, C., Aaronson, P. and Loutzenhiser, R. (1979) 'Sodium-Calcium Interactions in Mammalian Smooth Muscle', *Pharmacol. Rev.*, 30, 167–208

Vaughan, E.D., Buhler, F.R., Laragh, J.H., Sealey, J.E., Baer, L. and Bard, R.H. (1974) 'Renovascular Hypertension: Renin Measurements to Indicate Hypersecretion and Contra-lateral Suppression, Estimate Renal Plasma Flow and Score for Surgical Correctability', in J.H. Laragh (ed), *Manual of Hypertension*, Yorke Medical Books, New York, pp. 559–82

Vertes, V., Cangiano, J.L., Berman, L.B. and Gould, A. (1969) 'Hypertension in End-stage Renal Disease', *N. Engl. J. Med.*, 280, 978–81

Watkins, B.E., Davis, J.O., Hanson, R.C., Lohmeier, T.E. and Freeman, R.H. (1976) 'Incidence and Pathophysiological Changes in Chronic Two-kidney Hypertension in the Dog', *Am. J. Physiol.*, 231, 954–60

Watt, G.C.M., Edwards, C., Hart, J.T., Hart, M., Walton, P. and Foy, C.J.W. (1983) 'Dietary

Sodium Restriction for Mild Hypertension in General Practice', *Brit. Med. J.*, *286*, 432–6

Weidmann, P. and Maxwell M.H. (1975) 'The Renin-Angiotensin-Aldosterone System in Terminal Renal Failure', *Kidney Int.*, *8*, Suppl. 5, S219–34

Wiedmann, P., Beretta-Piccoli, L., Steffan, F., Blumberg, A. and Reubi, F.C. (1976) 'Hypertension in Terminal Renal Failure', *Kidney Int.*, *9*, 294–301

Wenting, G.J., Tan-Tjiong, H.L., Derx, F.H.M., de Bruyn, J.H.B., Man int' Veld, A.J., and Schalekamp, M.A.D.H. (1984) 'Split Renal Function after Captopril in Unilateral Renal Artery Stenosis', *Brit. Med. J.*, *288*, 886–90

Wiggins, R.C., Basar, I. and Slater, J.D.H. (1978) 'Effect of Adrenal Pressure and Inheritance on the Sodium Excretory Capacity of Normal Young Men', *Clin., Sci. Mol. Med.*, *54*, 639–47

Wilkinson, R., Scott, D.F., Uldall, P.R. and Kerr, D.N.S. (1970) 'Plasma Renin and Exchangeable Sodium in the Hypertension of Chronic Renal Failure', *J. Med.*, *39*, 377–94

Willassen, Y. and Ofstad, J. (1980) 'Renal Sodium Excretion and Peritubular Capillary Physical Factors in Essential Hypertension', *Hypertension*, *2*, 771–9

Winternitz, S.R. and Oparil, S. (1982) 'The Importance of the Renal Nerves in the Pathogenesis of Experimental Hypertension', *Hypertension*, *4*, Suppl. III, III108–14

Yagi, S., Kramsch, D.M., Madoff, I.M. and Hollander, W. (1968) 'Plasma Renin Activity in Hypertension Associated with Coarctation of the Aorta', *Am. J. Physiol*, *215*, 605–10

Zimmerman, B.G. (1981) 'Adrenergic Facilitation by Angiotensin: Does it Serve a Physiological Function?, *Clin Sci.*, *60*, 343–8

Zimmerman, B.G. and Mommsen, C. (1981) 'Renal Blood Flow Changes in Contralateral Kidney of Goldblatt Hypertensive Dog', *Am. J. Physiol.*, *241*, H145–8

Zusman, R.M. and Keiser, H.R. (1977) 'Prostaglandin Biosynthesis by Rabbit Renomedullary Interstitial Cells in Tissue Culture: Stimulation by Angiotensin II, Bradykinin and Arginine Vasopressin', *J. Clin. Invest.*, *60*, 215–23

9 RENAL FUNCTION IN PREGNANCY

Roger Green

Introduction

The purpose of this chapter is to discuss recent advances in knowledge of the physiological changes in renal function that occur during pregnancy. Pre-eclampsia and other changes that occur in abnormal or diseased states will not be considered, even though the high incidence of pre-eclampsia in primi-gravidae makes it almost 'normal'; interested readers should consult Aber (1983). Attention will be concentrated on those areas of renal function where significant advances have occurred over the last 8 to 10 years, so some topics, e.g. handling of amino acids by the kidney, are omitted.

For a variety of reasons most work has concentrated on human pregnancy, and until recently little has been known of pregnancy-induced renal changes in animals. This has meant that although plasma concentrations of solutes can be monitored, as can the urine output and composition, the kidney has to be treated very much as a 'black box' whose internal workings have not been probed. As a consequence, many of the changes are descriptive, and inform-ation of pregnancy-induced changes in underlying mechanisms is sparse.

Most work on the renal changes during pregnancy in animals has related to the rat. The normal length of gestation in the rat is 21-22 days, and some authors equate one week of rat pregnancy with one trimester of human pregnancy. Most of the changes so far described in the rat are qualitatively similar to those in women. There is one facet of rat physiology that has helped in our understanding of underlying mechanisms: the state of pseudopregnancy. Stimulation of the cervix with a glass rod, mating with a sterile male, or injecting either progesterone or prolactin, produces a physiological state resembling the early part of pregnancy and lasting for 10-12 days; there are no fetuses or placentae, so changes occurring in this state are likely to result from the changes in maternal hormones.

Kidney Growth

Maternal body weight increases during pregnancy in women and experimental animals. What has only recently been appreciated is that renal size probably increases as well. X-ray studies have shown that renal length probably increases by up to 1 cm in women (Bailey and Rolleston, 1971; Kaupilla *et al.*, 1972), and autopsies have shown that the weight of kidneys from pregnant women is greater than that from comparable controls. An increase in the size of glomeruli was also demonstrated (Sheenan and Lynch, 1973). Pollack and Nettles (1960) were unable to demonstrate any other microscopic changes in samples obtained by renal biopsy in patients undergoing caesarean section.

It is much easier to document changes in experimental animals. Mackay (1928) demonstrated that the increase in renal size was consonant with the increase in body size, and this has been amply confirmed since Garland *et al.*, (1978) showed that there was a 13 per cent increase in dry kidney weight in 7-day pregnant rats, although the difference between pregnant animals and virgin controls diminished as pregnancy progressed (Figure 9.1). Although confirmed by a number of studies from the same group (e.g. Arthur and Green, 1983), these results are at variance with those obtained by Davison and Lindheimer (1980), who found an increase in wet weight of the kidney, but no increase in dry weight, so the increased weight of the kidney was due to its increased water content. They also measured [^{14}C]choline uptake into phospholipids in the kidney and were unable to demonstrate an increased incorporation; this also led to the conclusion that the increased kidney weight was not due to growth. There is evidence in mice, however, that growth of tissues does occur; mice have a 25 per cent increase in kidney weight during pregnancy and an increased renal content of RNA. Since DNA content showed no significant change from virgin controls, it was concluded that mice at least showed cellular hypertrophy, but no hyperplasia (Matthews, 1977).

Figure 9.1: Changes in Kidney Weight and Proximal Tubular Length during Normal Rat Pregnancy. P = animals at 7, 12 and 19 days of pregnancy. V = virgin animals of the same age. Values are means ± SEM

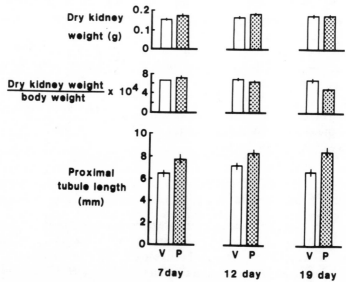

Reprinted with permission from Garland *et al.* (1978)

Rats do not increase the number of nephrons during pregnancy (Balmer *et al.*, 1977); in this they resemble humans. The length of the proximal convoluted tubule is increased early in pregnancy and by the end of the first week is 20-25 per cent longer than in comparably aged virgins (Figure 9.1; Garland *et al.*, 1978; Pirie, 1979; Atherton and Pirie, 1981). There is less information on other parts of the nephron but a general medullary hypertrophy has been described (Chang *et al.*, 1978).

The causes of these changes are not fully known. However, pseudo-pregnancy induced by mating with sterile rats produced an increased length of proximal tubule (Atherton *et al.*, 1982a), as did injections of prolactin if they induced a pseudopregnant state (El Karib *et al.*, 1983), but these were not accompanied by a significant change in kidney weight (El Karib, 1981). Chronic administration of progesterone resulted neither in elongation of the proximal tubule, nor in increased kidney weight (El Karib, 1981; El Karib *et al.*, 1983).

Renal Haemodynamics

Introduction

There are dramatic changes in the whole cardiovascular system during pregnancy. It is generally recognised that there is an early rise in cardiac output which is maintained throughout pregnancy. The increased blood flow is distributed mainly to the uterus (and its contents), the skin, mammary tissue, liver, gut and kidneys. In spite of the increased cardiac output, blood pressure, particularly diastolic blood pressure, usually decreases in normal pregnancy because of a dramatic fall in total peripheral resistance. A much more comprehensive review is given by de Swiet (1980).

As regards renal function, consideration needs to be given to renal plasma flow (or renal blood flow) and glomerular filtration rate. Renal plasma flow is one of the major determinants of glomerular filtration rate (Baylis and Brenner, 1978).

Changes in Glomerular Filtration Rate

More is known about changes in glomerular filtration rate (GFR) during pregnancy than about changes in renal plasma flow (RPF), mainly because it is much easier to measure. Measurement of GFR usually involves clearance techniques, and both inulin and creatinine clearance have been used in humans: most animal experiments have relied on inulin clearance.

Prior to 1960 there was much debate about the effect of pregnancy on GFR in humans but there is now general agreement on the pattern of changes. Most of the early studies were bedevilled by methodological problems or inconsistencies, but these have largely now been identified and overcome (Lindheimer and Katz, 1977; Chesley, 1978).

During the first trimester there is a rise in GFR (see Figure 9.2) which may be 50–100 per cent of the resting non-pregnant level (Dignam *et al.*, 1958; Sims and Krantz, 1958; Davison and Hytten, 1974; Davison and Dunlop, 1980). There is some evidence from sequential studies in single patients that GFR varies throughout the menstrual cycle, rising after ovulation; if conception occurs there is a further rise which is detectable within a few days (Davison and Noble, 1981). In the third trimester there is, in some studies, a fall in GRF, especially if measurements are made with the subject supine (Lindheimer and Katz, 1977; Chesley, 1978), possibly because the large uterus compromises venous return which decreases cardiac output and hence renal perfusion. Measurements made with patients in the left lateral position (Chesley and Sloan, 1964) or in the upright position (Dunlop, 1979) have suggested that there is no fall in GFR late in pregnancy. The position is not as clear as might be expected, however, since one study showed that posture did not affect GFR late in pregnancy (Dunlop, 1976).

Figure 9.2: Changes in Glomerular Filtration Rate, Effective Renal Plasma Flow and Filtration Fraction during Human Pregnancy

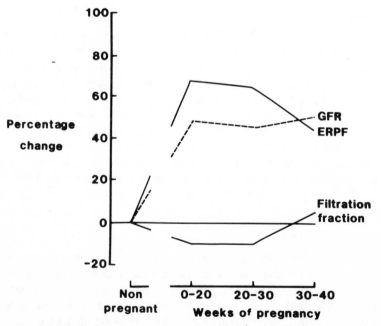

Reprinted with permission from Davison and Dunlop (1980) *Kidney International, 18,* p. 154

The majority of studies of renal haemodynamic changes in animals have been performed in the rat and there is general agreement that GFR rises by 25–50 per cent when compared with values in virgins. There is considerable

Figure 9.3: Changes in Glomerular Filtration Rate and Single Nephron Filtration Rate during Pregnancy in the Rat. Values are Mean ± SEM

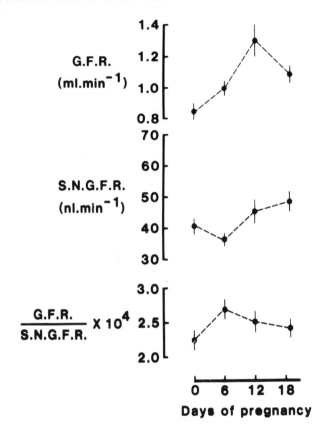

Reprinted with permission from Garland and Green (1982)

disagreement over *when* the changes occur, however. A number of reports suggest that the pattern of changes is similar to those occurring in humans (Figure 9.3). Thus in rats a rise has been demonstrated in GFR only two to three days after mating (Atherton and Pirie, 1981), which continues to the end of the first week. GFR is maintained for the second week and then stays constant or falls slightly towards the end of pregnancy (Matthews and Taylor, 1960; Lichton and Hugh, 1968; Atherton and Pirie, 1981; Garland and Green, 1982; Atherton, 1983). A number of workers have only been able to demonstrate a rise in GFR late in pregnancy (Lichton, 1963; Lindheimer and Katz, 1971; Davison and Lindheimer, 1980). The reasons for this discrepancy are not known. It was suggested (Davison and Lindheimer, 1980) that the difference might occur because of the anaesthetic used during the experiment, or because of the considerable amount of surgery which immediately preceded the experiment. Recently, however, studies in conscious animals that had had catheters implanted some days previously showed that the early rise in GFR was still demonstrable (Atherton, 1983; Conrad, 1983). Churchill *et al.* (1982) found that in their experiments the extensive surgery needed to prepare term-pregnant animals (i.e. animals just before delivery) for micropuncture reduced the GFR when compared with animals which were prepared only for clearance studies; indeed there was no significant difference between virgins and term-pregnant rats prepared for micropuncture. Garland and Green (1982) found no such effect. The difference may again be related to posture, since in the experiments of Churchill *et al.* (1982) the animals were supine, occasionally with some of the intestine displaced from the abdominal cavity, whereas Garland and Green (1982) used a left lateral approach to the kidney which allowed easier access to the kidney while the abdominal contents were not displaced.

Very few studies have measured the GFR in single nephrons (SNGFR). Churchill *et al.* (1982) found no significant change in SNGFR in term-pregnant animals, but since they found no change in GFR this is hardly surprising (see above). The changes described by Garland and Green (1982) were not easy to interpret, but they concluded that in superficially placed nephrons there were only small differences from virgins whereas in deeply placed juxtamedullary nephrons there was a much greater increase in blood flow. In addition they concluded that there was an increased tubuloglomerular feedback (see Chapter 4) occurring late in pregnancy. The significance of this for renal function during pregnancy is not readily apparent.

Changes in Renal Plasma Flow

Renal plasma flow is usually assessed from the clearance of *para*-amino-hippuric acid (PAH) which actually measures the plasma flow that goes to the glomeruli, i.e. the effective renal plasma flow (ERPF). This is not ideal since it depends on the assumption that PAH is extracted completely from plasma in one passage through the kidney, or that extraction of a similar fraction occurs in pregnant and non-pregnant alike. There is no evidence that this is so. Better information might become available from new imaging techniques for the kidney, but those currently in use, which depend on injection of isotopically labelled compounds, have not been used in pregnant women because of their possible effects on the fetus.

The early changes that occur in ERPF during pregnancy are similar to the changes that occur in GFR — a rapid rise during the first trimester in humans (Davison and Dunlop, 1980; Dunlop, 1981). Again there is a fall in ERPF during the third trimester, which has been attributed to postural effects during the measurement (Lindheimer and Katz, 1977; Chesley, 1978); there is good evidence, however, that even if the measurements are made with the woman in the left lateral position, there is still a highly significant fall in blood flow (Ezimokhai *et al.*, 1981).

Only a few studies have recorded changes in ERPF in rat pregnancy. In studies where an unusual pattern of GFR was recorded, no changes in ERPF were detected (Lindheimer and Katz, 1971; Davison and Lindheimer, 1980). In conscious animals a 20 per cent increase has been detected in pregnant animals with a fall towards term (Conrad, 1983). Baylis (1980a), calculating renal plasma flow from the inulin extraction ratio, showed an increase in 12 day pregnant animals, but towards term (19 days pregnant) it was not significantly elevated (Arthur and Green, 1983).

Since a significant redistribution of filtrate between superficial and deep nephrons has been demonstrated (Garland and Green, 1982), it might be expected that there would be an alteration of the distribution of blood flow during pregnancy. This has been examined directly using radioactively labelled microspheres (Figure 9.4). When rats were infused with 200 μl min^{-1} normal saline (comparable to the micropuncture studies), there was indeed a significantly different distribution in pregnant animals when compared with virgins (Walker, 1983; Garland and Walker, 1984). However, this was not because of a redistribution towards deep nephrons during pregnancy. Rather it arose because of the altered response of pregnant animals to saline infusion. When pregnant and virgin animals were infused at 20 μl min^{-1}, there was no significant difference in the ratio of blood flow to the superficial and deep nephrons in pregnant as compared with virgin animals. The response to increased saline infusion in virgin animals was to increase the blood flow to superficial (salt-losing) nephrons; pregnant animals were unable to offset this redistribution and so *relatively* more went to the deep (salt-retaining) nephrons than in the virgins.

Changes in Filtration Fraction

Filtration fraction is usually calculated as the ratio of GFR to ERPF. Only in studies where both have been measured can information be derived, and so little is known. Because of the relative changes of GFR and ERPF in humans (see Figure 9.2), there is a reduction in filtration fraction during the early part of pregnancy but towards term it increases. In rats no change is reported in the filtration fraction early in pregnancy although there is an increase towards term (Lindheimer and Katz, 1971; Davison and Lindheimer, 1980). It will be recalled that these studies, however, reported an unusual pattern for changes of GFR. The lack of change in filtration fraction has been confirmed in Munich-Wistar rats (Baylis, 1980a, b), but Arthur and Green (1983) report a small but significant decrease at term compared with virgins; they did not, however, measure filtration fraction at other times of pregnancy.

The best that can be said is that, as yet, in rats the data are not sufficient to give a clear picture.

Reasons for Haemodynamic Changes

It is not yet possible to be certain what are the underlying causes for the

Figure 9.4: Changes in Blood Flow Distribution during Pregnancy. In the upper figure the ratio of outer cortical blood flow is plotted for rats infused at either 20 μl min^{-1} saline (X) or 200 μl min^{-1} saline (Y). In the lower figure the ratio of the outer cortical blood flow to inner cortical blood flow at the high rate of infusion to that at the low rate of infusion, i.e. Y/X is presented

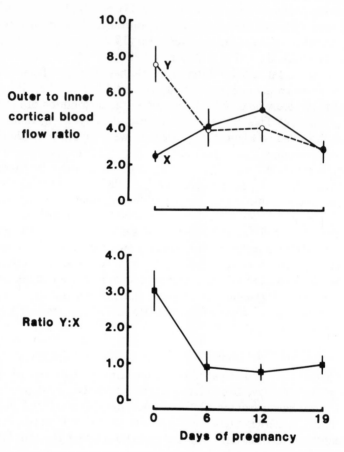

Data from Walker (1983)

changes in renal haemodynamics that occur during pregnancy. Certainly some of the changes are consequent on the overall change in cardiac output, but the changes in renal plasma flow are proportionately much greater than those in cardiac output.

Most of the changes in renal haemodynamics in pregnant rats also occur in pseudopregnant animals (Atherton *et al.*, 1982a). It appears likely, therefore, that the changes are hormonal in nature and do not depend on the presence of the fetus. Progesterone and prolactin are two hormones known to be elevated early in rat pregnancy and pseudopregnancy (Freeman *et al.*, 1974; Pepe and

Rothchild, 1974; Smith and Neill, 1976). It therefore seemed logical to test
the effects of these two hormones on renal haemodynamics.

When prolactin was administered for 7 days, with divided doses for the first
3 days to mimic the twice-daily prolactin surge (Smith and Neill, 1976),
significant increases in GFR occurred (Figure 9.5, El Karib *et al.*, 1983). On
the other hand, Munich-Wistar rats which do not have an early rise in prolactin
during pregnancy (H.O. Garland, J.C. Atherton, C. Baylis and M.R.A. Morgan,
unpublished) did not show the early rise in GFR which is common in Sprague-
Dawley rats (Baylis, 1980b). Progesterone administered for 12 days had no
effect on GFR (El Karib *et al.*, 1983).

Figure 9.5: Effects of Intramuscular Injection of Prolactin, 16 IU per Day in Divided Doses for
7 Days, on Renal Function and Proximal Tubular Length. C = Control animals injected with
saline; P = prolactin-treated animals

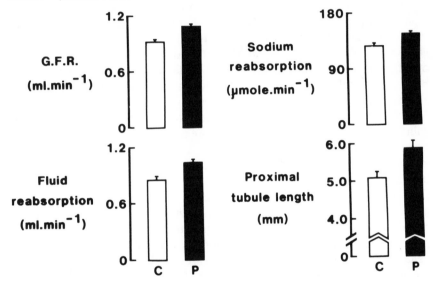

Reprinted with permission from El Karib *et al.* (1983)

It is not known whether prolactin exerts its effect directly on the glomerulus,
or whether it acts indirectly by increasing plasma volume (Atherton *et al.*,
1982b), which in turn may be a consequence of its action to increase drinking
behaviour (Kaufman, 1981). Although prolactin seems necessary for the
initial rise in GFR, its role in the maintenance of GFR is less certain. There is
some evidence that placentae are necessary to maintain the GFR at its raised
level even though the fetus may not be (Matthews and Taylor, 1960).
Presumably the action is dependent on one or other of the hormones which are
produced by the placenta. Recently it has been suggested that dopamine may
be important in modifying renal blood flow, and primigravid women have been
shown to have an increased urinary excretion of dopamine (Perkins *et al.*, 1981).

At the level of the single glomerulus, reasons for the changes in GFR are difficult to determine. In the only studies that have fully analysed the determinants of SNGFR, the increase in GFR was due solely to an increase in the renal plasma flow and there were no changes in glomerular capillary pressures, oncotic pressures or the permeability of the glomerular membranes (Baylis, 1980a, b). Similar results were found in pseudopregnant animals (Baylis, 1982).

Salt and Water

Introduction

Both women and rats gain weight during pregnancy and a large proportion of this is due to retention of fluid. In women there are obvious difficulties in monitoring normal weight gain because (a) of the wide range of weight gains that occur; (b) most have been subjected to 'advice' on the appropriate weight gain and modify their diet accordingly; (c) of poor record keeping, particularly over the first three months of pregnancy; (d) there is a very fine dividing line between normal weight gain and the abnormal gains that occur in pre-eclampsia. Nevertheless, two large series have been reported (Humphreys, 1954; Thomson and Billewicz, 1957), and both agree that the average weight gain is 11-12 kg after the 12th week of pregnancy. Of this total body water accounts for about 7.5 litres although there is considerable variation between individuals and between different series of results. Measurements of the increase in extracellular volume also vary widely, ranging from 6.9 litres (Röttger, 1953) to 3 litres (Friedman *et al.*, 1951). Much of the discrepancy may result from the use of different tracers in the measurement since for many of them it is not known whether they behave in pregnancy as they do in non-pregnant individuals. It is at present impossible to decide what are the 'correct' values. There are also concomitant increases in blood and plasma volumes (Miller *et al.*, 1915; Lund and Donovan, 1967; Taylor and Lind, 1979). Retention of sodium also occurs, and it is calculated that some 900 mmol is retained over the course of a normal pregnancy (Lindheimer *et al.*, 1977). Much of this is distributed in the increased extracellular fluid but some crosses the placenta for the fetus.

Rats gain proportionately more weight than women during pregnancy. At the end of gestation they may be up to 50 per cent heavier than comparably aged virgins (Garland *et al.*, 1978) and the increase in weight is detectable from early in gestation (Figure 9.6). There is also an increase in extracellular volume early in pregnancy (Atherton *et al.*, 1982b) and an increase in plasma volume (Baylis, 1980a; Atherton *et al.*, 1982b; Lindheimer *et al.*, 1983). Similar increases in plasma volume have also been reported in pregnant rabbits (Bjellin and Carter, 1977; Prince, 1982).

The increased fluid and salt retention that occurs during gestation might be due to an increased fluid and salt intake or to a decreased loss via the kidney. Whatever the cause, the body seems to reset its volume receptors so that the extracellular fluid volume is maintained at the new expanded level. The normal response to an expanded extracellular fluid compartment, i.e. excretion of increased amounts of salt and water, is lost.

Figure 9.6: Increases in Body Weight of Women and Rats during Pregnancy. A. Increases in weight of 2868 normotensive women during their first pregnancy. From Thomson and Billewicz, 1957. B. Percentage increases in body weight of a cohort of pregnant rats (●) and virgin controls (○). Data are expressed as percentage of body weight before the experiment, i.e. day−1

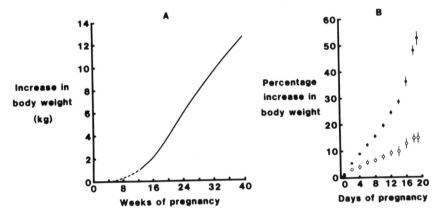

Reprinted with permission from Garland *et al.* (1978)

Increased Intake of Salt and Water

Balance experiments, where intake and output of fluid and sodium are monitored, are very difficult to perform in women but relatively easy to perform in virgin and pregnant rats which can be maintained in metabolic cages. There is an early rise in fluid intake and in food intake, presumably because of increased appetite (Churchill *et al.*, 1980; Al Modhefer, 1984). The increased fluid intake is balanced by an increased urine output during the first week of pregnancy in the rat, but during the second week, input exceeds output and retention of fluid occurs (Lichton, 1961; Kirksey and Pike, 1962; Churchill *et al.*, 1982; Atherton *et al.*, 1982b; Al Modhefer, 1984). Qualitatively similar results have been reported in humans (Francis, 1960) and goats (Olsson *et al.*, 1982).

It has been reported that the osmotic threshold necessary to stimulate thirst is decreased in pregnancy in both women and rats (Durr *et al.*, 1981, 1982). It is not known what causes the increased intake of fluid although chronic administration of progesterone will have that effect (El Karib, 1981). Prolactin is known to be dipsogenic (Kaufman, 1981) although the results of chronic administration did not indicate an increased intake.

In rats an increased intake of food (and hence sodium) may precede that of water (Atherton *et al.*, 1982b; Al Modhefer, 1984). Again this can be mimicked by prolactin and progesterone (El Karib *et al.*, 1983).

Changes in Kidney Function

The increased GFR during pregnancy results in increased delivery of sodium and water to the kidney, irrespective of any increased intakes. In humans this increase amounts to some 5–10 mol of sodium per day and 35–70 litres of fluid per day. This extra load must be reabsorbed otherwise massive sodium depletion would rapidly ensue.

In rats it can be shown that increased water and sodium reabsorption occur very early in pregnancy, certainly by the end of the first week (Atherton and Pirie, 1981; Garland and Green, 1982; Atherton, 1983) and that these are maintained throughout pregnancy (Figure 9.7). Other workers (those who were unable to detect changes in GFR) were unable to detect changes in salt and water reabsorption. However, since there is a tight link between GFR and reabsorption of salt and water, this is not surprising.

Changes in Single Nephron Function: Proximal Tubule

There have been few attempts to determine the sites in the nephron at which the increased salt and water reabsorption occurs during pregnancy. Experiments in women are not possible, and experiments in rats can only be performed in anaesthetised animals after they have undergone extensive surgical preparation; usually they also receive a high infusion rate of normal saline.

It might be expected on *a priori* grounds that the proximal convoluted tubule would be the site at which most of the increased load was absorbed since that is the site of greatest salt and water reabsorption. Experiments to measure the intrinsic reabsorptive capacity of proximal tubular epithelium (i.e. the rate of reabsorption per unit surface area) showed no significant change at any stage of pregnancy (Garland and Green, 1982). Collections from the *end* of the proximal convoluted tubule, however, indicated that, in the first and second weeks of pregnancy, although there was no alteration in the fraction of the filtered fluid reabsorbed, there was an increase in the total amount reabsorbed. In view of the similarity of the intrinsic reabsorption capacity, this means that the increased reabsorption capacity was a consequence of the increased length of the proximal tubule (see above) or that it was a flow-dependent reabsorption. Using indirect methods involving maximal diuretic water-loaded rats, Al Modhefer (1984) also came to the conclusion that increased proximal reabsorption of water occurred during pregnancy. Towards the end of pregnancy, total proximal tubular reabsorption was not dissimilar from that in virgins, and so the fractional reabsorption was considerably reduced (Garland and Green, 1982).

Reabsorption of fluid from the proximal tubule has been shown to depend on the rate of fluid flow along the nephron (Green *et al.*, 1981; Häberle and von

Figure 9.7: Changes in Glomerular Filtration Rate, Fluid Reabsorption and Sodium Reabsorption during Pregnancy in Rats. All animals were infused with 200 μl min^{-1} saline during the measurements

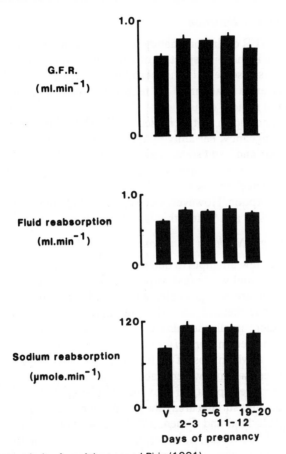

Reprinted with permission from Atherton and Pirie (1981)

Baeyer, 1983). This also occurs in virgin females, but in pregnancy, certainly in 12 day pregnant rats, proximal tubular reabsorption is no longer flow dependent (Figure 9.8, Walker, 1983; Garland *et al.*, 1984).

Changes in Single Nephron Function: Loop of Henle and More Distal Sites

However, when the delivery of fluid to the beginning of the distal tubule was considered, it was found that a constant fraction was delivered at all stages of pregnancy. This means that the loop of Henle has the capacity to reabsorb the excess delivered by the proximal tubule, and if more is delivered, then more is reabsorbed; presumably this is a flow-dependent phenomenon that persists in pregnancy. However, since a constant *fraction* is delivered to the distal

Figure 9.8: Reabsorption from Individual Proximal Tubules of Virgin (●—●) and 12 day Pregnant Rats (O---O) during Artificial Perfusion at Different Rates. Values are mean ± SEM

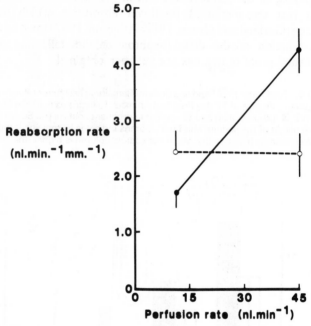

From Walker (1983)

nephron, this still means that it is more in absolute terms. So even in distal segments more fluid is reabsorbed during pregnancy since the amount of urine in the pregnant and virgin animals undergoing saline diuresis was similar (Garland and Green, 1982).

The sodium concentration in fluid at the end of the proximal tubule is similar to that in the glomerular filtrate, but thereafter sodium and water reabsorption are not as closely linked. Fluid delivered to the early part of the distal tubule has a reduced sodium concentration. Throughout pregnancy this is reduced even further because more sodium is reabsorbed in the loop of Henle in pregnancy (Garland and Green, 1982). Churchill *et al.* (1982), the only other workers to perform this experiment, were unable to show altered sodium handling, but it should be remembered that they were also unable to demonstrate an increased GFR, possibly because of the methods employed (see above). Direct perfusion of the loop of Henle at a constant rate indicates that sodium reabsorption was greater in pregnant than in virgin rats (R. Green, unpublished results).

Summary of Single Nephron Changes

Changes in reabsorption from different parts of the nephron are summarised in

Figure 9.9, which plots for 12 day pregnant rats and virgins the amount of fluid and sodium remaining at the glomerulus, the end of the proximal tubule, the beginning of the distal tubule and in the urine. From the diagram it is obvious that the increased fractional absorption which occurs during pregnancy (Garland and Green, 1982; Atherton, 1983) must be dependent on altered function of the distal nephron or the collecting ducts. Direct experimental proof of this has not yet been obtained.

Figure 9.9: Total Amount of Fluid and Sodium Remaining at Different Points along Nephrons in the Kidney of Virgin and 12 day Pregnant Animals: □ indicates fluid and ▨ sodium in virgin animals (V); ■ indicates fluid and ▨ sodium in pregnant animals (P). Scales are chosen such that equal height of the sodium and fluid columns indicates isotonicity. If the fluid column is higher, then there is hypotonicity, and if the sodium column is higher, the fluid is hypertonic

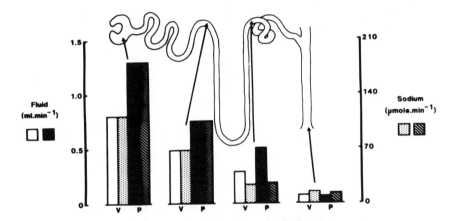

All the tubular changes described apply to superficial nephrons; there are no studies on juxtamedullary nephrons. Altered distribution to the deep (salt-retaining) nephrons at the expense of the superficial (salt-losing) nephrons may play some part in determining the final excretion of sodium. It may be pertinent that, on salt loading, virgin animals can redistribute their blood flow to more superficial nephrons whereas pregnant animals cannot (Garland and Walker, 1984).

Reasons for Renal Changes

In gross terms the reabsorption of sodium and water by the kidneys of pseudopregnant rats parallels that in pregnant animals (Atherton *et al.*, 1982a), and there would therefore appear to be a hormonal basis for many of the changes. Micropuncture experiments to determine reabsorption at single nephron level have not been performed in pseudopregnant animals.

Many hormones have been shown to have effects on salt and water handling. The plasma concentration of many of them is altered in pregnancy; however, there is no direct evidence that the altered plasma concentrations affect the altered renal function.

Oestrogens. Sodium is retained with little change in potassium excretion when oestrogens are chronically administered to human subjects (Dignam *et al.*, 1956; Reid *et al.*, 1972; Katz and Lindheimer, 1977) and to dogs (Christy and Shaver, 1974; Johnson and Davies, 1976) resulting in an increased extracellular volume (Aitken *et al.*, 1974). Acute administration had no effect. The effect of oestrogens in rats is controversial, some investigators finding a decrease in sodium excretion (De Vries *et al.*, 1972) whereas others found no effect (Simpson and Tait, 1952). However, whereas, in human pregnancy, oestrogens increase gradually (Klopper, 1980), predominantly derived from the placenta, oestrogens in rat pregnancy remain at a low level until day 4, peak sharply, are reduced to low levels again by day 5, and remain there until day 18, when they rise rapidly until parturition occurs (Yoshinaga *et al.*, 1969; Shaikh, 1971).

Progesterone. Progesterone has a natriuretic effect in man which may give rise to a compensatory rise in plasma aldosterone concentration (Oparil *et al.*, 1975) and it is suggested that it acts as a competitive inhibitor to aldosterone (Ehrlich and Lindheimer, 1972). However, it may have actions because it acts as a general vasodilator (Oparil *et al.*, 1975). In species other than humans there is no evidence that progesterone is natriuretic (Thorn and Engel, 1938; Fimognari *et al.*, 1967; O'Connell *et al.*, 1969; Lindheimer *et al.*, 1976; El Karib, 1981) although it may result in retention of potassium (El Karib, 1981). Both in women (Klopper, 1980) and in rats (Pepe and Rothchild, 1974) progesterone concentration has been shown to increase throughout pregnancy. Chronic and acute injections of progesterone into rats indicate that although some of the changes in pregnancy can be mimicked, the whole picture is not the same (El Karib, 1981; El Karib *et al.*, 1983).

Prolactin. Prolactin is concerned with volume and osmolal homeostasis in amphibians, birds and fish (see Ensor, 1978) but its role in mammals is less well defined. In man it causes salt and water retention (Horrobin *et al.*, 1971; Buckman *et al.*, 1976) but whether this has physiological significance is not known. Sodium and water excretion are reported to be reduced by prolactin in the conscious (Lockett and Nail, 1965; Bliss and Lote, 1982) and the anaesthetised rat (Lucci *et al.*, 1975), but this is not a universal finding and it has been reported that these effects may only occur after chronic but not after acute administration (El Karib *et al.*, 1983; Mills *et al.*, 1983). Walker and Garland (1982) reported a specific effect of chronic administration on proximal tubular reabsorption. During pregnancy in both women and rats there is an increase in prolactin concentration in the plasma shortly after conception (Freeman *et al.*, 1974; Smith and Neill, 1976; Rigg *et al.*, 1977), although it is not known whether women exhibit the twice-daily prolactin peak which is seen in rats. Chronic administration of prolactin in rats produced many of the early changes in pregnancy (El Karib, 1981; El Karib *et al.*, 1983).

Renin-Angiotensin-Aldosterone System. Renin is an enzyme that has no direct renal effects. Its action is directed towards plasma renin substrate from which angiotensin I and eventually angiotensin II are produced. Angiotensin II, or possibly a further derivative, angiotensin III, has a biphasic action in that at low doses in intact animals (Hall *et al.*, 1980) and in the isolated kidney (Borresen *et al.*, 1982) it causes sodium retention, probably because of a direct action on proximal tubular reabsorption (Harris and Young, 1977), and at higher doses proximal tubular reabsorption is inhibited (Harris and Young, 1977; Schuster *et al.*, 1982). It has also been suggested that angiotensin II might inhibit (Lowitz *et al.*, 1969) or stimulate sodium reabsorption in the distal nephron (Johnson and Malvin, 1977). Because it is a vasoconstrictor, angiotensin II is known to alter blood pressure and possibly also the filtration coefficient of the glomerular membrane (see Chapter 2). Both of these effects might have secondary consequences for sodium reabsorption by the kidney. One of the major actions of angiotensin II, however, is as a regulator of aldosterone secretion by the adrenal cortex. Aldosterone controls sodium reabsorption and potassium secretion in the distal convoluted tubules and collecting ducts, and so has a major influence on sodium homeostasis (Schwartz and Burg, 1978; Wright and Giebisch, 1978).

Renin is secreted in two forms, active and inactive. Plasma renin *concentration* reflects total renin concentration in the plasma, and plasma renin *activity* reflects the concentration of the active form. In women all components of the renin angiotensin-aldosterone system increase during pregnancy. Plasma renin activity and plasma renin concentration both rise early in pregnancy (Vallotton *et al.*, 1982) and there is also a rise in inactive renin concentration (Hsueh *et al.*, 1982). Plasma renin substrate increases early in pregnancy (Immonen *et al.*, 1982; Vallotton *et al.*, 1982), possibly induced by the rise in oestrogens during gestation (Immonen *et al.*, 1983). Together these effects result in a rise in angiotensin II concentration in the plasma (Godard *et al.*, 1976; Broughton-Pipkin and Symonds, 1977) although the expected rise in vascular resistance is prevented (Gant *et al.*, 1973). Aldosterone also rises during pregnancy (Wintour *et al.*, 1978; Vallotton *et al.*, 1982). Later in pregnancy, however, there is no correlation between plasma renin activity, angiotensin II, and aldosterone concentrations in plasma (Winberger *et al.*, 1976). It may be that other factors need to be considered.

In animals as well there are increased concentrations of plasma renin, even though plasma renin substrate is reduced (Whipp *et al.*, 1978). Angiotensin II has not been measured throughout pregnancy but aldosterone is raised in many species (Wintour *et al.*, 1976; Whipp *et al.*, 1978; Churchill *et al.*, 1981).

Other Hormones. A number of other substances whose plasma concentrations alter during pregnancy also have renal actions. There is little if any evidence for their effects in pregnancy and their physiological significance is doubtful. They include prostaglandins, thyroxine, and oxytocin. Antidiuretic hormone is considered later.

Osmoregulation

Changes in Plasma Osmolality

So far we have considered only the total amounts of fluid and sodium excreted and retained. Their concentration in plasma may be equally important during pregnancy. Normally the osmolality of plasma is closely monitored by the osmoreceptors in the hypothalamus; in turn they control the amount of antidiuretic hormone (ADH) secreted by the posterior lobe of the pituitary gland. ADH has marked effects on the volume and osmolality of the urine by controlling water reabsorption from distal parts of the nephron.

During pregnancy in humans, plasma osmolality is reduced by some 8–10 mOsmol per kilogram of water (McDonald and Good, 1971; McDonald *et al.*, 1976; Davison *et al.*, 1981, 1983). Changes have been reported as early as the second week after conception and they persist until term (Davison *et al.*, 1981, 1983).

In rats also, plasma osmolality is reduced during pregnancy (Lichton, 1961; Durr *et al.*, 1981; Atherton *et al.*, 1982b; Al Modhefer, 1984) but this is not common to all species. Sheep (Wintour *et al.*, 1976) and goats (Olsson *et al.*, 1982) go through pregnancy with no detectable changes in plasma osmolality.

The major cause of the reduction in plasma osmolality that occurs in both humans and rats is a reduction in the plasma concentration of sodium.

Changes in Antidiuretic Hormone

Since changes in plasma osmolality are a major determinant of ADH secretion, it might be expected that in pregnancy the secretion of ADH and its plasma concentration would be reduced in both humans and rats. This is not the case. Such studies as have been performed indicate that plasma concentrations of ADH are similar during pregnancy to those obtained in non-pregnant controls (Durr *et al.*, 1981; Al Modhefer, 1984; Davison *et al.*, 1984), and that increases of osmolality above the new plasma concentration in pregnancy produced significant rises in ADH (Figure 9.10; Durr *et al.*, 1981).

To account for this apparently altered relationship it has been proposed that during pregnancy the osmoreceptors (as occured with the volume receptors — see earlier) are reset so that the lower osmolality and the higher extracellular volume are regarded as normal. Control mechanisms are activated to hold the osmolality about this new set point. The underlying cause of the change of the set point is not known.

Figure 9.10: The Relationship between the Plasma Osmolality and Plasma Concentrations of Antidiuretic Hormone during a 2 h Infusion of 5% Saline in Human Pregnancy. Data are derived during the third trimester of pregnancy (●) or 6-8 weeks after delivery (○). The lines for best fit are shown; for pregnant $P_{ADH} = 0.32$ $(P_{osm} = 279)$ $r = 0.79$; post partum $P_{ADH} = 0.38$ $(P_{osm} = 285)$ $r = 0.86$

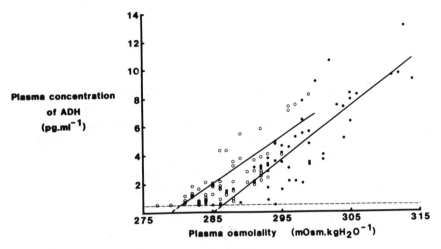

Reprinted with permission from Davison *et al.* (1984)

Urine Osmolality

Reports suggest that there are no changes in urine osmolality in human pregnancy (Davison *et al.*, 1981) but this appears not to be the case in other species. Goats decrease urine osmolality gradually throughout pregnancy (Olsson *et al.*, 1982). The picture is less clear in rats. Durr *et al.* (1981) reported that there was no difference in the urine osmolality of rats during pregnancy, but the data showed considerable variability and this might have masked some of the changes. On the other hand a number of workers in our laboratories have clearly demonstrated a reduction of urine osmolality, perhaps as early as the second day after conception, and this was maintained till the end of pregnancy when the difference amounted to some 400–500 mOsmol kg^{-1}water (Figure 9.11). This was caused by a reduction of sodium, potassium chloride and urea concentration in the urine, probably because of increased water intake and hence excretion (Pirie, 1979; Atherton *et al.*, 1982; Al Modhefer, 1984). When rats were subjected to water deprivation, however, pregnant animals were able to raise their urine osmolality to the same level as virgins (Al Modhefer, 1984).

The causes of dilute urine production are not clear. There was no alteration in ADH secretion (see above) but there is a decrease in the concentrations of solutes in the renal medulla (Al Modhefer, 1984) which thus resulted in a decreased gradient to drive water reabsorption from the collecting ducts. Whether the reduced solute concentration in the medulla is a consequence of

Figure 9.11: Changes in Water Intake, Urine Output and Urine Osmolality during Pregnancy in the Rat. Animals were maintained in individual metabolic cages and followed through pregnancy. Pregnant animals are shown (●) and virgin animals (○). Control data are the means (± SEM) of both groups prior to the induction of pregnancy

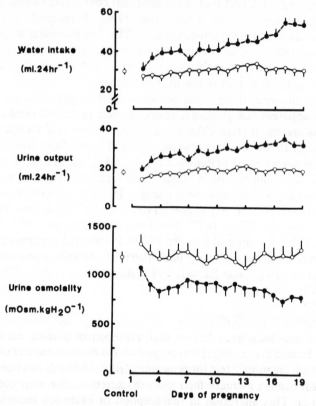

From Al Modhefer (1984)

increased blood flow in medullary blood vessels which would dissipate the gradient, or whether increased reabsorption of water from distal parts of the nephron dilutes the medulla, is not known. Because of increased flow rates in the distal parts of the nephron, it may be that fluid passing along the collecting ducts does not have sufficient time to achieve osmotic equilibrium with the medulla (Al Modhefer, 1984). Alterations in blood flow have not been investigated.

Glucose

Normal Glucose Handling

To understand the alterations to glucose handling that occur in pregnancy it is necessary to briefly review the reabsorption of glucose by the kidney in non-pregnant animals. The conventional description of glucose reabsorption is oversimplified. Glucose is said to be reabsorbed by a secondary active-transport process in the first part of the proximal convoluted tubule, until the limit of reabsorptive capacity of the system (Tm_G) is reached. Any excess glucose then passes out in the urine (Smith, 1951). Any glucose that appears in the urine would result either because of an increase in the amount of glucose filtered at the glomerulus, or because there is a defect in the transport mechanisms in the first part of the proximal tubule.

Recently, with better chemical detection methods for glucose in the urine, it has become apparent that glucose is always present in normal urine although the amounts are small (Renschler *et al.*, 1966; Rohde and Deetjen, 1968; Fröhnert *et al.*, 1970; von Baeyer *et al.*, 1973). This confirms what Benedict discovered many years ago (Benedict *et al.*, 1918). In addition it has been shown that the concept of a Tm_G is ill-founded. Tubular maximum reabsorption for glucose varies with changes in GFR, sodium reabsorption and extracellular volume expansion (Baines, 1971; Keyes and Swanson, 1971; Kurtzman and Pillay, 1973; Morel and de Rouffignac, 1973; Schultze and Berger, 1973; Kwong and Bennett, 1974). Parts of the nephron other than the first part of the proximal tubule have also been shown to reabsorb glucose (Fröhnert *et al.*, 1970; von Baeyer, 1975; Bishop *et al.*, 1981; Bishop and Green, 1983).

Glucose Excretion in Pregnancy

In women it has long been known that excretion of glucose increases in pregnancy. Indeed at one time it was suggested that measurement of glucose in the urine was a diagnostic test for pregnancy (Blot, 1856)! It has been shown that pregnant women increase their glucose excretion soon after conception (Figure 9.12). This alteration in reabsorption or excretion becomes more apparent if the reabsorption mechanisms are stressed by infusing glucose (Davison and Hytten, 1975). Normal patterns of glucose excretion are regained within a week of the end of pregnancy (Davison and Lovedale, 1974). When tested using conventional 'dipsticks', the increased glucose excretion appears to be intermittent, but it should be remembered that these are not very sensitive and in any case measure concentration, not total amount. Thus variations in the amount of water excreted would be expected to influence the results.

Pregnant rats also excrete more glucose than their virgin controls (Bishop and Green, 1980; Wen and McSherry, 1982). At normal concentrations of plasma glucose this was about twice the excretion in virgins. When the animals were stressed by infusing glucose to make them grossly hyperglycaemic (plasma glucose > 20 mmol litre^{-1}), rather surprisingly the pregnant animals excreted *less* glucose than virgins (Bishop and Green, 1980).

The explanations usually given for the increased glucose excretion mainly

Figure 9.12: Glucose Excretion in Pregnant Women. Data are derived from 20 normal pregnancies reported by Lind and Hytten (1972) which had at least one measurement prior to pregnancy and in each trimester. Multiple measurements are averaged. Bars indicate standard error

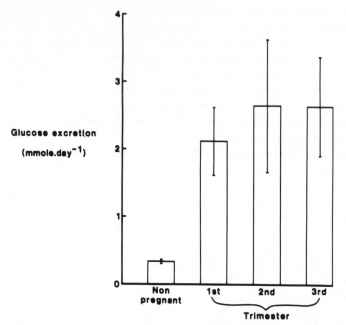

depend on the older concepts of glucose reabsorption. From the earlier description it will be obvious that an increased filtered load of glucose (presumably consequent on the increased GFR) or a defect in tubular reabsorption of glucose must be prime candidates (Christiansen, 1958; Welsh and Sims, 1960). It has recently been suggested that previous undetected urinary tract infections may have damaged the kidneys and that this causes or adds to the increased glucose excretion (Davison and Hytten, 1975).

It has not proved possible to test any of these hypotheses directly in women, but a number of investigations have now been performed in rats where reabsorption of glucose, rather than excretion, has been measured.

Glucose Reabsorption in Single Nephrons

When reabsorption and filtered load of glucose were measured in single nephrons in anaesthetised 7–8 day pregnant Sprague-Dawley rats, it was shown that the filtered load was increased. This resulted from an increase in GFR with no change in the plasma glucose concentration (Bishop and Green, 1981). However, contrary to what might be predicted, the absolute amount of glucose reabsorbed was greater in pregnant animals than in virgins. Although Tm_G, with measurement of glucose reabsorption at many plasma glucose concentrations, was not estimated, nevertheless at high glucose concentrations, with filtered loads four to five times normal and heavy loss of glucose in the urine, pregnant animals reabsorbed considerably more glucose in their proximal tubules than did virgin controls. Thus, while the evidence for an *increased* Tm_G in pregnancy is poor, there is no evidence for the decreased Tm_G as has been predicted (Christiansen, 1958; Welsh and Sims, 1960).

The only inference that can be drawn from the above results is that proximal reabsorption of glucose is not impaired in pregnancy, and so the altered reabsorption must occur in more distal parts of the nephron which normally reabsorbs some 5–8 per cent of the filtered glucose (Bishop *et al.*, 1981). In a preliminary communication, however, Wen and McSherry (1982) came to the conclusion that at 11–12 days of pregnancy in rats the increased glucose excretion could be explained by decreased proximal tubular reabsorption. Final comments on this must await the publication of a full paper.

Using a variety of micropuncture techniques Bishop and Green (1983) have been able to show that at normal plasma glucose concentrations pregnant animals reabsorbed slightly less of a glucose load presented directly to the loop of Henle than did virgins. When the system was stressed by infusion of glucose intravenously, however, the picture was not as clear. Pregnant animals reabsorbed less when net reabsorption was considered, although the unidirectional reabsorption flux was *greater* in pregnant animals. This was explained by postulating a leak of glucose into the loop of Henle which became significant only in hyperglycaemic pregnant animals (Bishop and Green, 1983). The existence of such a leak has been documented previously (Bishop *et al.*, 1981). It is not known whether cellular metabolism of glucose in the loop of Henle is a significant factor, nor whether it can be altered in pregnancy.

Results of microinjection studies into late distal tubules are easier to interpret. At both normal and high plasma glucose concentrations, pregnant animals were able to reabsorb less of a delivered load of glucose (Bishop and Green, 1983). It is postulated that this contributes significantly to the increased glucose excretion that occurs in pregnancy.

Summary of Glucose Reabsorption by the Nephron

Taking all the data presented by Bishop and Green (1980, 1981, 1983) it is possible to construct a composite model for glucose reabsorption in pregnancy. The data values are, of course, only approximate.

At normal plasma glucose concentrations (Figure 9.13) the abnormality of glucose reabsorption occurs in distal portions of the nephron. Increased filtration of glucose is matched by increased reabsorption in the proximal tubule, and because so little is delivered to the loop of Henle the differences in reabsorption there are not significant.

In hyperglycaemic animals (Figure 9.14) much more glucose is reabsorbed from the proximal tubules in pregnant animals than in virgin controls. (Because a constant infusion of glucose was used, the rise of plasma glucose

Figure 9.13: Glucose Reabsorption along a Single Idealised Nephron for Virgin and Pregnant Rats Maintained at Normal Glucose Concentration. Figures within the outline of the nephron indicate the amount of glucose remaining at that point and passing on to the next segment of nephron. Net reabsorption or secretory fluxes are shown outside the nephron, with an arrow indicating the direction of movement. Values are picomoles of glucose per minute

Glucose reabsorption at Normal Glucose concentration

Virgin

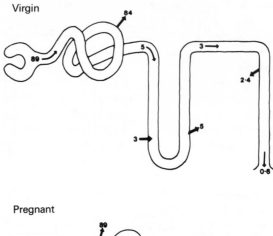

Pregnant

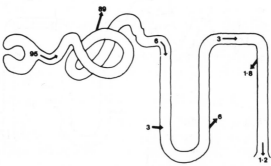

concentration in pregnant animals was less than that of age-matched controls and, by chance, the filtered loads were similar.) This means that less glucose is passed to the loop of Henle in pregnant rats. The net effect of the reabsorption and back-leak into the loop of Henle is less glucose reabsorption in pregnant animals, but more glucose is still delivered to the distal tubules in virgins than in pregnant animals. Even though more reabsorption occurs thereafter in the virgins, this cannot compensate for the increased delivery to the distal tubules so more glucose is excreted by the virgins.

Whether the same model can be applied to humans is not known. Direct experimental evidence of the sort obtained in rats can never be obtained. The best that can be said is that in humans there is, at present, no evidence that would refute the above hypothesis.

Figure 9.14: Glucose Reabsorption along a Single Idealised Nephron for Virgin and Pregnant Rats which Were Made Hyperglycaemic by Infusion of 5% Glucose. Other details as Figure 9.13

Glucose reabsorption at High Glucose concentration

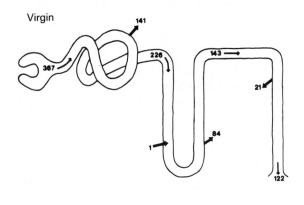

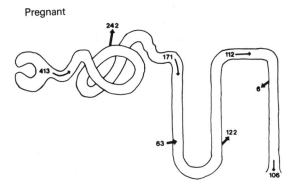

Uric Acid

Obstetricians have been interested in the renal handling of uric acid for a number of years. Normal pregnancy is associated with a reduced serum uric acid concentration (Semple *et al.*, 1974; Dunlop and Davison, 1977; Egwuatu, 1983; Lind *et al.*, 1984) and hyperuricaemia is associated with the delivery of small-for-dates infants (Dunlop *et al.*, 1978) and pre-eclampsia (Lancet and Fisher, 1956) in which it correlates well with the severity of the conditions, the findings on renal biopsy (Pollack and Nettles, 1960) and fetal prognosis (Redman *et al.*, 1976). It is thought that the increased plasma uric acid concentration results from reduced renal excretion (Seitchik *et al.*, 1958).

There is little information about the normal handling of uric acid in pregnancy other than two studies in humans which are at variance in some respects (Semple *et al.*, 1974; Dunlop and Davison, 1977). No studies have been performed in pregnant animals. Both the human studies agree that plasma uric acid concentration is low in the first trimester of pregnancy, and that this is caused by, or at least accompanied by, an increased clearance of uric acid by the kidney. There is also an increased fractional excretion of uric acid. Towards the end of pregnancy, Dunlop and Davison (1977) reported that there was an increase in plasma uric acid concentration which approached normal non-pregnant levels, and a concomitant decrease in the uric acid clearance by the kidney. Semple *et al.* (1974) found no such changes at the end of pregnancy. The reasons for this discrepancy are not known but may relate to methodological differences; the infusion rate of fluid was ten times that used by Semple *et al.* (1974) in the Dunlop and Davison (1977) study. Later data (Lind *et al.*, 1984) have shown that the rise in plasma uric acid concentration did not occur till after 32 weeks of gestation, and it may be that the patients reported by Semple *et al.* (1974) were monitored before this time (no precise data on time of sampling are given).

If renal handling of uric acid is such an important prognostic tool, it would seem to be essential that further studies be done to clarify the normal pattern of urate handling in pregnancy. To this end, experiments in animals may help to clarify the situation, although, since the amount of uric acid excreted depends on the filtered load and at least two reabsorptive and secretory processes (Lang, 1981), the final pattern emerging is likely to be complex.

Summary

In recent years a number of advances have taken place in our understanding of the changes that occur in normal renal function during pregnancy. Most of these have arisen because closely controlled experiments can be performed in animals, usually rats, whereas investigations in pregnant women, where much of the earlier work was done, cannot be adequately controlled. In addition some experiments have now been performed looking at changes in single nephron function. If the mechanism underlying the changes in pregnancy are ever to be understood, more of these investigations must be performed.

So far, most attention has been given to changes in renal haemodynamics, salt and water handling, osmoregulation and glucose handling, and recent advances in these fields are included in some detail. In other areas, e.g. handling of uric acid, potassium, calcium and acid-base balance, there has been little recent work, but these await our efforts in the future.

References

Aber, G. (1983) 'The Kidney in Pregnancy', in N.F. Jones and D.K. Peters (eds) *Advances in Renal Medicine,*, Churchill Livingstone, Edinburgh, pp. 177–95

Aitken, J.M., Lindsay, R. and Hart, D.M. (1974) 'The Redistribution of Body Sodium in Women on Long Term Oestrogen Therapy', *Clin. Sci. Mol. Med.*, 47, 179–87

Al Modhefer, A.K.J. (1984) 'Renal Function, Osmoregulation and Volume Homeostasis during Pregnancy in the Conscious Rat', PhD Thesis, University of Manchester

Arthur, S.K. and Green, R. (1983) 'Renal Function during Lactation in the Rat', *J. Physiol. (Lond.)*, 334, 379–93

Atherton, J.C. (1983) 'Glomerular Filtration Rate and Salt and Water Reabsorption during Pregnancy in the Conscious Rat', *J. Physiol. (Lond.)*, 334, 493–504

Atherton, J.C. and Pirie, S.C. (1981) 'The Effect of Pregnancy on GFR and Sodium Reabsorption in the Rat Kidney', *J. Physiol. (Lond.)*, 319, 153–64

Atherton, J.C., Bu'Lock, D. and Pirie, S.C. (1982a) 'The Effect of Pseudo-pregnancy on Glomerular Filtration Rate and Salt and Water Reabsorption in the Rat', *J. Physiol. (Lond.)* 324, 11–20

Atherton, J.C., Dark, J.M., Garland, H.O., Morgan, M.R.A., Pidgeon, J. and Soni, S. (1982b) 'Changes in Water and Electrolyte Balance, Plasma Volume and Composition during Pregnancy in the Rat', *J. Physiol. (Lond.)*, 330, 81–93

Bailey, R.R. and Rolleston, G.L. (1971) 'Kidney Length and Ureteric Dilatation in the Puerperium', *J. Obstet. Gynaecol. Brit. Commw.*, 78, 55–61

Baines, A.D. (1971) 'Effect of Extracellular Fluid Volume Expansion on Maximum Glucose Reabsorption Rate and Glomerular Tubular Balance in Single Rat Nephrons', *J. Clin. Invest.*, 50, 2414–25

Balmer, B.D., Garland, H.O., Green, R., Moriarty, R.J. and Richardson, S. (1977) 'The Effect of Pregnancy on Proximal Tubular Lengths and Total Numbers of Nephrons in the Rat Kidney', *J. Physiol. (Lond.)*, 273, 83–4P

Baylis, C. (1980a) 'The Mechanisms of the Increase in Glomerular Filtration Rate in the 12-day Pregnant Rat', *J. Physiol. (Lond.)*, 305, 405–14

Baylis, C. (1980b) 'The Effect of Early Pregnancy on Glomerular Filtration Rate and Plasma Volume in the Rat', *Renal Physiol.*, 2, 333–9

Baylis, C. (1982) 'Glomerular Ultrafiltration in the Pseudopregnant Rat', *Am. J. Physiol.*, 234, F300–6

Baylis, C. and Brenner, B.M. (1978) 'Physiologic Determinants of Glomerular Ultrafiltration', *Rev. Physiol. Biochem. Pharmacol.*, 80, 1–46

Benedict, S.R., Osterberg, E. and Neuwirth, I. (1918) 'Studies in Carbohydrate Metabolism. II. A Study of the Urinary Sugar Excretion in Two Normal Men', *J. Biol. Chem.*, 34, 217–62

Bishop, J.H.V. and Green, R. (1980) 'Effects of Pregnancy on Glucose Handling by Rat Kidney', *J. Physiol. (Lond.)*, 307, 491–502

Bishop, J.H.V. and Green, R. (1981) 'Effects of Pregnancy on Glucose Reabsorption by the Proximal Convoluted Tubule in the Rat', *J. Physiol. (Lond.)*, 319, 271–85

Bishop, J.H.V. and Green, R. (1983) 'Glucose Handling by Distal Portions of the Nephron during Pregnancy in the Rat', *J. Physiol. (Lond.)*, 336, 131–42

Bishop, J.H.V, Green, R. and Thomas, S. (1981) 'Glucose Transport by Short Loops of Henle in the Rat', *J. Physiol. (Lond.)*, 320, 127–38

Bjellin, L. and Carter, A.M. (1977) 'Circulatory Adjustments to Pregnancy in the Rabbit', *Biol. Reprod.*, 16, 112–16

Bliss, D.J. and Lote, C.J. (1982) 'Effect of Prolactin on Urinary Excretion and Renal Haemodynamics in Conscious Rats', *J. Physiol. (Lond.)*, 322, 399–407

Blot, H.G. (1856) 'De la glycosurie physiologique chez les femmes en couches, les nourrices et un certain nombre de femmes enceintes', *Gaz. Hôp. Civils Militaire*, 29, 482–4

Borresen, H.C., Rorvik, S., Gulduog, I. and Aakvaag, A. (1982) 'Angiotensin II and Renal Excretion of Sodium and Potassium in Unanaesthetised Dogs', *Scand. J. Clin. Lab. Invest.*, 42, 87–92

Broughton-Pipkin, F. and Symonds, E.M. (1977) 'The Renin Angiotensin System in the Maternal and Fetal Circulation in Pregnancy Hypertension', *Clin. Obst. Gynaecol.*, 4, 651–64

Buckman, M.T., Peake, G.T. and Robertson, G. (1976) 'Hyperprolactinaemia Influences Renal Function in Man', *Metabolism*, 25, 509–16

Chang, C., Pike, R.L. and Clagett, C.O. (1978) 'Progressive Gross Changes in Renal Medullary Composition in Pregnant Rats', *Lipids, 13*, 167–73

Chesley, L.C. (1978), *Hypertensive Disorders in Pregnancy*, Appleton-Century-Crofts, New York

Chesley, L.C. and Sloan, D.M. (1964) 'The Effect of Posture on Renal Function in Late Pregnancy', *Am. J. Obst. Gynaecol., 89*, 754–9

Christiansen, P.J. (1958) 'Tubular Reabsorption of Glucose during Pregnancy', *Scand. J. Clin. Lab. Invest., 10*, 364–71

Christy, N.P. and Shaver, J.C. (1974) 'Estrogens and the Kidney', *Kidney Int., 6*, 366–76

Churchill, S.E., Bengele, H.H. and Alexander, E.A. (1980) 'Sodium Balance during Pregnancy in the Rat', *Am. J. Physiol., 239*, R143–8

Churchill, S.E., Bengele, H.H. and Alexander, E.A. (1982) 'Renal Function in the Term-pregnant Rat: a Micropuncture Study', *Renal Physiol., 5*, 1–9

Churchill, S.E., Bengele, H.H., Melby, J.C. and Alexander, E.A. (1981) 'Role of Aldosterone in Sodium Retention in the Rat', *Am. J. Physiol., 240*, R175–81

Conrad, K.P. (1983) 'Renal Haemodynamics increase Significantly during Pregnancy in Trained Chronically Catheterised Conscious Rats', *Clin. Res., 31*, 514A

Davison, J.M. and Dunlop, W. (1980) 'Renal Haemodynamics and Tubular Function in Normal Human Pregnancy', *Kidney Int., 18*, 152–61

Davison, J.M. and Hytten, F.E. (1974) 'Glomerular Filtration during and after Pregnancy', *J. Obstet. Gynaecol. Brit. Commw., 81*, 585–95

Davison, J.M. and Hytten, F.E. (1975) 'The Effect of Pregnancy on the Renal Handling of Glucose', *Brit. J. Obstet. Gynaecol., 82*, 374–81

Davison, J.M. and Lindheimer, M.D. (1980) 'Changes in Renal Haemodynamics and Kidney Weight during Pregnancy in the Unanaesthetised Rat', *J. Physiol. (Lond.), 301*, 129–36

Davison, J.M. and Lovedale, C. (1974) 'The Excretion of Glucose during Normal Pregnancy and after Delivery', *J. Obstet. Gynaecol. Brit. Commw. 81*, 30–4

Davison, J.M. and Noble, M.C.B. (1981) 'Serial Changes in 24-hour Creatinine Clearance during Normal Menstrual Cycles and the First Trimester of Pregnancy', *Brit. J. Obstet. Gynaecol., 88*, 10–17

Davison, J.M., Vallotton, M.B. and Lindheimer, M.D. (1981) 'Plasma Osmolality and Urinary Concentration and Dilution during and after Pregnancy: Evidence that Lateral Recumbency Inhibits Maximal Urinary Concentrating Ability', *Brit. J. Obstet. Gynaecol., 88*, 472–9

Davison, J.M., Robertson, G.L. and Lindheimer, M.D. (1983) 'Evidence that the Osmotic Thresholds for Vasopressin (AVP) Release and Thirst Decrease in Human Pregnancy', *Clin. Res., 31*, 427A

Davison, J.M., Gilmore, E.A., Durr, J.A., Robertson, G.L. and Lindheimer, M.D. (1984) 'Altered Osmotic Thresholds for Vasopressin Secretion and Thirst in Human Pregnancy', *Am. J. Physiol., 246*, F105–9

de Swiet, M. (1980) 'The Cardiovascular System', in F.E. Hytten and G. Chamberlain (eds) *Clinical Physiology in Obstetrics*, Blackwell Scientific, Oxford, pp. 3–42

De Vries, J.R., Ludens, J.H. and Fanestil, D.D. (1972) 'Estradiol Renal Receptor Molecules and Estradiol-dependent Antinatriuresis', *Kidney Int., 2*, 95–100

Dignam, W.J., Voskian, J. and Assali, N.S. (1956) 'Effects of Estrogens on Renal Haemodynamics and Excretion of Electrolytes in Human Subjects', *J. Clin. Endocrinol., 16*, 1032–42

Dignam, W.J., Titus, P and Assali, N.S. (1958) 'Renal Function in Human Pregnancy. 1. Changes in Glomerular Filtration Rate and Renal Plasma Flow', *Proc. Soc. Exp. Biol., 97*, 512–14

Dunlop, W. (1976) 'Investigations into the Influence of Posture on Renal Plasma Flow and Glomerular Filtration Rate during Late Pregnancy', *Brit. J. Obstet. Gynaecol., 83*, 17–23

Dunlop, W. (1979) 'Renal Physiology in Pregnancy', *Postgrad. Med. J., 55*, 329–32

Dunlop, W. (1981) 'Serial Changes in Renal Haemodynamics in Normal Human Pregnancy', *Brit. J. Obstet. Gynaecol., 88*, 1–9

Dunlop, W. and Davison, J.M. (1977) 'The Effect of Normal Pregnancy on the Renal Handling of Uric Acid', *Brit. J. Obstet. Gynaecol., 84*, 13–21

Dunlop, W., Furness, C. and Hill, L.M. (1978) 'Maternal Haemoglobin Concentration, Haematocrit and Renal Handling of Urate in Pregnancies Ending in the Births of Small for

Date Infants', *Brit. J. Obstet. Gynaecol.*, *85*, 938–40

Durr, J.A., Stamoutsos, B. and Lindheimer, M.D. (1981) 'Osmoregulation during Pregnancy in the Rat', *J. Clin. Invest.*, *68*, 337–46

Durr, J.A., Stamoutsos, B., Barrow, W.M. and Lindheimer, M.D. (1982) 'Osmoregulation in the Pregnant Brattleboro Rat', *Ann. NY Acad. Sci.*, *394*, 481–90

Egwuatu, V.E. (1983) 'Plasma Urate, Urea and Creatinine Levels during Pregnancy and after the Puerperium in Normal Primigravid Nigerians', *Brit. J. Obstet. Gynaecol.*, *90*, 21–5

Ehrlich, E.N. and Lindheimer, M.D. (1972) 'Effect of Administered Mineralocorticoids on ACTH in Pregnant Women', *J. Clin. Invest.*, *51*, 1301–9

El Karib, A.O. (1981) 'Effects of Progesterone and Prolactin on Renal Function in the Rat', PhD Thesis, University of Manchester

El Karib, A.O., Garland, H.O. and Green, R. (1983) 'Acute and Chronic Effects of Progesterone and Prolactin on Renal Function in the Rat', *J. Physiol.*, *337*, 389–400

Ensor, D.M. (1978) *Comparative Endocrinology of Prolactin*, Chapman & Hall, London

Ezimokhai, M., Davison, J.M., Philips, P.R. and Dunlop, W. (1981) 'Non-postural Serial Changes in Renal Function during the Third Trimester of Normal Human Pregnancy', *Brit. J. Obstet. Gynaecol.*, *88*, 465–71

Fimognari, G.M., Fanestil, J.D. and Edelman, I.S. (1967) 'Induction of RNA and Protein Synthesis in the Action of Aldosterone in the Rat', *Am. J. Physiol.*, *213*, 954–62

Francis, W.J.A. (1960) 'Disturbances of Bladder Function in Relation to Pregnancy', *J. Obstet. Gynaecol. Brit. Emp.*, *67*, 353–66

Freeman, M.E., Smith, M.S., Nazian, S.J. and Neill, J.D. (1974) 'Ovarian and Hypothalamic Control of the Daily Surges of Prolactin Secretion during Pseudopregnancy in the Rat', *Endocrinology*, *94*, 875–82

Friedman, M.M., Goodfriend, M.J., Berlin, P.F. and Goldstein, T. (1951) 'Extracellular Fluid in Normal Pregnancy', *Am. J. Obstet. Gynaecol.*, *61*, 609–14

Fröhnert, P.P., Hohmann, H., Zweibel, R. and Baumann, K. (1970) 'Free Flow Micropuncture Studies of Glucose Transport in the Rat Nephron', *Pflügers Arch.*, *315*, 66–85

Gant, N.F., Daley, G.L., Chand, S., Whalley, P.S. and McDonald, P.C. (1973) 'A Study of Angiotensin II Pressor Response throughout Primigravid Pregnancy', *J. Clin. Invest.*, *52*, 2682–9

Garland, H.O. and Green, R. (1982) 'Micropuncture Study of Changes in Glomerular Filtration and Ion and Water Handling by the Rat Kidney during Pregnancy', *J. Physiol. (Lond.)*, *329*, 389–409

Garland, H.O. and Walker, J. (1984) 'Intrarenal Blood Flow Distribution Following Acute Saline Loading in the Pregnant Rat', *J. Physiol. (Lond.)*, *354*, 67P

Garland, H.O., Green, R. and Moriarty, R.J. (1978) 'Changes in Body Weight, Kidney Weight and Proximal Tubular Length during Pregnancy in the Rat', *Renal Physiol.*, *1*, 42–7

Godard, C., Gaillard, R. and Vallotton, M.B. (1976) 'The Renin Angiotensin Aldosterone System in Mother and Fetus at Term', *Nephron*, *17*, 351–61

Green, R., Moriarty, R.J. and Giebisch, G. (1981) 'Ionic Requirements of Proximal Tubular Fluid Reabsorption: Flow Dependence of Transport', *Kidney Int.*, *20*, 580–3

Häberle, D.A. and von Baeyer, H. (1983) 'Characteristics of Glomerular Tubular Balance', *Am. J. Physiol.*, *240*, F355–66

Hall, J.E., Guyton, A.C., Smith, M.J. and Coleman, T.G. (1980) 'Blood Pressure and Renal Function during Chronic Changes in Sodium Intake: Role of Angiotensin', *Am. J. Physiol.*, *239*, F271–80

Harris, P.F. and Young, J.A. (1977) 'Dose Dependent Stimulation and Inhibition of Proximal Tubular Sodium Reabsorption by Angiotensin II in the Rat Kidney', *Pflügers Arch.*, *367*, 295–7

Horrobin, D.F., Lloyd, I.J., Lipton, A., Burstyn, P.G., Durkin, N. and Muiruri, K.L. (1971) 'Actions of Prolactin on Human Renal Function', *Lancet*, *ii*, 352–4

Hsueh, W.A., Luetscher, J.A., Carlson, E.N., Grislis, G., Fraze, E. and McHargue, A. (1982) 'Changes in Active and Inactive Renin throughout Pregnancy', *J. Clin. Endocrinol. Metab.*, *54*, 1010–16

Humphreys, R.C. (1954) 'An Analysis of the Maternal and Fetal Weight in Normal Pregnancy', *J. Obstet. Gynaecol. Brit. Emp.*, *61*, 764–71

Immonen, I., Lammintausta, R., Fyhrquist, F., Erkkola, R., Punnonen, R. and Rauramo, L.

(1982) 'Bilateral Oopherectomy and Plasma Renin Substrate Concentration', *Int. J. Clin. Pharmacol. Toxicol.*, *20*, 287–8

Immonen, I., Siimes, A., Stenman, U.H., Karrkainen, J. and Fyhrquist, F. (1983) 'Plasma Renin Substrate and Oestrogens in Normal Pregnancy', *Scand. J. Clin. Lab. Invest.*, *43*, 61–5

Johnson, J.A. and Davis, J.D. (1976) 'The Effect of Estrogens on Renal Sodium Excretion in the Dog', in M.D. Lindheimer, A.I. Katz and F.P Zuspan (eds), *Hypertension in Pregnancy*, Wiley, New York, pp. 239–48

Johnson, M.D. and Malvin, R.L. (1977) 'Stimulation of Renal Sodium Reabsorption by Angiotensin II', *Am. J. Physiol.*, *232*, F298–306

Katz, A.I. and Lindheimer, M.D. (1977) 'Actions of Hormones on the Kidney', *Ann Rev. Physiol.*, *39*, 97–133

Kaufman, S. (1981) 'The Dipsogenic Activity of Prolactin in Male and Female Rats', *J. Physiol.*, *310*, 435–44

Kaupilla, A., Satuli, R. and Vuorinin, P. (1972) 'Ureteric Dilatation and Renal Cortical Index after Normal and Preeclamptic Pregnancies', *Acta Obstet. Gynaecol. Scand.*, *51*, 147–53

Keyes, J.L. and Swanson, R.E. (1971) 'Dependence of Glucose T_m on GFR and Tubular Volume in the Dog Kidney', *Am. J. Physiol.*, *221*, 1–7

Kirksey, A. Pike, R.L. (1962) 'Some Effects of High and Low Sodium Intake during Pregnancy in the Rat. I. Food Consumption, Weight Gain, Reproductive Performances, Electrolyte Balances, Plasma Total Protein and Protein Fractions in Normal Pregnancy', *J. Nutr.*, *77*, 33–42

Klopper, A. (1980) 'Placental Metabolism', in F.E. Hytten and G. Chamberlain (eds), *Clinical Physiology in Obstetrics*, Blackwell, Oxford, pp. 441–67

Kurtzman, N.A. and Pillay, V.K.G. (1973) 'Renal Reabsorption of Glucose in Health and Disease', *Arch. Int. Med.*, *131*, 901–4

Kwong, T.F. and Bennett, C.M. (1974) 'Relationship between Glomerular Filtration Rate and Maximum Tubular Reasorption Rate in Glucose', *Kidney Int.*, *5*, 23–9

Lancet, M. and Fisher, I.L. (1956) 'The Value of Blood Uric Acid Levels in Toxaemia of Pregnancy', *J. Obstet. Gynaecol. Brit. Commw.*, *63*, 116–19

Lang, F. (1981) 'Renal Handling of Urate', in R. Greger, F. Lang and S. Silbernagl (eds), *Renal Transport of Organic Substances*, Springer-Verlag, Berlin, pp. 234–61

Lichton, I.J. (1961) 'Salt Saving in the Pregnant Rat', *Am. J. Physiol.*, *201*, 765–8

Lichton, I.J. (1963) 'Urinary Excretion of Water, Sodium and Total Solutes by the Pregnant Rat', *Am. J. Physiol.*, *201*, 563–7

Lichton, I.J. and Hugh, J.E. (1968) 'Renal Clearance of Water Solutes by Pregnant Rats Treated with Spironolactone', *Proc. Soc. Exp. Biol. Med.*, *129*, 312–15

Lind, T. and Hytten, F.E. (1972) 'The Excretion of Glucose during Normal Pregnancy', *J. Obstet. Gynaecol. Brit. Commw.*, *79*, 961–5

Lind, T., Godfrey, K.A. and Otun, H. (1984) 'Changes in Serum Uric Acid Concentrations during Normal Pregnancy', *Brit. J. Obstet. Gynaecol.*, *91*, 128–32

Lindheimer, M.D. and Katz, A.I. (1971) 'Kidney Function in the Pregnant Rat', *J. Lab. Clin. Med.*, *78*, 633–41

Lindheimer, M.D. and Katz, A.I. (1977) *Kidney Function and Disease in Pregnancy*, Lea & Febiger, Philadelphia

Lindheimer, M.D., Koeppen, B. and Katz, A.I. (1976) 'Renal Function in Normal and Hypertensive Pregnant Rats', in M.D. Lindheimer, A.I. Katz and F.P. Zuspan (eds), *Hypertension and Pregnancy*, Wiley, New York, pp. 217–28

Lindheimer, M.D., Katz, A.I., Nolten, W.E., Oparil, S. and Ehrlich, E.N. (1977) 'Sodium and Mineralocorticoids in Normal and Abnormal Pregnancy', *Adv. Nephrol.*, *7*, 33–45

Lindheimer, M.D., Katz, A.I., Koeppen, B.M., Ordonez, N.G. and Oparil, S. (1983) 'Kidney Function and Sodium Handling in the Pregnant Spontaneously Hypertensive Rat', *Hypertension*, *5*, 498–66

Lockett, M.F. and Nail, B. (1965) 'A Comparative Study of the Renal Actions of Growth and Lactogenic Hormones in Rats', *J. Physiol. (Lond.)*, *180*, 147–56

Lowitz, H.D., Stumpe, K.O. and Ochwadt, B. (1969) 'Micropuncture Study of the Action of Angiotensin II on Tubular Sodium and Water Reabsorption in the Rat', *Nephron*, *6*, 173–87

Lucci, M.S., Bengele, H.H. and Solomon, S. (1975) 'Supressive Action of Prolactin on Renal Response to Volume Expansion', *Am. J. Physiol.*, *229*, 81–5

Lund, C.J. and Donovan, J.C. (1967) 'Blood Volume during Pregnancy', *Am. J. Obstet. Gynaecol.*, *98*, 393–403

Mackay, L.L. (1928) 'Factors which Determine Renal Weight. IV. Pregnancy and Lactation', *Am. J. Physiol.*, *86*, 215–24

Matthews, B.F. (1977) 'Growth of Maternal Kidneys in Pregnant Mice', *J. Physiol. (Lond.)*, *273*, 84P

Matthews, B.F. and Taylor, D.W. (1960) 'Effects of Pregnancy on Inulin and *para*-aminohippurate Clearances in the Anaesthetised Rat', *J. Physiol. (Lond.)*, *151*, 385–9

McDonald, H.N. and Good, N. (1971) 'Changes in Plasma Sodium, Potassium and Chloride Concentration in Pregnancy and the Puerperium with Plasma and Serum Osmolality', *J. Obstet. Gynaecol. Brit. Commw.*, *78*, 798–803

McDonald, H.N., Good, H. and Hancock, K.W. (1976) 'Plasma Solute Concentrations during Gonadotrophin-induced Ovulation', *Brit. J. Obstet. Gynaecol.*, *83*, 137–41

Miller, J.R., Keith, N.M. and Rowntree, L.G. (1915) 'Plasma and Blood Volume in Pregnancy', *J. Am. Med. Assoc.*, *65*, 779–82

Mills, D.E., Buckman, M.T. and Peake, G.T. (1983) 'Mineralocorticoid Modulation of Prolactin Effect on Renal Solute Excretion in the Rat', *Endocrinology*, *112*, 823–8

Morel, F.F. and de Rouffignac, C. (1973) 'Kidney', *Ann. Rev. Physiol.*, *35*, 17–54

O'Connell, J.M., Boonshaft, B., Hayes, J.M. and Schreiner, G.E. (1969) 'Metabolic Effects of Progesterone in the Dog', *Proc. Soc. Exp. Biol. Med.*, *132*, 862–4

Olsson, K., Benlamlih, S., Dahlborn, K. and Orberg, J. (1982) 'A Serial Study of Fluid Balance during Pregnancy, Lactation and Anoestrus in Goats', *Acta Physiol. Scand.*, *115*, 39–45

Oparil, S., Ehrlich, E.N. and Lindheimer, M.D. (1975) 'Effect of Progesterone on Renal Sodium Handling in Man: Relation to Aldosterone Excretion and Plasma Renin Activity', *Clin. Sci. Mol. Med.*, *49*, 139–47

Pepe, G.J. and Rothchild, I. (1974) 'A Comparative Study of Serum Progesterone Levels in Pregnancy and Various Types of Pseudopregnancy in the Rat', *Endocrinology*, *95*, 275–9

Perkins, C.M., Hancock, K.W., Cope, G.F. and Lee, M.R. (1981) 'Urine Free Dopamine in Normal Primigravid Pregnancy and Women Taking Oral Contraceptives', *Clin. Sci.*, *61*, 423–8

Pirie, S.C. (1979) 'Altered Renal Function in Pregnancy in the Rat', PhD Thesis, University of Manchester

Pollack, V.E. and Nettles, J.B. (1960) 'The Kidney in Toxaemia of Pregnancy. A Clinical and Pathological Study Based on Renal Biopsies', *Medicine*, *39*, 469–526

Prince, H. (1982) 'Blood Volume in the Pregnant Rabbit', *Q. J. Exp. Physiol.*, *67*, 87–95

Redman, C.W.G., Beilin, L.J., Bonnar, J. and Wilkinson, R.H. (1976) 'Plasma Urate Measurements in Predicting Fetal Death in Hypertensive Pregnancy', *Lancet*, *i*, 1370–3

Reid, I.A., Schrier, R.W. and Earley, L.E. (1972) 'An Effect of Extra Renal Beta-adrenergic Stimulation on the Release of Renin', *J. Clin. Invest.*, *51*, 1861–9

Renschler, H.E., Bach, H.G. and von Baeyer, H. (1966) 'Die Ausscheidung von Glucose in Urin bei normaler Schwangershaft', *Dtsch. Med. Wochenschr.*, *91*, 1673–6

Rigg, L.A, Lein, A. and Yen, S.S.C. (1977) 'Pattern of Increase in Circulating Prolactin Levels during Human Gestation', *Am. J. Obstet. Gynaecol.*, *129*, 454–6

Rohde, R. and Deetjen, P. (1968) 'Die Glucose Resorption in der Rattenniere', *Pflügers Arch.*, *302*, 219–323

Röttger, H. (1953) 'Uber den Wasserhaushalt in der physiologischen und toxischen Schwangerschaft. 1. Der Wasserhaushalt in der physiologischen Schwangerschaft', *Arch. Gynaekol.*, *184*, 59–65

Schultze, R.G. and Berger, H. (1973) 'The Influence of GFR and Saline Expansion on Tm_G of the Dog Kidney', *Kidney Int.*, *3*, 291–7

Schuster, V.L., Kokko, J.P. and Jacobson, H.R. (1982) 'Angiotensin II Directly Inhibits Sodium Reabsorption in the Isolated Perfused Proximal Tubule', *Clin. Res.*, *30*, 462A

Schwartz, G.J. and Burg, M.B. (1978) 'Mineralocorticoid Effects on Cation Transport by Cortical Collecting Tubules *in vitro*', *Am. J. Physiol.*, *235*, F576–85

Seitchik, J., Szutka, A. and Alper, C. (1958) 'Further Studies on the Metabolism of N^{15}-labelled Uric Acid in Normal and Toxaemic Pregnant Women', *Am. J. Obstet. Gynaecol.*, *76*, 1151–5

Semple, P.F., Carswell, W. and Boyle, J.A. (1974) 'Serial Studies of the Renal Clearance of

Urate and Inulin during Pregnancy and after the Puerperium in Normal Women', *Clin. Sci. Mol. Med.*, *47*, 559–65

Shaikh, A.A. (1971) 'Estrone and Estradiol Levels in the Ovarian Venous Blood from Rats during the Estrous Cycle and Pregnancy', *Biol. Reprod.*, *5*, 297–300

Sheenan, H.L. and Lynch, J.B. (1973) *Pathology of Toxaemia of Pregnancy*, Churchill Livingstone, Edinburgh, p. 47

Simpson, S.A. and Tait, J.F. (1952) 'A Quantitative Method for the Bioassay of the Effects of Adrenal Cortical Steroids on Mineral Metabolism', *Endocrinology*, *50*, 150–61

Sims, E.A.H. and Krantz, K.E. (1958) 'Serial Studies of Renal Function during Pregnancy and in the Puerperium in Normal Women', *J. Clin. Invest.*, *37*, 1764–74

Smith, H.W. (1951) *'The Kidney: Structure and Function in Health and Disease*, Oxford University Press, New York

Smith, M.S. and Neill, J.D. (1976) 'Termination at Mid-pregnancy of the Two Daily Surges of Plasma Prolactin Initiated by Mating in the Rat', *Endocrinology*, *98*, 696–701

Taylor, D.J. and Lind, T. (1979) 'Red Cell Mass during and after Normal Pregnancy', *Brit. J. Obstet. Gynaecol.*, *86*, 364–70

Thomson, A.M. and Billewicz, W.Z. (1957) 'Clinical Significance of Weight Trends during Pregnancy', *Brit. Med. J. 1*, 243–7

Thorn, G.W. and Engel, L.L. (1938) 'The Effect of Sex Hormones on the Renal Excretion of Electrolytes', *J. Exp. Med.*, *68*, 299–312

Vallotton, M.B., Davison, J.M., Rondell, A.M. and Lindheimer, M.D. (1982) 'Response of the Renin Aldosterone System and Antidiuretic Hormone to Oral Water Loading and Hypertonic Saline Infusion during and after Pregnancy', *Clin. Exp. Hypertension (B)*, *1*, 385–400

von Baeyer, H. (1975) 'Glucose Transport in the Short Loop of Henle of the Rat Kidney', *Pflügers Arch.*, *357*, 317–23

von Baeyer, H., von Conta, C., Haberle, D. and Deetjen, jP. (1973) 'Determination of Transport Constants for Glucose in Proximal Tubules of the Rat Kidney', *Pflügers Arch.*, *343*, 273–86

Walker, J. (1983) 'Renal Function in the Female Rat during Various Reproductive States', PhD Thesis, University of Manchester

Walker, J. and Garland, H.O. (1982) 'Renal Tubular Function in the Prolactin Induced Pseudopregnant Rat', *J. Endocrinol.*, *94* (Suppl.), 81

Weinberger, M.H., Kramer, N.J., Petersen, L.P., Cleary, R.E. and Young, P.C.M. (1976) 'Sequential Changes in the Renin Angiotensin-Aldosterone Systems and Plasma Progesterone Concentrations in Normal and Abnormal Human Pregnancy', in M.D. Lindheimer, A.I. Katz and F.P. Zuspan (eds), *Hypertension in Pregnancy*, John Wiley, New York, pp. 263–70

Welsh, G.W. and Sims, E.A.H. (1960) 'The Mechanism of Renal Glycosuria in Pregnancy', *Diabetes*, *9*, 363–9

Wen, S.F. and and McSherry, N.R. (1982) 'Renal Glucose Transport in Pregnant Rats', *Proc. 15th Ann. Meeting Am. Soc. Nephrol.*, 177A

Whipp, G.T., Coghlan, J.P., Shulkes, A.A., Skinner, S.L. and Wintour, E.M. (1978) 'Regulation of Aldosterone in the Rat. Effect of Oestrous Cycle, Pregnancy and Sodium Status', *Aust. J. Exp. Biol. Med. Sci.*, *56*, 545–51

Wintour, E.M., Blair-West, J.R., Brown, E.H., Coghlan, J.P., Denton, D.A., Nelson, J., Oddie, C.J., Scoggins, B.A., Whipp, G.T. and Wright, R.D. (1976) 'The Effect of Pregnancy on Mineralo- and Gluco-corticoid Secretion in the Sheep', *Clin. Exp. Pharmacol. Physiol.*, *3*, 331–42

Wintour, E.M., Coghlan, J.P., Oddie, C.J., Scoggins, B.A. and Walters, H.A.W. (1978) 'A Sequential Study of Adrenocorticoid Level in Human Pregnancy', *Clin. Exp. Pharmacol. Physiol.*, *5*, 399–403

Wright, F.S. and Giebisch, G. (1978) 'Renal Potassium Transport: Contributions of Individual Nephron Segments and Populations', *Am. J. Physiol.*, *235*, F515–27

Yoshinaga, K., Hawkins, R.A. and Stocker, J.F. (1969) 'Estrogen Secretion by the Rat Ovary *in vivo* during the Estrous Cycle and Pregnancy', *Endocrinology*, *85*, 103–12

INDEX

A 23187 143
ACE *see* Angiotensin converting enzyme
Acetazolamide
  and prostaglandin excretion 148
  see also Carbonic anhydrase inhibition
Acetylcholine
  and Atrial Natriuretic Factor release
    205
  and glomerular dynamics 69
Acidosis and prostaglandin excretion
  146–9
Active transport *see individual substances*
  e.g. sodium, chloride *etc.*
Adenylate cyclase
  and atrial natriuretic factor release 205
  in thick ascending limb of Henle
    103–4
  in thin ascending limb of Henle 96
ADH *see* vasopressin
Adrenal steroids *see* Aldosterone
Adrenaline and Atrial Natriuretic Factor
  release 205
Adrenergic receptors
  and dopamine 232, 241
  and prostaglandins 154
  α-receptors 206; and atrial natriuretic
    factor release 205; and renin release
    154; blockade 72
  β-receptors 241; and atrial natriuretic
    factor release 204–5; and renin
    release 152–4
Afferent arterioles 34, 50–1
  and angiotensin II 61–7
Albumin 232
  filtration of 5–27 *passim*
  pI value 6
  prostaglandin binding to 143
Alcian blue 4, 25
Aldosterone 272
  and dopamine 238
  and prostaglandins 165
  'escape' 180–1
  in pregnancy 313–14
Aldosteronism 268
Alkalosis and prostaglandin excretion
  146–8
Ammoniagenesis and prostaglandins 148
Angiotensin II 60–7
  and afferent arteriole 61–7
  and arachidonic acid 139
  and autoregulation 57–8
  and calcium 64

and dopamine 232–3
and efferent arteriole 61–7
and filtration coefficient 62
and hypertension 268–81
and manganese 64
and mesangial cells 71
and prostaglandins 62, 151, 155
and proteinuria 19
and renal nerves 73
and single nephron glomerular filtration
  rate 61–7, 69–72
and sympathetic nervous system 272–3
glomerular binding 64
in pregnancy 313–14
receptors 71, 257
slow pressor response 271–4
Angiotensin converting enzyme 275
  inhibition 66–7, 275
Anions
  and glomerular filtration 4–27 *passim*
  in pars recta 87
  prostaglandins as 147
  see also individual ions, chloride *etc.*
ANP *see* Atrial natriuretic factor
Antidiuretic hormone *see* vasopressin
Antihypertensive polar renomedullary
  lipids 166, 279–81
APRL 279–81
Arachidonic acid 138–66 *passim*
  and angiotensin II 139
  and prostaglandin synthesis 138–43
  dietary 138
  release 141
Arterioles
  afferent *see* afferent arterioles
  efferent *see* efferent arterioles
Autoregulation 57–60
  and myogenic reflex 57
  of glomerular filtration rate 57–60
  of renal blood flow 57–60
Atrial extracts 197–200
Atrial granules 195–7
Atrial natriuretic factor(s) 195–208
  and calcium 201
  effect on glomerular filtration and renal
    blood flow 200
  effect on $(Na^+ + K^+)$ ATPase 202
  effect on smooth muscle 202
  in hypertension 206–7
  release 204–6; and adrenaline 205; and
    adenylate cyclase 205; and
    vasopressin 205

Renin-secreting tumours 268
Renomedullary lipids 280–1
Reptation 8

Saralasin 65–7, 69, 275, 277
Shark rectal gland 102–3
Single nephron glomerular filtration rate
   (SNGFR) 36–57 *passim*
   and acetylcholine 69–70
   and angiotensin II 61–7
   and bradykinin 69–70
   and cyclic AMP 69–70
   and pregnancy 302
   and prostaglandins 62, 67–8
Slit diaphragm 18
Slow-reacting substance 143
Sodium
   and macula densa 119
   dietary 65–6, 123–9, 159, 180–1, 230,
      236, 253–6, 272
   excretion 180–208; and hypertension
      249–56; and prostaglandins 152–60
   permeability of pars recta 86
   transport in pars recta 88–91
Sodium-Calcium exchange 265–7
Sodium-Hydrogen exchange 89
Sodium-Potassium ATPase
   and atrial natriuretic factor 202
   endogenous inhibitors of 188–95, 207,
      266
   in pars recta 88–91
   in thick ascending limb of Henle 100–5
   in thin ascending limb of Henle 94
   in thin descending limb of Henle 93–4
SRS-A 143
Star vessels 33
Stop-flow technique 39
Sulphate 89
Sympathetic nerves
   and angiotensin II 73, 272–3
   see also Renal nerves

Teprotide 275
Thick ascending limb of Henle *see* Loop of
   Henle
Thick descending limb of Henle *see* Pars
   Recta
Thin ascending and descending limbs of
   Henle *see* Loop of Henle
Thromboxane A$_2$ 139, 140, 149

Transepithelial potential difference 88,
   92–3, 97–103
Tubuloglomerular feedback 57–60, 114–30
   and angiotensin II 57–8
   and volume expansion 123–9

Ultrafiltration coefficient (Kf) 45–8, 53–5,
   61–72, 114–18
   and angiotensin II 62–7
   and calcium 62–7
   and histamine 69
   and papaverine 69
   and parathyroid hormone 70
   and prostaglandins 62, 69, 154
   and vasopressin 67–8
   in diabetes 54–5
   in glomerulonephritis 54
   in ischaemic damage 54
   in toxic injury 54
Urea
   and prostaglandin synthesis 161, 165
   permeability 87, 95, 97
Uric acid, in pregnancy 321–2

Vasopressin 67–8
   and arachidonic acid 139
   and atrial peptides 205
   and Kf 67–8
   and loop of Henle 96, 103, 162
   and mesangial cells 67
   and pregnancy 314–15
   and prostaglandin synthesis 151, 161–4
Volume expansion
   and natriuretic hormone 182–5
   and prostaglandins 159
   and tubuloglomerular feedback 123–9
   in pregnancy 306–14

Water diuresis, proximal tubule pressure
   115
Water excretion
   and hypertension 259–65
   and prostaglandins 161–4
Water permeability
   and ultrafiltration coefficient 46
   and vasopressin 96, 103–4
   of glomerular capillaries 1, 18, 46–7
   of loop of Henle 91–3, 95–7, 103–4
   of pars recta 85–91